DICTIONARY
OF
ANTHROPOLOGY

DICTIONARY
OF
ANTHROPOLOGY

Charlotte Seymour-Smith

G.K.HALL &CO.

70 LINCOLN STREET, BOSTON, MASS.

Published 1986 in the United States of America
by G.K. Hall & Co., 70 Lincoln Street,
Boston, Massachusetts 02111, U.S.A.

Published 1986 in Great Britain by
The Macmillan Press Ltd., London and Basingstoke

Library of Congress Cataloging-in-Publication Data

Dictionary of anthropology.

    1.   Anthropology—Dictionaries.   I. Seymour-Smith,
Charlotte.
GN11.D48   1986   306′.03′21   86–214
ISBN 0–8161–8817–3

Printed in Great Britain.

Foreword

There are few fixed definitions in anthropology. Instead, ours is a discipline which advances by constantly revising and interrogating current concepts and their use. This Dictionary is intended to convey the critical spirit of anthropological enquiry to students of social and cultural anthropology and to the interested lay reader. Emphasis is placed on theoretical and conceptual issues, as well as on the clarification of technical terms which sometimes confuse the uninitiated. The aim of the Dictionary is thus to provide the reader with the basic information necessary in order to understand and critically assess anthropological texts and material, as well as to furnish a starting point for the student, who may wish to go further by following up the references on any given topic.

Entries on individual anthropologists are brief and limited. Only those authors born before 1920 are included – references to the works of younger scholars will be found under the entries relating to the topics to which they have contributed. Similarly, for reasons of space it is impossible to explore all the interdisciplinary ramifications of anthropology, and the reader will not find coverage here of the fields of linguistics, physical anthropology, archaeology and so on.

In order to use this book most fruitfully the reader is advised to follow up the cross-referencing, which is designed to counteract the necessarily fragmented dictionary format.

Finally, this is perhaps not a dictionary in the strictest sense of the term. Many entries here are not 'definitive': they are designed instead to open up the debate.

CSS, June 1986

Acknowledgements

The author wishes to acknowledge the assistance of the following persons who made the completion of this work possible: Shaie Selzer and Martin Seymour-Smith, who came up with the idea of the book; John Hodgson, Penelope Allport and Ravi Mirchandani, for editorial support at Macmillan Press; Felicity Edholm, for valuable suggestions and revisions; and, finally, Hamilton Mencher, for generously providing word-processing facilities in Metasistemas SA, Iquitos, Peru.

Contributors

I would also like to thank Maurice Bloch, Michael Chibnik, Britt Krause and Norman Whitten who contributed a number of entries to the Dictionary.

How to use the Dictionary

Alphabetization

In entry headings in the text where more than one word forms part of the heading, the words are alphabetized as if continuous up to the first mark of punctuation, then again after the comma.

Cross-references

Cross-references are distinguished by the use of SMALL CAPITALS; large capitals appear in cross-references where the entry is a proper name (e.g. LEVI-STRAUSS). In a cross-reference to another entry within the Dictionary the word 'see' is printed in *italics*. Where the word 'see' is printed in roman type the reference is to another publication.

Cross-references are of two basic kinds. First, there are those 'cross-reference' entries that direct the reader to where he can find the entry he is seeking; thus:

childhood. *See* AGE, ANTHROPOLOGY OF.

The other type of cross-reference is that within an article. Some cross-references will be found at the end of short articles, or at the end of paragraphs, directing the reader to another entry where further information relevant to the subject he is reading about may be found (these may, as appropriate, embody such formulae as '*see*' or '*see also*'). Further cross-references will be found in running text to direct the reader to places where he can find further information on the topic. However, cross-references are used selectively, so it is always worth looking up a related term elsewhere in the Dictionary.

Bibliographical references

Throughout the text bibliographical references have been given with the name of the author/editor and the date of publication. Readers should refer to the Bibliography beginning on page 293.

The Bibliography is arranged in alphabetical order by author/editor, and chronologically under the author's/editor's name. Where a work has been published originally in a language other than English, the original date of publication and date of English translation have been given, where known. In the case of specific references to chapters in a book with more than one contributor, the reader will find a cross-reference within the Bibliography to the editor of the publication concerned.

Abbreviations

For kinship terminology the reader is advised to consult the article **abbreviations in kinship** on page 1. The abbreviation BP refers to dates 'before present'.

A

abbreviations in kinship. In order to express KINSHIP relations more economically in anthropological writing and tables, it is common to use the following abbreviations:

Fa or F	=	Father
Mo or M	=	Mother
Si or Z	=	Sister
Br or B	=	Brother
So or S	=	Son
Da or D	=	Daughter
Sb	=	Sibling
Ne	=	Nephew
Ni	=	Niece
Pa	=	Parent
Ch	=	Child
Hu or H	=	Husband
Wi or W	=	Wife
Sp	=	Spouse
La	=	In-law
Gf	=	Grandfather
Gm	=	Grandmother
Gp	=	Grandparent

Thus, for example, 'father's sister's son's daughter' may be abbreviated as FZSD or FaSiSoDa.

ablineal. In kinship studies, synonymous with COLLATERAL.

aboriginal. Indigenous or pertaining to the original population of a given region. When capitalized, refers to Australian Aborigines.

abortion. *See* CONTRACEPTION AND ABORTION.

accommodation. A process or state of adjustment to a situation of conflict, where overt strife is avoided and compensatory advantages are gained by the parties or groups involved. (*See* ACCULTURATION; CHANGE.)

acculturation. This term has been used since the 19th century to describe processes of ACCOMMODATION and CHANGE in culture contact, but during the 1930s it came to be used increasingly by US anthropologists interested in the study of cultural and social change and the problems of social disorientation and cultural decline. They defined acculturation as 'those phenomena which result when groups of individuals having different cultures come into first hand contact, with subsequent changes in the original cultural patterns of both groups'. Starting from a CULTURAL BASELINE of pre-contact culture patterns, acculturation studies then attempted to describe and analyse the process of change. In practice, they concentrated almost exclusively on contact between industrial societies and native populations, emphasizing the one-way influence of the former on the latter, and its implications for APPLIED ANTHROPOLOGY. They have accordingly been criticized for their open attitude towards the DEVELOPMENT process and towards the culture of the dominant group and the changes arising in it as a result of new political, economic and social forms. Specific points of research within the acculturation perspective included the study of mechanisms of change and resistance to change, and the creation of typologies of results of change: ASSIMILATION, reinterpretation, SYNCRETISM, REVITAZLIATION etc. More recent studies of change have tended to move away from explanations in terms of cultural pattern and towards the analysis of social, economic and political structures of dominance or of ETHNIC interaction, and the strategic use of cultural elements in contact situations.

acephalous. Literally 'headless', referring to societies which do not possess centralized political authority. The term is generally employed to refer to societies which within

1

an evolutionary scheme are classified as BANDS or TRIBES, and in which the political system may be of the SEGMENTARY type, decentralized or 'multicentric' (also 'polycentric'). An alternative term is 'stateless societies'. In such groups, the unity of the society as a whole is given by the common ethnic or cultural identity of its member communities, but not by a centralized political system. (*See* POLITICAL ANTHROPOLOGY.)

achievement and ascription. The distinction between achieved and ascribed ROLES or STATUSES is one which was developed by the anthropologist LINTON, and refers to the criteria by which the individual is considered to be eligible for a particular status or role in society. The ascribed role or status is one which is assigned by virtue of factors outside the individual's control such as sex, age, kinship relationship, race etc. Linton (1936) points out that this type of status or role is predominant in traditional societies. The achieved role, on the other hand, depends on individual effort or ability (in other words, it is a role for which one must compete), and Linton argues that this type of status or role is predominant in modern society and is consonant with democratic or egalitarian ideologies. A good example of an achieved role in modern society is the occupational or professional role, which involves the exercise of effort and choice, as well as an element of competition, to occupy a given position. However it is important to recall that there is still a large area of industrial society which is governed by role or status ascription: we are, in modern society, allocated certain functions or positions by virtue of being male or female, young or old, black or white, and so on. Similarly, there are roles which are competed for and achieved in traditional societies, as the study of political organization in these societies amply demonstrates. Like social MOBILITY, the concept of achieved status or role is one which has a strong ideological component: it corresponds to the egalitarian ideals of a 'democratic' society but not necessarily to the reality of social relations, which continue to rely heavily on status and role ascription. In addition, it should be remembered that it is not always possible to maintain a rigid distinction bet-

ween roles or statuses which are achieved and those which are ascribed: social class, for example, is ascribed at birth but is subject to change during a person's lifetime in accordance with achievements.

achievement motivation. A configuration of personality traits linked to the entrepreneurial role which it is argued will favour economic DEVELOPMENT in populations where the achievement oriented personality is common. Many anthropologists and sociologists would argue that such a psychological measure cannot be cited as a causal factor in social CHANGE, and would seek instead to establish what are the social and economic forces which are favouring or shaping the 'achieving personality'.

action anthropology. *See* APPLIED ANTHROPOLOGY.

action theory. Under this term we may include studies of society generally, and those of political systems in particular, which focus on individual actors and their strategies within a given sociopolitical context. Theoretical frameworks of action theory have included those focusing on TRANSACTIONS, SYSTEMS ANALYSIS and GAME THEORY. Action theory in anthropology locates the individual within the framework of social organization and then analyses political action and interaction. Within POLITICAL ANTHROPOLOGY, action theory is distinguished by its attention to political processes and formations such as FACTIONS, interest groups, and so on, and by its fieldwork method, which concentrates on face-to-face interactions within given sociopolitical contexts. In part, action theory was a reaction to the tendency of STRUCTURAL FUNCTIONALISM to reify political structures and concentrate on corporate groups and the moral/jural dimension of political systems. Action theory emphasizes dynamic modes of political behaviour such as strategy, decision making and maximization. In the works of Mair, FIRTH and LEACH the foundations for an action-oriented approach to anthropology were already laid. During the 1950s and 1960s action theory was further developed by Bailey, Barth, TURNER, Boissevain, A.P. Cohen and others. Themes included the study of political and economic change and the structural principles ordering political action, and comparative/historical analysis. Thus Bailey (1969) developed a tool kit for the analysis of competitive political action, while Boissevain (1974) suggested a classification of noncorporate political action sets. Barth (1961), after developing a transactional model of political analysis, has moved on to explore the possibilities of combining action theory with other theoretical approaches in order to complete the study of the structural and symbolic as well as strategic dimensions of social systems. Others such as Turner have focused on the 'manipulation of symbols' in political systems. Action theory has influenced the anthropological study of ETHNICITY as well as a broad range of other areas where action-oriented approaches have been fruitfully incorporated in combination with other methodological and theoretical approaches.

A general criticism of action-oriented theories is that they tend to focus on competitive intraclass behaviour while neglecting power relations and conflict between social classes. Also, they rely on notions such as that of the maximizing individual decision maker and the 'rational man', notions which have been criticized as ETHNOCENTRIC. Critics of action theories have claimed that by focusing on individuals it is impossible to apprehend the nature of a political system or a power structure. Both action theorists themselves and critics of the approach have tried to overcome these problems and to generate new models which incorporate both individual and structural elements: thus A. Cohen in his work on ethnicity (1974) attempts to reconcile action theory and structuralism by stressing the dialectical relationship between power and symbolism, as does Turner in his theory (1974) which interrelates the manipulation of symbols and the struggle for power.

actor. A concept which has been increasingly called upon in modern anthropology, both in the field of ACTION THEORY, where the notion of the actor or decision maker is crucial, and also in the modern study of ROLE. In the second field, the notion of the actor is important in the sense that it suggests the distance which exists between the person and the role he or she adopts. Roles are not passively accepted or learned by individuals; instead, they may 'play' them in a variety of ways, comment upon them, innovate and switch from role to role.

adaptation. A concept which is used in biological theories of genetic EVOLUTION to refer to physiological or behavioural changes which result in increased chances of survival in a given environment. In biology, the term has two distinct senses: individual responses acting to maintain homeostasis, and evolutionary adaptation or change over generations in the direction of increased 'fitness'. By extension, the term has been applied to human behaviour and to socio-cultural evolution. If the use of the concept is not to be circular (traits which exist are adaptive, adaptive traits are those which exist), then it must be linked to an independent measure or theory of 'fitness'. (*See* ADAPTIVE STRATEGY; CULTURAL ECOLOGY.)

adaptive strategy. The concept of adaptive strategy refers to a plan of action carried out over a specified time period by a specific group or aggregate of people to allow them to adjust to or cope with internal or external constraints. Adaptive strategies may or may not be made explicit by an actor in a given social situation, but they are not ever conscious for all actors. Actors may give contradictory statements about what they are doing, planning, and thinking. The construct 'adaptive strategy' is a generalized statement developed by disciplined observers of human behaviour to understand repetitive and unique outcomes of social action with careful attention to external and internal constraints on such action. Constraints themselves are forever being imposed from outside a given group or aggregate of people, and they are also the inevitable consequence of the strategies developed to attain a goal.

An adaptive strategy such as a predatory expansion of one group into the territory of another is disruptive to the social relations of another social grouping. It is impossible to study the adaptive strategies of any particular social grouping without considering the various symmetrical and asymmetrical relationships between groupings and between individuals and subgroupings. Accordingly, the concept of reciprocity is fundamental to the analysis of adaptive strategies. Because adaptive strategy analysis is oriented toward understanding both continuity and change, it is an essential complement to the study of ecological patterns, economic growth and decline, social structure, political process, or ideological presentations. The concept of adaptive strategy allows us to view structure dynamically. Adaptive strategy analysis sees humans as always coping with the structures that they create, and continually altering in a systematic way that which they seek to maintain.

Through time certain adaptive strategies become part of the world-view or ideology of a given people, or group of people, as well as being manifest in patterned social relationships vis-à-vis internal or external constraints. A given people, or members of a given society, may describe to the researcher a desirable and effective strategy that cannot be maintained, initiated or completed due to extant constraints and due to lack of options. When studying adaptive strategies, the researcher must understand the availability of options and the consequence for environment, society and culture of selecting one option over another. DECISION THEORY deals with this facet of strategy analysis by constructing sophisticated cognitive maps that reflect the way by which options and constraints are weighed by actors in specific situations.

Alternative adaptive strategies may be deployed by different individuals and groupings within the same system. The concept of adaptive strategy does not imply success in a given social, ecological, economic, political or ideological movement. It simply allows one to develop a model from observed and analysed data so as to allow the investigator to condense concepts developed at different levels of analysis and to introduce the notion of aggregate plans of reciprocating action carried out over specified time periods vis-à-vis constraints and options. The concept is of value to the analysis of conflict and may treat conflict and social disruption as system-maintaining activities or system-changing activities. One goal of adaptive strategy analysis is predictability of outcomes when competition is a key to continuing adaptation.

adelphic polyandry. Synonymous with FRATERNAL POLYANDRY, a form of POLYANDRY in which the co-husbands are brothers. It may be regarded as an extreme form of the tendency, present in many societies, for some kind of extension of the MARRIAGE alliance to the husbands' brothers or male kin: either in the form of sexual licence or of rights to claim the widow in marriage (see LEVIRATE). The extent to which this and other forms of repeated alliance are practised in a given society may be related to demographic and/or political factors.

adhesion. A term coined by TYLOR in a pioneering study of CROSS-CULTURAL COMPARISON. Adhesions, which would be called correlations in modern statistical terminology, are traits which are consistently found together, indicating the possibility of functional interrelations.

adjudication. In the anthropology of LAW, we may distinguish between different modes of DISPUTE SETTLEMENT which are characteristic of specific societies or types of society. Adjudication is the intervention, in a dispute or a case of violation of law, of a third person (or other persons) vested with special authority within a formal legal system. We may contrast MEDIATION, where the third party is not vested with legal authority and may be of high or low status in relation to the disputing parties, and NEGOTIATION where the disputing parties or their representatives come to a direct agreement without the intervention of a third party. Adjudication, or the formal legal mode of social control, is characteristic of societies with considerable specialization of roles. According to WEBER, the development of capitalist society implies and requires the development of a system of legal rationality, including specialized legal institutions.

administration. See POLICY AND ANTHROPOLOGY.

adolescence. In our society, a stage between the attainment of physical maturity (puberty) and adult status. It is not a recognized AGE GRADE in all societies, as in many the change from childhood to adult status is direct, being marked either by INITIATION rites or by marriage. The prolonging of adolescence in Western society due to such factors as late marriage and long periods of education has led to a pronounced liminal phase characterized by intergenerational conflict. The presence or absence of such conflict in other societies is related to the smoothness of the transition from child to adult status and also to the degree of conflict which exists between generations over access to resources (inheritance, land, wives, houses) and roles of responsibility or authority. (*See* AGE, ANTHROPOLOGY OF.)

adoption. A form of FICTIVE KINSHIP which may be regarded as a social mechanism through which imbalances or deficiencies in the natural (biological) process of reproduction may be adjusted to fit with the norms of kinship ideology. Adopted kinsmen thus fill the role of true kinsmen whom nature has not supplied, and in our own culture it is taboo even to mention the 'natural' origin of an adopted child. At the other extreme, adoption merges with certain forms of peonage or SLAVERY, where the adopted child may be received as payment of a debt or taken in as a servant and not as a full family member. This should perhaps be regarded as an EXTENSION OF KINSHIP TERMS rather than as adoption proper.

adultery. Sexual relations by married persons other than those with their legitimate spouse. (Sexual relations between unmarried persons is called 'fornication'.) In many cultures, these relations are forbidden and severely sanctioned, though this varies with the nature of the MARRIAGE relationship itself: in some, sexual fidelity is a key feature of the marriage relationship, in others it may be of secondary importance. A double standard is common, particularly in societies characterized by male dominance and an ideology of male control over female sexual and reproductive activity. In other cultures, neither biological paternity nor adultery may be of great importance.

adulthood. The attainment of maturity – for anthropological purposes defined as social maturity – that is the acquiring of full rights and responsibilities to the extent to which

these are age-structured. This often occurs along with marriage or parenthood. (*See* AGE, ANTHROPOLOGY OF.)

aesthetics. The notion of the aesthetic, which defines the concepts of beauty and evocativeness, is of course a culture-bound one, and may, like notions of the artistic, be quite different in cultural contexts other than our own. Aesthetic experience involves both emotion and cognition: d'Azevedo (1958) defines the 'aesthetic effect' as the 'shock of recognition emerging from the correspondences perceived between the qualities of an aesthetic object and their affinities in the subjective experience of the individual'. Art is itself a social construction out of aesthetic elements (*see* ART, ANTHROPOLOGY OF). Ethnoaesthetic research seeks to reconstruct native aesthetic categories and principles. It has been suggested that there are certain formal principles which are universal to all aesthetic systems: for example, the principles of symmetry, of proportion and balance, and so on.

affect. Generally used to refer to emotion or feeling attached to an idea or system of ideas. Anthropological approaches to the study of affect have included the CULTURE AND PERSONALITY school. In general the study of affect has received little explicit attention other than in PSYCHOLOGICAL ANTHROPOLOGY, but many anthropological theories rely implicitly on supposed regularities in affective systems (the theory of the extension of sentiments, for example, in kinship studies).

affinity. In kinship studies, an affine is a person related to Ego by a MARRIAGE link. Sometimes the term KINSHIP is used in such a way as to include both consanguineal and affinal relations, and at other times anthropologists oppose these two categories in order to contrast relations of consanguinity with those established by marriage. In kinship studies dominated by LINEAGE THEORY, relatively little importance was attached to affinal relationships, since consanguineal and descent ties were regarded as constituting the backbone of the social order. ALLIANCE THEORY however gives priority to the examination of the affinal relationships which link individuals or groups, and the affinal categories and relationships between them in KINSHIP TERMINOLOGY.

agamy. The absence of a marriage rule (that is, a system which is neither ENDOGAMOUS nor EXAGAMOUS).

age, anthropology of. Age as a principle of social organization has not received systematic anthropological attention, nor have the different conditions for types of age differentiation been examined cross-culturally. Most studies of age grouping have focused on young men's AGE SETS, though there may be other kinds of AGE GROUPS which are important. Many anthropologists have relied on elderly informants in the field, but fewer have examined the mechanisms by which the old acquire and maintain wisdom or superior knowledge, and the relationship between this and sociopolitical power. Keith, in a review of this topic (1980), distinguishes various dimensions of age differentiation which require anthropological investigation. One of these is the cognitive dimension: is age a salient feature of social classification, and if so in what contexts, and how are age differences perceived? How do people distinguish age borders and their markers, and does this vary according to the sex, age or status of the subject? Another dimension is the ideological one. Age appropriate behaviour is related to specialized roles (such as that of creator or guardian of norms and values often ascribed to the old), and this in turn relates to the structure of political roles. A further dimension is the interactional, which comprises the manner in which age peer groups are organized, and the way in which they relate to interactions which cross-cut age boundaries: for example, the relationship which exists between age groupings and the vertical principles of descent. Finally Keith distinguishes the corporate dimension, that is, the use of age principles as means of recruiting people to associations or corporate groups.

Considerable attention has been focused in modern society on the question of age conflict. Anthropological evidence shows that just as age itself is differentially defined and employed in different societies, so the type and degree of conflict between age groups is highly variable. This depends upon the definition of the generation, on the spatial or organizational separation of age groups, and on the patterns of property and power holding and transmission in each society. (*See* ADOLESCENCE, GERONTOCRACY.)

age-area hypothesis. A theory developed by WISSLER and widely accepted by the CULTURE HISTORICAL school. Wissler (1923) claimed that DIFFUSION usually proceeded at a uniform rate, thus those TRAITS which were most widely distributed were the oldest (this included elements of material culture as well as other ethnographic features). Analysis of distribution patterns enables the determination of centres of cultural innovation and diffusion. Unlike BOAS, however, Wissler's theory did not postulate functional interrelations of traits, but considered each as an independent variable.

age classes. *See* AGE GRADES.

age grades. Unlike AGE SETS, age grades are not corporate groups but consist of a series of statuses through which the individual moves over time. The distinction between age grades and age sets is one originally made by RADCLIFFE-BROWN. Like age sets, age grades may be important elements of social stratification, initiation or transition from one stage to the next giving access to knowledge, resources, social position etc. (*See* AGE, ANTHROPOLOGY OF.)

age groups. A generic term which includes both AGE GRADES and AGE SETS.

age sets. In many tribal societies, especially in East Africa, central Brazil and parts of New Guinea, there exist age-based social groupings which cross-cut kinship and descent ties. In age set systems, young people (often men only but sometimes men and women) are grouped into a named unit which has elements of corporate identity. Some age set systems are cyclical, in that names reappear after a given number of generations, while others are progressive in the sense that they continually create new names. There may be correlations in the world view and concept of time of the cultures which display cyclical and progressive age set systems respectively. Some age set systems involve the physical segregation of the age set during adolescence or before marriage: often it is the warrior age grade of young men who live apart in a MEN'S HOUSE. In other societies age sets are not residential groups, but are characterized by other types of ceremonial, social or politico-economic obligations. Age sets, by cross-cutting kinship ties, play an important part in regulating the relationships between kin groups. They also serve to regulate relationships between different generational groups, and the transmission of or access to valuables, resources and social status in societies where these are structured according to age. (*See* INITIATION; AGE, ANTHROPOLOGY OF.)

age villages. This is an unusual type of age-based organization in which the age set stays together after marriage and forms the basis of the local community. WILSON has described the Nyakyusa age-villages of Central Africa as products of an extreme opposition and separation of consecutive generations.

agnatic. Agnates, in Roman law, were persons descended from a common male ancestor. In modern usage, they are those persons who are related to one another by links through males only. Agnatic descent is therefore the equivalent of PATRILINEAL descent.

agrarian reform. *See* LAND REFORM.

agribusiness. The industrialization of agricultural production, often in the hands of transnational or multinational corporations. Wheat production in the Midwestern region of the United States is perhaps the best-known example of agribusiness on a massive scale. The so-called 'GREEN REVOLUTION' which took place mainly in the developed world from the 1960s on involved the development of higher yield varieties of food grains, and intensification of the use of fertilizers and mechanized farming techniques. The agricultural sector in the developed world thus became more capital intensive as well as more productive, and as the scale of farming increased so did the participation of large corporations at the expense of the small farmer. Agribusiness took hold in some regions of the developing

nations, controlled by the multinational and transnational corporations and taking advantage of the availability of a cheap local labour force producing cash crops for export. The green revolution and the growth of industrialized agriculture both in the developed and developing nations has had the net effect of increasing the dependence of Third World countries on food imports or food aid, and discouraging the development of small-scale agriculture devoted to subsistence needs. The industrialization and capital intensification of agricultural production is an integral part of Third World dependency, as we may observe in many parts of the world where much of the best land is in use for the cultivation of cash crops for export at prices determined by world markets and by the transnational corporations, while at the same time the local population goes short of subsistence crops. The encouragement of agribusiness by Third World governments also tends to increase the differences in wealth and power between social classes as land and agricultural production pass out of the control of tribal or peasant communities and are concentrated in the hands of a local middle or upper class who can afford the investment in capital intensive farming techniques and products, many of these in turn being imports from the developed world (farm machinery, fertilizers).

agriculture. This term is often used generally to refer to all systems of cultivation of plants for food, but sometimes it is restricted to refer to large-scale cultivation of fields using the plough and draught animals. In the latter, restricted, sense, the term is contrasted with HORTICULTURE which is the more primitive system of garden cultivation using the hoe or the digging stick. In the archaeological record, the domestication and cultivation of plants is associated with the domestication of animals, and these two activities constitute a major shift in subsistence strategies of prehistoric peoples. This shift away from HUNTING AND GATHERING subsistence strategies and towards dependence on domesticated plants and animals was termed the 'Neolithic Revolution' by the archaeologist CHILDE.

Plant cultivation was independently invented in three different areas of the world (and possibly in more): the Near East, Southeast Asia, and Mesoamerica. The reasons for the adoption of new subsistence strategies (and for the failure to adopt them among certain peoples even though they may have had access to or knowledge of agricultural techniques) have been the subject of intense debate among archaeologists and anthropologists with competing theories of cultural evolution or cultural change. The advent of new food-producing technology in the Neolithic Revolution effected a transformation in large areas of the world, establishing the foundations for population growth, increased social complexity and division of labour, and the origins of URBANISM and of STATE formation. But the relationship between the different factors involved – technology, demography, environment, social organization and culture – are matters of considerable debate.

In the Near East, the agricultural tradition based on the cultivation of grains (wheat, barley, rye and others) and the domestication of animals (sheep, goats, pigs and later cattle) developed between 10,000 and 6000 BP. Some authors emphasize the role of climatic changes at the end of the Pleistocene epoch, changes which may have played a part in forcing late Pleistocene hunters and gatherers into greater dependence on a decreasing range of plants and animals, a process culminating in the domestication of the selected species. L.R. Binford has suggested that semisedentary or sedentary communities of hunter gatherers first emerged in areas such as Palestine and Syria which were favoured by late Pleistocene climatic changes and which presented extremely rich environments in wild grains and herd animals. Population increase in these ecologically rich zones may have caused growing populations to migrate out of the ecologically favoured zones into marginal or less rich environments where they started to sow the wild grains in an attempt to reproduce the dense stands of grain of the richer areas. A further expansion of agricultural production took place around 5000 BP with the development of IRRIGATION in the hitherto marginal and arid lowlands which were to become the centre for the emergence of Near Eastern civilization.

It is frequently assumed that the adoption

of agriculture leads to a 'population explosion', but we should beware of a simplistic cause-and-effect explanation. Many authors have in fact suggested that population increases may precede rather than follow advances in agricultural technology. Demographic increases may force populations either to migrate to marginal areas where their subsistence strategies may have to be modified, or in the absence of the possibility of migration to intensify food production by the use of new techniques. The factors contributing to population increase are also complex. Hunting and gathering peoples maintain a relatively stable population level by virtue of a combination of strategies for spacing births and limiting family size: the factors influencing the abandonment of these strategies and the increasing fertility of sedentary and agricultural populations are likely to be a combination of biological, environmental and sociocultural elements. Another interesting area of study within this topic is the comparison of evidence from different parts of the world, and the attempt to explain how and why the Neolithic Revolution took a different course with different characteristics in the New World and in Asia. Evidence from Southeast Asia is scanty, though it seems probable that the earliest farmers were located in Thailand around 9000 BP, with the later development of sedentary farming in China before 3000 BP with millet as the principal crop. In the New World, we have considerably more information about the origins of cultivation in Mesoamerica, and probably also independently in Peru around 5000 BP. The first Mesoamerican crops were probably beans, squash and maize, the latter spreading to Peru by 750 BP where it joined the range of crops already being cultivated there which included squash, beans, gourds, cotton and chillies.

It is important to remember that the Neolithic Revolution should not be considered solely as a technological revolution, but first and foremost as a social revolution, which implied a transformation in social organization from the nomadic or seminomadic hunting and gathering band to the sedentary farming community, and with this, the origin of the social group which with the rise of urbanism and civilization is to become the first great social class: the PEASANTRY.

aid. *See* DEVELOPMENT.

alcohol. *See* DRINKING.

alienation. In the philosophy of Hegel, the concept of alienation refers to man's consciousness of the gulf which exists between the real world and the ideal. Marx, when he used the concept, argued that rather than being a necessary product of man's 'being in the world', alienation should be considered as historically specific to the capitalist mode of production, where it arises out of the alienated labour process in which man views his labour and therefore himself as an object, producing goods not for their use VALUE but for their exchange value. This concept has greater importance in the early works of Marx than in the later ones, though the concept of COMMODITY FETISHISM in *Capital* may be seen as a continuation of Marx's concern with alienation. In Freudian theory, the term has another sense: for Freud, it was a psychological phenomenon arising out of the imposition of civilization on man's instinctive being. Compare ANOMIE.

alliance theory. Alliance theory is associated with the pioneering works of the STRUCTU-RALIST anthropologist LEVI-STRAUSS and with subsequent developments in the theory of KINSHIP and MARRIAGE which stress the structural and organizational importance of alliance rather than of DESCENT. Levi-Strauss in his *Elementary Structures of Kinship* delineated the major elements of alliance theory at a general level, concerning himself with the structural properties and evolutionary implications of different types of alliance rule. He postulated a distinction between ELEMENTARY STRUCTURES where a positive marriage rule exists (i.e. the marriageable category is defined by kin status) and COMPLEX STRUCTURES where the choice of marriage partner is based on non-kin criteria. In the first edition of *Elementary Structures* at least Levi-Strauss did not categorically oppose alliance and descent, and conceived of alliance relations as being between local descent groups which exchanged women. Subsequent debate between alliance and descent theory however led to a hardening of positions, and alliance theorists argued that the positive marriage

rule referred not to kin categories but to alliance categories. In recent years, anthropologists have moved away from programmatic assertions of the importance of alliance or descent and towards the recognition of the empirical diversity of kinship and marriage systems in different ethnographic contexts – some of which employ descent as their primary organizational principle, others alliance, and others a combination of the two. Alliance theory has consistently been linked to structural anthropology and its concern for the tracing of the logic of RECIPROCITY and EXCHANGE in sociocultural systems. The debate between alliance and descent theory has also been linked to that between Anglophone EMPIRICIST and Francophone structuralist approaches in anthropology. Thus alliance theory was an important element in the 'rethinking' of British and US anthropology during the 1960s and 1970s. However many of Levi-Strauss' British and US followers were still too empiricist for Levi-Strauss himself, generating uncomfortable exchanges such as Levi-Strauss' discrepant reply to Needham's (1962; 1971) defence of his theory of marriage PRESCRIPTION. However much of the debate regarding the interpretation of Levi-Straussian theories results from a confusion of analytical levels, failing to distinguish between the general philosophical explanatory aims of Levi-Strauss and the attempts by his Anglophone followers to trace the more detailed working out of these general principles at the level of local social organization.

One of the major areas of study within alliance theory has been the implications of different types of positive marriage rules in real-life social and political systems. Thus it has been shown that the formal models of DIRECT EXCHANGE, of MATRILATERAL CROSS-COUSIN MARRIAGE, of PATRILATERAL CROSS-COUSIN MARRIAGE and so on, with their implications of MOIETIES, of 'marrying in a circle' or of 'delayed reciprocity' respectively are far from sufficient accounts of real marriage systems. In practice the marriage rules and associated kinship terminologies may or may not coincide with the empirical existence of the appropriate system of wife-exchanging local groups (*see* DRAVIDIAN KINSHIP SYSTEMS). Modern kinship studies have increasingly shown that the degree of flexibility and adaptability of kinship terms and marriage norms is such that few if any features of social organization can be predicted from knowledge of the marriage rule in its terminological expression alone. Thus the analysis of the formal properties of kinship terminologies and the structure of a hypothetical alliance model in accordance with terminological equivalences is regarded as only one aspect of the total analysis, which must take into account both the possibility of historical change and adaptation in kinship and marriage systems and the existence at any one time of multiple, contradictory and inconsistent 'ideal models'. Another important area of modern alliance theory is the broadening of the study of marriage alliance systems to those societies where there is apparently no positive marriage rule but where nevertheless we may discern patterns of repeated or reciprocal alliance which replicate the same structural principles as are found in the so-called 'elementary' systems.

Opposition to alliance theory came both from conventional descent theory and from some proponents of new techniques of formal analysis within COGNITIVE ANTHROPOLOGY. Thus Scheffler and Lounsbury employed formal semantic analysis in order to demonstrate their hypothesis of the extension of sentiments, in opposition to interpretations of kin terms as category terms proposed by alliance theorists. However formal analysis has also been employed to class kin terms as category terms, and there is general agreement that the formal technique cannot be held to prove basic assumptions which the analyst builds in to his study as *a priori* conditions.

allopathic medicine. The tradition of medical practice which holds that therapy should use substances whose effects are different from those of the disease being treated. This is the dominant mode in 'conventional' or 'Western' medicine. Other medical disciplines are the '*homeopathic*' which treats 'like with like', and the '*osteopathic*' or manipulative system. (*See* ALTERNATIVE MEDICINE.)

alphabet. The alphabetic system of writing represents each sound in the language with a letter, though the PHONEME-to-symbol cor-

respondence is not absolute and varies from language to language, as the same sound may be represented by more than one letter or each letter may have more than one possible pronunciation depending upon its context. Compared to other writing systems, the alphabetic system is relatively efficient and easy to learn in the sense that it employs a very restricted range of symbols. The use of an alphabetic writing system may thus favour the spread of literacy to a larger sector of the population under given historical circumstances. Alphabetic writing was first used in the Near East before 2000 BP. (*See* LITERACY.)

altered states of consciousness. Also called 'non-ordinary' states, variations from ordinary waking consciousness and perception take many forms and may be related either to increases or decreases in sensory stimuli, activity or emotion; to abnormal or pathological psycho-physiological conditions; and to drugs or other agents. They may take the form of increased arousal (e.g. hallucinations) or decreased arousal (e.g. meditation). These changes, which modern psychology locates in consciousness itself, are explained in many other cultures in terms of changes in reality (mystical or 'otherworld' knowledge and perception). Thus there is a frequent link between these states and religious belief. They may be used culturally and socially: as when dreams are interpreted, or trance states are sought by healers or religious specialists (*see* SHAMANISM). It has been suggested that one of the effects of altered states of consciousness is to prepare people for new learning or behaviour by reducing the effects of previous learning and thought habits.

alternative medicine. This term is usually used to refer to a range of therapeutic or healing practices not included within the formal professional training of conventional Western medicine. Such therapies or practices may have their roots in traditional or folk medicine, local or imported, and may be more or less formalized as far as the training and qualifications of their practitioners is concerned. Some 'alternative' therapies are in fact well developed medical systems in their countries or regions of origin: for example, acupuncture is regarded as alternative therapy in the West but in China is practised as part of recognized professional medicine. The medical profession, both in developed and developing countries, is often resistant to the incorporation of traditional or alternative therapies, and to collaboration with their practitioners, though some innovative primary health care projects have demonstrated the utility and importance which traditional healers and therapists can have in the extension of health care to the rural and urban population of the developing countries. In the developed world, the broad current of popular support for a wide range of alternative therapies perhaps reflects a feeling of discontent with conventional 'high technology' medicine, as well as the search for therapies applicable to complaints not dealt with successfully by the official medical practitioner. (*See* MEDICAL ANTHROPOLOGY.)

alternative technology. *See* APPROPRIATE TECHNOLOGY.

Althusser, Louis (1918–   ). This often controversial French intellectual has had considerable influence on Marxist theory in anthropology as well as in other disciplines. His works address themselves principally to issues relating to the interpretation of Marx and Marxist thought in modern philosophy and social science, and have been the focus of much disagreement and division among Marxist scholars, particularly the interpretation of key concepts such as socioeconomic formation, mode of production, and the nature of economic or infrastructural determinism. Althusser maintains that different spheres such as the economic, the political and the ideological possess a relative degree of autonomy and independence, and that the base or INFRASTRUCTURE is only determinant of the totality 'in the last instance'. Thus within a given mode of production different historical 'conjunctures' give rise to a number of different social formations subject to the influence of a range of determining factors. This interpretation of economic determinism stands in opposition both to vulgar materialism and to CRITICAL THEORY with its emphasis on the early 'Hegelian' Marx.

altruism. Behaviour which cannot be explained in terms of individual self-interest but which is intended to further the interests of others. FORTES spoke of 'prescriptive altruism' or 'amity' as a basic norm of kinship behaviour. Altruistic behaviour, as a category, is problematic for those theories of behaviour or of society which rely on the model of the rational self-seeking individual or ECONOMIC MAN. SOCIOBIOLOGY has explored the significance of 'kin altruism' for evolutionary theory.

ambilineal. *See* BILINEAL.

ambilocal. A residence pattern which allows a choice of VIRILOCAL or UXORILOCAL residence.

amoral familism. A term coined by Edward Banfield (1958) in his study of behaviour in a South Italian PEASANT community. He defines 'amoral familism' as the belief that each person should 'maximize the material, short term advantage of the nuclear family; assume that all others will do likewise'. This is intended as a generalization which explains and predicts a wide range of behaviour (similar to the 'familistic individualism' postulated by KLUCKHOHN as an underlying premise of Navaho philosophy and values). According to Banfield's model, social life outside the family lacks moral constraints. Like the concepts of limited good and the CULTURE OF POVERTY Banfield's model has been considerably criticized for its attribution to the system of values or attitudes of phenomena which should rather be understood in terms of the structural features of peasant society and its relation to the dominant politico-economic system.

anarchism. Anarchism as a political philosophy is characterized by its rejection of the State, which is considered to be intrinsically evil. Right-wing anarchism advocates the replacement of the functions of the State by free enterprise within a system of private property and individual liberty, while left-wing anarchism advocates collectivism.

anarcho-syndicalism. A political movement associated principally with Sorel and Guillaume, who advocated the violent overthrow of the state and of organized religion.

The basis both of the social revolution and for the construction of the future society was to be the trade union organization and the 'collective', an autonomous political, social and economic unit.

ancestor.   Ancestors and ancestor worship had been the subject of some attention in 19th- and early 20th-century anthropology: for example, TYLOR gave ancestor worship an important place in his ANIMISTIC theory of the origin of religion. The study of ancestors and ancestor worship came to the forefront, however, in the LINEAGE THEORY of social organization. According to the structural functionalist interpretation given to ancestor worship, ancestors were seen as an extension of the contemporary social structure. Thus FORTES' (1945; 1949) classic accounts of the Tallensi argue that ancestors are significant points of genealogical unification/differentiation which serve to identify segments of the lineage system, while at the same time they also serve as repositories of moral authority. Since the ancestors are idealized impersonal figures, the interpretation or divination of their 'will' both reflects motivations among the living and provides a means of reinforcing authority within kin groups. For Fortes, therefore, the authority of ancestors is an expression of kinship morality and of social organization based on the segmentary lineage system.

Later theorists have argued that this model of ancestor worship is unduly restricted: Keesing (1970), for example, points out that Fortes paid too little attention to cognatic ancestors in his analysis. Kopytoff, in a more radical critique (1971), attacks the whole distinction of living/dead kinsmen as 'ethnocentric'. He argues that in many African cultures and languages there is no distinction between elder and ancestor, and that ancestors should be seen as part of the category 'elder', and ancestor worship as an integral part of the eldership complex. Other studies have focused on the symbolic elements of ancestor cults, apart from their sociological referents, showing that their symbolic range is wider and more complex than a simple reflection of the structure of the segmentary lineage. The political implications of ancestor worship may also be more complex than Fortes suggested: ancestors are not only foci of consensus and

authority, but are part of political processes which may be characterized by conflict and dissensus, and which are often more open-ended than the Fortesian model implies.

androcentrism. 'Male bias', or the tendency to underestimate or ignore the female perspective. (*See* FEMINIST ANTHROPOLOGY; GENDER; WOMEN AND ANTHROPOLOGY.)

animatism. This term refers to the belief that the world is inhabited or animated by an impersonal force which may manifest itself both in living things and in non-living objects. The most famous example of this type of belief is the Melanesian concept of *mana*. The concept of animatism was employed by R.R. Marrett (1900) in his theory of primitive RELIGION, which stressed the role of awe at the extraordinary and inexplicable in the origin of religious beliefs. Marrett, opposing TYLOR's theory of ANIMISM, used the ethnographic example of *mana* to demonstrate the tendency of primitive thought to endow any surprising or unusual event which caught its attention with supernatural powers. He claimed that this generalized tendency to animatize or personalize inanimate objects and natural phenomena was a stage prior to animism.

animism.   The belief that natural phenomena are endowed with 'life' or 'spirit', or the tendency to attribute supernatural or spiritual characteristics to plants, geological features, climatic phenomena and so on. It also refers to a theory of RELIGION associated with SPENCER and TYLOR. Spencer opposed the theory of religion advanced by MCLENNAN, who had suggested that the earliest form of religious belief was TOTEMISM. Rather, Spencer claimed that the origin of the universal religious notion of the dual nature of man (his natural and his spiritual aspects) lay in the experience of dreaming. The association of the 'other' or dream self with the soul or ghost gave rise in turn to primitive religious beliefs and practices centred on ANCESTOR worship. Tylor (1871) similarly located the origin of religion in man's reflections on his experiences of waking, dreaming, loss of consciousness and so on. According to Tylor, these experiences gave rise to the concept of the personal soul which inhabits the body during life and becomes a ghost at death. This concept then became the basis for the beliefs in spiritual beings which for Tylor constituted religion. The term 'animism' is also widely employed to refer to the traditional religious beliefs of African peoples.

anisogamy. Asymmetric marriage alliance, that is to say, the marriage of persons of different social status. This takes two forms: HYPERGAMY and HYPOGAMY.

annual cycle. In many human groups the alternation or cycle of seasons is accompanied by periodic changes in economic activities, settlement patterns and social life. This phenomenon may be observed clearly in nomadic or semi-nomadic populations who change their location according to the availability of natural resources, and also among horticulturalists and agriculturalists where there is a marked seasonal alteration in activities related to cultivation. But it extends too to industrial and urban societies where the pattern of work and recreation may be shaped by a seasonal cycle. In a pioneering study, MAUSS (1925) argued that the relationship between seasonal alternation and 'social morphology' among the Eskimo was not to be viewed in terms of simple environmental determinism, but rather as a complex and systematic opposition to be understood above all at the level of social life. This study was very influential particularly in the development of the British STRUCTURAL FUNCTIONALIST approach to the relationship between human groups and their environment, which stressed the importance of the social interpretation of natural elements and their incorporation into native models of social structure.

anomie. A term first used by DURKHEIM, referring to a state of 'normlessness': that is, the absence of a collective morality or a state of conflicting norms in society. The term was adopted by MERTON, who defined it as a state in which socially prescribed goals and the norms governing the means of attaining them are incompatible. According to FUNCTIONALIST social theory, the absence of collective norms or the conflict between incompatible norms is related to the degree of DEVIANCE found in society. Durkheim

related the rate of SUICIDE to the existence of anomie in given social settings.

anthropometry. In PHYSICAL ANTHROPOLOGY, the measurement of physical types in different human populations.

anthropomorphism. The attribution of human characteristics to non-human phenomena (deities, animals, natural phenomena). A feature of many cosmological systems which posit a unity between human, natural and supernatural domains.

apartheid. An extreme form of INSTITUTIONAL RACISM, practised in the Republic of South Africa, whereby different racial groups are rigidly distinguished and separated in all aspects of social interaction. This separation is enforced by law. By means of the apartheid system, a minority white population maintains effective political and economic control over a majority population of blacks, Asians and mixed race groups, each of whom has a legally established status and limitations on residence, marriage, employment and the use of public facilities. The apartheid system has been compared to the Indian CASTE system, as two examples of extremely rigid systems of social STRATIFICATION based on ASCRIPTION of status. In the case of apartheid, however, we do not find the degree of ideological elaboration and justification associated with the caste system, and it is evident that the maintenance of the apartheid system is largely dependent on the use of force and political repression by the white minority.

apical ancestor/ancestress. In ANCESTOR-focused descent systems, the ancestor from whom a group traces its common membership, and who thus stands at the apex of a triangle of descendants.

applied anthropology. This area of study developed particularly in the USA after World War II, due to postwar involvement in administration and development policy in the Third World. In general, applied anthropologists accepted the need for change and the desire for DEVELOPMENT in the Third World. Overall, they tended to view the dominant national and international political structure as basically benevolent, and they devoted their efforts to the minimization of clashes of values between different cultural elements, and to the creation of a more positive relationship between the 'underdeveloped' and the 'developers'. The most famous test case of applied anthropology is Cornell University's Vicos project in Peru, where an anthropological team under the direction of A. Holmberg stepped into the role of 'patron' in a large estate and carried out what has often been criticized as a basically paternalistic reform plan aimed at ultimately devolving power to the producer. Applied anthropologists in other settings addressed themselves especially to the problems of cultural interpretation, and misinterpretation, and of suggesting creative syntheses of traditional and modern institutions, technologies, and so on.

Van Willigen in a recent survey of this field (1986) traces the development of applied anthropology through stages which he calls the 'applied ethnology stage', the 'Federal Service stage', the 'role extension, value-explicit stage' and the 'policy research stage'. In addition he reviews the offshoots of applied anthropology which have resulted from different theoretical and ideological stances: the 'action anthropology' proposed by Sol Tax, 'research and development anthropology' epitomized by the Cornell–Peru project, the community development approach and the more recent approaches of advocacy anthropology and cultural brokerage.

Applied anthropology has been criticized particularly for its apolitical stance, by those who call for a more broadly based 'development anthropology' with greater political awareness. According to these critics, applied anthropology by focusing on cultural differences merely obscures the fact that it is structures of social and politico-economic dominance which create development problems. Similarly, those anthropologists who have criticized the influence of colonial power structures within the discipline view applied anthropology as a paternalistic extension of neo-colonialism, a kind of public relations exercise which detracts attention from the real problems of dependence and underdevelopment, and which involves the anthropologist in alleviating the symptoms of conflict and thus serving the interests of a dominant group by reducing the revolutionary potential of the subordinate population. These criticisms have resulted in part from some of the more notorious involvements of anthropology in politically sensitive situations: Project Camelot, for example, involved US government attempts to use university research in order to gauge anti-communist feeling in Chile. This and other examples such as the anthropological involvement in Vietnam and Thailand have to some extent forced more awareness of the political aspects of the role of the 'applied anthropologist'.

In response to these critiques several attempts have been made to develop applied anthropology in a direction which is more sensitive both to the political implications of the discipline and to the possible conflicts of interest which may become focused upon an anthropological intervention. Many of the new developments in applied anthropology have taken place 'at home'. The field of MEDICAL ANTHROPOLOGY for example has been the focus of many recent advances in the methodology and theory of applied anthropology. In modern applied anthropology disciplinary boundaries (for example between sociology and anthropology) are less evident, as anthropologists seek to expand their methodological toolkit beyond the traditional PARTICIPANT OBSERVATION method, in search not only of increasing methodological sophistication but also of models and methods capable of taking into account the macrodimensions of sociocultural process. In the context of Third World nations, modern developments in CRITICAL ANTHROPOLOGY and MARXIST ANTHROPOLOGY increasingly erode the theoretical division between pure and applied anthropology, showing that all anthropological research and intervention is based implicitly or explicitly on ideological and political criteria. However the practical problems of intervention in DEVELOPMENT situations, of contract research and of the relationship between anthropology and POLICY have yet to be dealt with systematically other than at a very general or programmatic level. (*See* COLONIALISM; DEVELOPMENT.)

appropriate technology. This is technology designed with local factors in mind: for example, it may be more labour-intensive and less capital-intensive than technology designed for the developed countries. A related concept is that of alternative technology which implies the minimal use of non-renewable resources, minimum interference with the environment, and maximum self-sufficiency of the producing/consuming unit. There is also INTERMEDIATE TECHNOLOGY, a concept pioneered by E.F. Schumacher, and which refers to a technology intermediate between the capital-intensive Western pattern and the indigenous one. (*See* DEVELOPMENT.)

arbitration. A mode of DISPUTE SETTLE-MENT which is characterized by the intervention of a third party where the disputing parties agree to submit to the decision of the third party. Arbitration thus differs from MEDIATION, where the disputing parties do not formally agree to abide by the mediator's decision, and from ADJUDICATION, where the third party represents a legal authority empowered to enforce a decision. (*See* LAW, ANTHROPOLOGY OF.)

archaeology and anthropology. Archaeology may be divided into two principal traditions: classical and prehistoric. Classical archaeology is concerned mainly with the study of the civilizations of Ancient Greece and Rome, while prehistoric archaeology has a greater range both temporally and geographically, since it reconstructs the ways of life of peoples in all parts of the world from the emergence of man to the advent of written history. Prehistoric archaeology is above all a social science, since the archaeologist seeks an understanding not only of the physical remains he studies, but of the social and cultural tradition which created them, and attempts to reconstruct the social processes leading to the change of one form of society into another. There are many links both in theory and method between prehistoric archaeology and anthropological studies and these links have multiplied in the last two decades as archaeologists studying topics such as URBANISM and STATE formation have made increasingly sophisticated use of social science theory. This 'New Archaeology' does not limit itself to the description and classification of material remains in chronological and regional sequences, but rather adopts a systemic view of past populations in adaptation to their environments, and of processes of sociocultural change and development. In this new perspective, ecological and demographic theories, as well as sociological and anthropological ones, will play as important a part as the traditional techniques of excavation and classification which we generally associate with the archaeologist. At the same time, new scientific techniques for the dating of prehistoric remains (radiocarbon dating being perhaps the best known of a range of new techniques) enable the prehistoric archaeologist to determine the age of his finds with greater precision. The greater sophistication of mathematical models, including the use of computers, of systems analysis and other innovative analytical techniques, has also increased the archaeologist's ability to extract information from the limited data which he possesses. The modern archaeologist is thus able to construct far richer and more sophisticated theories and models of past ways of life and their development than his predecessor was.

archaic. In archaeology, used to designate a stage in the development of regional sequences. This term, which has sometimes been used to refer to PRIMITIVE or 'simple' societies, implies that they are representatives of earlier evolutionary stages who have failed to continue the evolutionary process. As Levi-Strauss argues in his essay on the concept (1963), since every society has a history and development, there is no such thing as an authentic archaism or SURVIVAL from the most primitive stage of development.

archetypes. In Jungian psychology, the images which form the content of the collective unconscious. The term has also been used somewhat more broadly in the study of art and of SYMBOLISM with the meaning of basic common symbolic images. In STRUCTURAL ANTHROPOLOGY, the notion of archetypes or common contents to the unconscious mind is rejected in favour of the notion of common symbolic forms or patterns which place order on the variety of possible contents.

architecture and anthropology. Explorations

into the relationship between architecture and anthropology have been relatively few, in spite of the fact that this is a field of great potential interest for the anthropologist, representing as it does an interface between ideology and technology. Man's dwellings and the layout of his settlements reflect both the constraints and necessities imposed by the environment and his mode of subsistence, and his concept of individual, family and communal life. Architectural design both reflects and shapes public expectation regarding the environment and man's use of resources, and it may be used to translate political dogmas or ideas into a relatively public and permanent form. Among peoples with relatively little technological development dwellings and communities may be more impermanent than a modern city, but we may examine here too the dynamic interplay between materials, environment and man's ideal models of family and social life. In traditional societies architectural design as such may apparently not exist, the form and design of a building or a house emerging 'as the work goes along'. However these improvised constructions do reflect culturally standardized models of the distribution and activities of their inhabitants, as well as possessing in many cases a special symbolism identifying, the house, for example, with a human body, a lineage, and so on. Thus the orientation, position and internal relations between the parts of the house acquire symbolic significance, and ethnoarchitectural principles reflect important social and cultural categories and relationships.

arena. In ACTION THEORY of political systems, this refers to the domain within which conflict or competition for power takes place. Such arenas may be small-scale (the village, the tribe etc.) or large-scale (e.g. the state). (*See* FIELD.)

Arensberg, Conrad M. (1910–). US anthropologist with a broad range of ethnographic and theoretical interests. Arensberg was associated with the Yankee City studies carried out by WARNER which brought anthropological fieldwork methods to the study of an urban community. Arensberg's study of Irish rural life (1968) has been influential in the COMMUNITY STUDY tradi-

tion, and he has also undertaken research in India. His broad theoretical interests have embraced fields as diverse as ECONOMIC ANTHROPOLOGY (where he is associated with the substantivist school inspired by POLANYI), industrial anthropology, and the study of DEVIANCE.

aristocracy. From the Greek 'rule by the best'. Aristotle contrasted aristocracy with OLIGARCHY, which is rule by the wealthiest. In modern usage the term refers to a hereditary ruling and property-holding group with special privileges and titles. Typically this is accompanied by a MONARCHY, and historically and cross-culturally we may observe varying degrees of opposition and separation between the crown and the aristocracy. The aristocracy, with its hereditary entitlement to land, property and political office, is an expression of the FEUDAL or feudal-type MODE OF PRODUCTION, where the dominant class is that which controls property in land.

army. *See* WARFARE.

art, anthropology of. Anthropologists have focused on the study of the art of preliterate societies, and also of artistic traditions belonging to FOLK cultures or ethnic minorities within a dominant literate culture. More attention has been paid to plastic and graphic arts than to performing arts, the latter often being subsumed under the study of RITUAL. Few preliterate societies have specialized artists, and some scarcely differentiate the artist's role at all, since artistic production may be general to a large proportion of the population. Our distinction between art and craft often does not apply, since many of these societies do not distinguish the concepts of 'function' and 'beauty' in artistic production. Similarly, concepts of creativity and innovation are subject to tremendous cross-cultural variation. In general, ethnic art is more conservative (less innovative, though not therefore less creative) than Western art which is generally highly specialized and encourages both innovation and sophisticated comment on style itself.

   Some anthropologists have used artistic data to address questions of cross-cultural variation or universals. Thus artistic style, which is the recurrence of clusters of formal features in art, was used along with other cultural traits as evidence of general hypotheses concerning evolution and diffusion in 19th- and early 20th-century anthropological theory. BOAS introduced an early concern with the psychic and symbolic aspects of art styles, and KROEBER attempted to relate the historical development of artistic style to the development of civilizations. The cross-cultural approach to art attempts to establish broad correlations between art styles or forms and social or social-psychological factors. Thus Fischer argues, using statistical evidence, that egalitarian societies are characterized by graphic designs which repeat simple elements, while hierarchical societies produce designs integrating a number of dissimilar elements. Such analysis rests on the notion of a MODAL PERSONALITY shared by all members of society, and assumes the artists' conformity to social norms. It has been criticized on the grounds that both values and artistic styles vary within a single sociocultural context.

Anthropological studies of the SYMBOLISM of art have followed a variety of approaches ranging from psychological or psycho-analytic to structuralist perspectives. Neo-Freudian interpretations relate artistic symbolism to classic psychoanalytic themes involving the resolution of individual psychic conflicts, but studies such as that by Forge (1973) provide a demonstration that it is equally possible to analyse sexual symbolism in art in terms of wider cosmological and technoenvironmental contexts without resort to the Freudian model.

The theories of LEVI-STRAUSS have been influential in the anthropology of art. Munn (1972) follows up Levi-Strauss' suggestions as to how the underlying structural principles of artistic production reflect the structural patterns underlying the functioning of society. He suggests that in Walbiri graphic art the design patternings parallel the ordering principles which govern the totemic system and other cosmological theories. Graphic designs thus become visual models for abstract principles of social and cosmological ordering.

Another approach, which Silver terms 'ethnoart' (1979) (cf. ETHNOSCIENCE) concentrates on the study of art from an EMIC perspective, and the reconstruction of native artistic categories and principles. This contrasts with those studies which focus on the social function of art. These tie in with the study of ritual and religion, and emphasize the power of symbolism in social action, rather than examining the content of artistic production.

articulation of modes of production. This concept is an important one in MARXIST ANTHROPOLOGY, where it refers to the interaction and interrelationship of different MODES OF PRODUCTION or different institutional arrangements for the organization of the economic process. It has been claimed that Marxist theory, in its emphasis on the historical transformation of modes of production and the transition from one SOCIO-ECONOMIC FORMATION to another, pays insufficient attention to the simultaneous existence of different modes of production within a single regional or national social system. These situations of contact and interaction between different productive systems are of course commonly encountered in anthropological studies, and Marxist anthropology has devoted considerable attention to the interpenetration of capitalist and pre-capitalist relations of production in colonial and post-colonial settings. (*See* DEPENDENCY; WORLD SYSTEMS.)

ascription. *See* ACHIEVEMENT AND ASCRIPTION.

Asiatic mode of production. In the writings of MARX this refers to self-sufficient village economies with minimal division of labour and with productive systems which are ossified around traditional forms. There is a centralized state BUREAUCRACY and military force, controlled by a ruling elite of surplus takers. Marx considered it to be an exception to the general tendency for productive forces to evolve and develop. In *Capital* (New York, 1906) Marx says: 'The simplicity of the organization for production in these self-sufficing communities...supplies the key to the secret of the unchange-ableness of Asiatic societies...in such striking contrast with the constant dissolution and refounding of Asiatic states, and the never-ceasing changes of dynasty'. The theory of ORIENTAL DESPOTISM developed by Wittfogel (1957) is related to the concept of the Asiatic mode of production, but Wittfogel emphasizes the importance of centralized control over water supplies in the formation of 'irrigation civilizations'. The Asiatic mode of production is a category which has been left on one side by many Marxist scholars, perhaps because the suggestion of a special geographical category appears to go against the general contention of Marxist theory that the stages of evolution of socioeconomic formations are universally applicable.

assimilation. One of the outcomes of the ACCULTURATION process, in which the subordinate or smaller group is absorbed into the larger or dominant one and becomes indistinguishable from it in cultural terms. The concept of assimilation has been widely questioned in modern anthropology, and most writers now argue for a more careful examination of the different dimensions of cultural interchange and social dominance in situations of contact between different sociocultural systems.

association. Associations, which are groups of persons who join together or are joined together for a particular activity, interest or purpose, have been classified along a number of different dimensions: for example, contractual versus non-contractual, voluntary versus involuntary, with or without explicit purpose, incorporated or unincorporated, formal or informal, open or restricted, to name only the most common dichotomies. The term has often been used to translate TONNIES' concept of *Gesellschaft*, contrasted with that of *Gemeinschaft* or 'community'. The exploration of associations and the classification of the forms they adopt has been developed more fully in sociology than in anthropology, where the study of social groups with a shared purpose or interest is often subsumed under other headings. In simple or traditional societies the range of social activities and organization which is covered by special purpose associations is comparatively small, while in modern industrial society they are the dominant mode of organization in many sectors and their range of forms is far greater.

asymmetric/symmetric alliance. This dichotomy, which may also be referred to as that between indirect and direct exchange, or between generalized and restricted exchange, is an important element in LEVI-STRAUSS' theory of ELEMENTARY STRUCTURES and in ALLIANCE THEORY in general. Symmetric, direct or restricted systems are those characterized by a pattern or rule of MARRIAGE alliance involving the exchange of women between two kin groups (it may also be conceptualized as the exchange of men between two kin groups, though this latter interpretation has been less fully explored). The most elementary example of direct exchange is the rule of bilateral cross-cousin marriage, where the children of a brother and sister are prescribed or preferred spouses. However the pattern of direct exchange may be detected in systems where actual bilateral cross-cousin marriage is not the rule, or even where this is prohibited between cousins of the first degree, but where nevertheless marriages follow some kind of pattern of direct exchange between groups. Asymmetric, indirect or generalized systems on the other hand are those where wife-givers are distinguished from wife-takers and direct marriage exchanges are proscribed. The two model types of indirect exchange are MATRILATERAL CROSS-COUSIN MARRIAGE and PATRILATERAL CROSS-COUSIN MARRIAGE, though again it should be mentioned that the structural principles of indirect exchange do not require strict adherence to these genealogical categories. Levi-Strauss in his theory of elementary structures speculated about the evolutionary consequences of these types of exchange, suggesting that the symmetric or direct form is both more stable and at the same time less integrative. Since it involves the participation of only two wife-exchanging units or kin groups in order to complete the system, he argues, the symmetric alliance system tends towards the breakdown of society into such independent units. Indirect systems however may be conceived of as chains or circles which may link together any number of local or kin groups, though by their asymmetric nature they are also inherently unstable. The consequences of this inherent instability and the functions of asymmetric marriage alliance have been widely debated and explored in the anthropology of India and Southeast Asia in particular. (*See* HYPERGAMY; HYPOGAMY.)

atom of kinship. A model proposed by LEVI-STRAUSS in opposition to conventional theories of the nuclear FAMILY and the AVUNCULATE. Levi-Strauss (1963) argues that it is not sufficient to consider the relations F/S and MB/ZS as an opposed pair. They must be treated instead as part of a total system of relations: B/Z, H/W, F/S and MB/ZS. This set of four relations will always contain two positive and two negative ones, such that MB/ZS:B/Z::F/S:H/W (the relation between MB and ZS is to the relation between B and Z as the relation between F and S is to that between H and W). This model of the elementary unit of kinship was important within ALLIANCE THEORY because it challenged the conventional consanguineous model of the nuclear family, arguing for the inclusion of the alliance relationship in the atom of kinship and interpreting the avunculate also in terms of affinal ties. However the formulation of the model has been criticized both in terms of its empirical accuracy and by those who claim that it is arbitrary to delimit these four relationships as universally constituting the basic structure of kinship systems. Critics have argued that in different kinship systems the atom of kinship may be differently constituted and that more empirical investigation is necessary before arriving at general conclusions.

attitudes. In studies of KINSHIP, it is common to distinguish the system of TERMINOLOGY from the system of attitudes, such as feelings of respect or familiarity, affection or hostility, rights or obligations by which people feel bound and which will manifest themselves in certain patterns of behaviour. RADCLIFFE-BROWN argued that attitudes were a transposition or reflection of terminology at the affective level, but subsequent critics, including LEVI-STRAUSS, have pointed out that there are often discrepancies between terminological classifications and attitudes. Levi-Strauss suggests that the system of attitudes should be regarded as a dynamic integration of the terminological system. Stylised or prescribed attitudes towards certain categories of kin,

he argues, may serve to resolve the contradictions inherent in the terminology.

authority. Authority, as distinct from POWER, is the social attribution of the right to control the actions or decisions of others in certain social situations. It is therefore essentially a collective phenomenon vested in an individual by the group, though at the level of ideologies and political philosophies it is often represented as extra-social in origin: that is, as either natural or divine. DURKHEIM viewed authority as an expression of the conscience collective which was also the origin of RELIGION. WEBER contrasts traditional authority, which is based on the LEGITIMACY of a set of norms which are fixed and sacred, with rational-legal authority. In the rational-legal type, which is impersonal by nature, authority resides not in the person but in the office. A third type of authority is the CHARISMATIC type, which depends on the characteristics of an individual leader. The Weberian scheme has been much debated and developed in POLITICAL ANTHROPOLOGY. In the study of simple or traditional societies, it is evident that the Weberian notion should be modified to the extent that authority may be viewed not so much as proceeding from a fixed set of norms as emerging out of a process of social interaction and dialogue. M. Bloch has suggested that an important element in authority relations in traditional societies may be located at the linguistic level, where social actors are committed to stylised or ritual exchanges which limit their ability to suggest innovative or alternative interpretations and outcomes to social situations.

autochthonous. Greek: 'from the earth itself'; sometimes used to refer to the original inhabitants of a region.

autocracy. Literally 'self-rule', used to mean arbitrary and absolute power or rule by one person.

auto-ethnography. The anthropological study of a sociocultural system by a member of the society concerned. In the USA this has become increasingly common in recent years, and involves a process of critical appraisal (both professional and personal) which has been documented by a number of researchers, notably Messerschmidt (1981). Problematic aspects of carrying out research in the USA include the relationship between involvement as a citizen or as a political actor and professional involvement as an anthropologist (*see* POLICY), and the need for the researcher to rethink his or her previous assumptions of 'belonging' to US society or culture in order to make way for an anthropological analysis. Indeed it is evident that within the USA there exists a wide variety of different sociocultural systems or subsystems, the penetration and analysis of which may be as difficult for the ethnographer as that of a tribal society in a Third World nation.

The problems of auto-ethnography within Third World nations have been less fully explored, though they are in many respects similar to those which have been discussed in the case of the USA. The Third World scholar is likely to be a middle-class intellectual who in order to study rural or urban popular sectors of his own society must overcome his own class (and/or racial) prejudice. Even in those cases where members of native or peasant communities themselves are involved in anthropological research it is necessary to examine with great care the models and approaches they are employing, who is orienting them, and the extent to which their involvement is separating them from the social and cultural system of origin. Above all it is necessary to analyse critically the implicit and explicit politico-ideological bases of auto-ethnography in the same fashion as we examine those of conventional ethnographic research. Thus CRITICAL ANTHROPOLOGY in Latin America and other regions has documented the manner in which anthropological studies carried out by national scholars tend to perpetuate NEO-COLONIAL political and ideological structures and to justify ETHNOCIDAL national policies, where these studies are not accompanied by analyses of the wider problematic of interethnic relations and DEVELOPMENT.

autonym. Name applied to a person independent of his relation to others. (*See* NECRONYM; TEKNONYMY.)

avoidance. It is common for certain relationships to be consistently marked out by avoidance behaviour, the most well-known case being mother-in-law avoidance which is practised to some degree in a very large range of societies. Naturally enough, functional explanations of avoidance behaviour have treated the avoidance relationship as an expression of tensions created by social and kinship structures – in other words, as a mechanism which both expresses and diverts potential conflicts. A structuralist approach to avoidance behaviour would examine not only the avoidance relationship itself but its position with regard to other relationships which together form the structure of kin attitudes and behaviour: an avoidance relationship may exist not so much because of tensions inherent in the relationship itself as because it forms a structural opposition to another relationship (*see* ATOM OF KINSHIP).

The terms 'avoidance' or 'avoidance behaviour' have been employed as substitutes for TABOO in modern anthropology, since the unitary conception and explanation of the phenomenon of taboo has been widely questioned. Avoidance behaviours in modern anthropology are studied as part of the total SYMBOLIC system of which they form a part, and have been interpreted by writers following M. Douglas as sociopsychological responses to phenomena which are anomalous in terms of systems of CLASSIFICATION.

avunculate. A special relationship with the maternal uncle, which may be one of indulgence or alternatively one of authority. RADCLIFFE-BROWN suggested that there are two different sets of roles relating to the mother's brother/sister's son relationship, and that the incidence of these sets was determined by the rule of descent. In matrilineal societies the MB is an authority figure and the relationship with the father is characterized by greater freedom and affection, while in patrilineal systems the roles are reversed. This theory was criticized by LEVI-STRAUSS in his formulation of the concept of the ATOM OF KINSHIP.

avunculocal. Also viri-avunculocal. Refers to the rule of residence in some matrilineal societies whereby a man and his wife take up residence with the man's maternal uncle.

B

Bachofen, Johann Jacob (1815–87). A Swiss lawyer and classicist, Bachofen was inspired by his studies of classical mythology to develop a theory of the evolution of kinship systems. He postulated that an early stage of primitive promiscuity was characterized by MATRIARCHY or mother right, which was replaced by PATRILINEALITY at a later stage of development (e.g. 1861). The emergence of patrilineality was related in Bachofen's theory to the development of private property and the corresponding desire of men to pass this on to their children. MORGAN, basing his argument on the analysis of kinship terminology, agreed with Bachofen that the matrilineal preceded the patrilineal stage in social evolution.

band. In the evolutionary scheme commonly employed in US anthropology, one of the major stages of sociocultural evolution (band, TRIBE, CHIEFDOM and STATE). Band organization is typical of HUNTING AND GATHERING societies. The band is a small group of some 50–300 persons, defined by its simplicity and flexibility of structure, the absence of a formal leadership role, and the absence of significant social stratification. These characteristics are generally related by anthropologists to the absence of significant property relationships or the impossibility of concentration of control over resources or productive relationships.

bandits. Banditry is a special form of crime combined with political rebellion which is particularly evident historically where a territorial state is in the process of incorporating and subjugating formerly autonomous local communities. Bandits often enjoy the support of the local community, and their labelling at the level of national politics as 'criminals' may mask the fact that locally they are legitimate defenders of traditional territorial rights or political autonomy. Banditry emerges where there is a disjunction of NORMS of legitimacy between the state and the local community, and also where there is a breakdown of traditional communal social, economic and political structures.

baptism. *See* COMPADRAZGO; RITUAL KINSHIP.

barbarism. Part of the evolutionary scheme first employed by MONTESQUIEU: hunting or savagery, herding or barbarism and civilization were the three stages of this scheme, which became very popular among 19th-century social theorists. Among others, MORGAN adopted this scheme, as did TYLOR. Barbarism was distinguished from savagery by the development of agriculture and pastoralism, and the emergence of certain crafts such as metalworking and pottery.

barter. The exchange of goods for goods, without the intervention of MONEY. Barter is generally found in conjunction with a SUBSISTENCE economy, and economic systems with large surpluses or a high degree of specialization in the division of labour tend to make use of the more flexible system of money exchange. However this is not to say that a barter economy is necessarily extremely simple, as the studies of SPHERES OF EXCHANGE have shown that within these economies there are complex mechanisms of equivalence and of insulation of certain domains of production, consumption and exchange. Barter as a type of non-money exchange may be characterized as relatively impersonal, as compared to the generalized RECIPROCITY of exchanges with close kin, or the balanced reciprocity of ceremonial or GIFT exchange. Barter is a type of exchange where economic rather than social considerations are primary.

base. *See* INFRASTRUCTURE.

baseline. *See* CULTURAL BASELINE.

basic personality. This term was used by the psychoanalytically-oriented anthropologist A. Kardiner in his study of the relationship between CULTURE AND PERSONALITY. According to Kardiner, the PRIMARY INSTITUTIONS of a society, which include socialization practices and subsistence patterns, form the typical set of attitudes and orientations of its members, or the basic personality. Through social interaction, this basic personality type then in turn shapes the secondary institutions of society.

Bastian, Adolf (1826–1905). A German trained in law, science and medicine, he served as curator in a Berlin museum. He had travelled widely and was impressed by the similarities in customs in different locations, a phenomenon which he attributed to the 'psychic unity of mankind' or *Elementargedanken* (e.g. 1860). He claimed that this unity, rather than a process of diffusion, accounted for similar cultural manifestations in different places. Though Bastian's theory was not an evolutionary one, since it rested on innate psychological givens, his ideas were adopted by CULTURAL EVOLUTIONISTS.

Bateson, Gregory (1904–80). US scholar who brought his training in biology and psychology to his distinctive and innovative anthropological work, and developed also an interest in the relationship between COMMUNICATION science and anthropology, introducing several concepts from CYBERNETIC theory into anthropological studies. His ethnographic study *Naven* (1958) pioneers many areas which were later to become central to the study of SYMBOLISM in anthropology. In this work, Bateson uses the concepts of *ethos* and *eidos* to designate the general principles which give coherence to a belief system and those which give coherence to a value system respectively. These concepts were widely adopted in US cultural anthropology, particularly that of *ethos*. Other influential concepts introduced by Bateson include SCHISMOGENESIS, which describes the manner in which the cumulative tensions produced by social and linguistic interaction culminate in the fission

of groups; that of double bind, a condition of inconsistent or contradictory demands on the individual which has been linked by some theorists with the development of schizophrenia; and that of META-COMMUNICATION, which refers to 'messages about messages' or the 'framing' of linguistic behaviour. The relationship between communications theory, ecological theory and SYSTEMS THEORY is explored in Bateson's stimulating *Steps to an Ecology of Mind* (1972).

Beattie, John Hugh Marshall (1915–). British social anthropologist who has published extensively on the Bunyoro of Uganda (e.g.1960), and who has also made substantial contributions to the study of the relationship between philosophy and anthropological theory and method.

beauty. *See* AESTHETICS.

behaviourism. This term is generally associated with the behavioural school of psychology which is rooted in the classical CONDITIONING theory of the Russian psychologist Pavlov. In the United States, where behaviourism was pioneered by the psychologist J.B. Watson, the leading modern exponent is B.F. Skinner, who has described another form of conditioning known as operant. In general, behaviourism is characterized by its focus on learning, and by its rejection of the study of subjective mental states as the basis for a scientific psychology. In Great Britain, the psychologist H.J. Eysenck has been an often controversial exponent and popularizer of behaviourist psychology, though Eysenck places greater emphasis on the role of genetic factors (for example, in differences in intelligence) than do the majority of his colleagues. When applied to linguistics and the social sciences, behaviourism can be used as a method of accounting for most, if not all, of human social behaviour. The behaviourist assesses the cumulative outcomes of learning processes, which are themselves based on conditioning via the association of positive or negative reinforcement with parts of behaviour. Behaviourist theory holds that the only truly scientific study is that which limits itself to what may be measured and observed (that is, behaviour), and that we should not postulate models or theories of 'consciousness', which is unobservable, in order to account for what we observe. The scientist is thus limited to the observation of chains of stimulus, response and reinforcement. This perspective became dominant in experimental psychology, especially in the USA, but the influence of behaviourist theory on other disciplines and specifically on anthropology has been slight. Important challenges to behaviourist theory have come from transformational linguistics and from cognitive and developmental psychology. These critiques have shown the inability of behaviourist theory to account for large areas of human conduct and above all for the complex organization of language, cognition and behaviour. In one of the better known critiques of behaviourism, the linguist N. Chomsky points out that the conditioning model of language acquisition cannot account for the phenomenon of linguistic creativity (the ability to create new utterances, not merely repeat those already heard), and claims that it is necessary to posit an innate linguistic capacity or 'programming' in the child which primes him to learn language once exposed to it. Behaviouristic psychology has of course reacted to these criticisms, giving rise to various neo-behaviourist accounts of learning which take into account cognitive schemata mediating between the stimulus and the response. (*See* COGNITION).

belief. This term, and that of belief system, have been widely used in the anthropology of RELIGION and in cultural and social anthropology in general, but often with no precise definition of what constitutes a 'belief' at the level of a sociocultural system, or in what manner beliefs are integrated to form a 'system'. It is evidently problematic to attribute a 'belief' (ultimately an individual and psychological phenomenon) to a group, community or society. In US cultural anthropology influenced by the CULTURE AND PERSONALITY school, it was commonly assumed that the beliefs of a group could be viewed as a single integrated system. BATESON introduced the term 'eidos' to describe the general principles or premises which give coherence to a belief system (this parallels the 'ethos' which gives coherence to

the VALUE system). Similarly KLUCKHOHN describes the 'implicit philosophy' of the Navaho. The British STRUCTURAL FUNCTIONALIST anthropologists similarly tended to assume uniformity of belief throughout a society and to formulate their theories of the correspondence between social structure and belief systems accordingly. More recently, COGNITIVE ANTHROPOLOGY has refined the anthropological approach to the cultural organization of KNOWLEDGE and beliefs. It is important to retain the distinction between CLASSIFICATION and belief, since the classification of two phenomena in the same linguistic or supralinguistic category does not necessarily imply a 'belief' in their equivalence or identity other than for the purposes of that specific classification. An important area of investigation is the differential distribution of beliefs among different members of society or different groups and classes. This topic has been explored with relation to the study of IDEOLOGY and the anthropology of knowledge by Marxist anthropologists and others concerned with the social and political mechanisms influencing organization and distribution of both knowledge and belief. Such explorations call into question earlier generalizations regarding 'belief systems' considered as uniform throughout social or cultural groups. (*See* WORLD VIEW; COSMOLOGY.)

Benedict, Ruth Fulton (1887–1948). US scholar who entered anthropology from a background in philosophy and literature. As a student of BOAS and a close associate of SAPIR her particular interest was in the area of CULTURE AND PERSONALITY. She developed the theory that personality types and criteria of psychological 'normality' were culturally moulded. In *Patterns of Culture* (1934) she attempted to elaborate culturally specific master plans or dominant personality types.

bifurcation. In KINSHIP TERMINOLOGY, the lineal distinction between kin of the maternal and paternal sides. Thus the 'bifurcate merging' terminology distinguishes maternal from paternal kin but does not recognize collateral distinctions, grouping together F and FB, M and MZ; while the 'bifurcate collateral' system recognizes both lineal and collateral distinctions, giving separate terms for M, F, MB, FZ, MZ, and FB.

big man. This term is used in Melanesian ethnography to describe a kind of political leader, and also a kind of political system. The big man is a leader within a relatively unstable FACTIONAL political system, and his position depends largely on his ability to maintain his personal prestige and the prestige of his group. He is thus in constant competition with other big men, attempting to maintain and enhance his faction at the expense of others. Unlike a true CHIEF, the big man has no position of formal AUTHORITY, and the anthropologist M. Sahlins (1963) has characterized the big man system as one in which LEGITIMACY, though constantly pursued, is rarely achieved by a political leader. Sahlins has also pointed out that to a certain extent the competition between big men and between factions may be regarded as a mechanism by which big men as a group maintain some degree of dominance over their respective faction members. The phenomenon of the big man may be considered to be intermediate between a BAND-type political system where leadership is highly informal and where the leader is characterized by his obligation to give away all he obtains rather than by his accumulation or prestige consumption of goods, and the true chiefly system. Like the prestige exchanges of traditional chiefdoms (e.g. POTLATCH) the big man system stimulates production over and above domestic subsistence needs. And like a true chief, the big man acts as a focal point for the exchange of goods between local communities. But the difference lies in the fact that the big man system is in Sahlins' words one of 'open status competition' in which the leader must construct his following and his position, whereas a chief steps in to an already existing OFFICE. Comparisons have been made between the Melanesian big man system and other systems of informal factional politics, for example in the Amazonian region.

bilateral. Bilateral kinship reckoning is that which recognizes links through both sexes. (*See* KINDRED.)

bilineal, ambilineal. Bilineal kinship reckoning is that which traces DESCENT through both male and female links. (*See* NON-UNILINEAL DESCENT.)

bilingualism. The existence, in a given individual's linguistic capability or in a given community, of two or more languages (multilingualism being as a rule included under the general category of bilingualism). Like the boundaries between SOCIETIES or CULTURES, those between languages and between SPEECH COMMUNITIES are often hard to define, and bilingualism is both a common and extremely complex phenomenon which has caused linguists to revise many of their traditional concepts of language acquisition and language use. The importance of bilingualism in terms of anthropological study is mainly in terms of the way in which language serves as an expression of cultural and ethnic identity, and also as a vehicle for the imposition of a dominant culture or for the expression of relations of political and social dominance. Language may be used as a vehicle for the imposition of a dominant national culture, as in many educational systems both in developed and Third World nations which fail to take into account local and regional languages and rather attempt to impose a uniform national language and educational curriculum. Bilingual education programmes in such contexts are often a focus of political opposition and debate, since they represent the attempt to incorporate local needs and expressive systems into the formal educational system. Language use may also on the other hand be exclusive in the sense of denying access to a national or elite language in order to deny access to political power. Thus, bilingual education programmes may fall into the trap of perpetuating marginality if they deny to local populations an adequate education in the language of the dominant group.

binary opposition. A relationship of opposition or contrast between two elements. A binary CODE is at once a simple and very powerful tool for the performance of logical operations, and is the basis of the modern digital computer. The notion of binary oppositions is important in STRUCTURALIST theory.

biological anthropology. This term has come into use in recent years to indicate the study of the relationship between biology and sociocultural systems, including the biological basis and consequences of human behaviour. It thus embraces the concerns of PHYSICAL ANTHROPOLOGY as well as areas of PSYCHOLOGICAL ANTHROPOLOGY and CULTURAL ECOLOGY.

birth. Every society possesses what might be referred to as a social organization of the LIFE CRISIS which the birth of a new member constitutes. This includes a series of accepted behaviours both for the mother and her kin and affines, observances relating to the birth itself and to the newborn baby. Some of these observances are ritual in nature, others are designed to protect the health of mother and baby, and some may combine these functions. The birth of a baby in traditional societies may be attended by the mother's own kinswomen (her mother, for example) or by her affines (such as her mother-in-law), and/or by a specialist traditional birth attendant who is generally a woman. In some societies the father may be excluded from the birth, while in others he may be present and play an active part in the proceedings. A well-known example of the extent of male participation in birth is the COUVADE, which refers to the ritual observance by the father of rest and seclusion when his wife gives birth. Commonly both father and mother of the newborn baby must observe certain avoidances relating to food, physical activities and contact with potentially magically dangerous substances in order to protect the child from harm. In the majority of traditional societies, most of the ritual observances surrounding childbirth are comparatively private in nature, and are restricted to the protection of the mother and child against harmful influences or disease. In many of these societies however, the image of birth is central in other rituals concerning the individual life-cycle or the ceremonial/religious life of the group as a whole. In many of these rituals a second, superior 'social' birth is created, borrowing the imagery of the natural birth but transferring control from women to men, who thus assert their function as socializers of the children that women naturally create (see COMPADRAZGO; RITUAL SEXUAL SYM-

METRY; INITIATION.) Thus the natural birth itself receives little public attention, and the custom of not allotting full 'human' or social status, including a name to a very young child which is sometimes attributed to high infant mortality rates also relates to the ritual negation of women's part in creating members of society: the child is not 'complete' until it has received its social identity in a second ritual birth.

In the more affluent industrial nations birth is nowadays generally managed by the medical profession, effectively preventing family and community from participating in it, and involving some practices which are medically useless or counterproductive (for example, the separation of mother and baby in the first days of life, the discouragement of breast-feeding) and which tend towards de-emphasizing or replacing the 'natural' aspects of childbirth where possible. These practices, experienced by many mothers and families as 'de-humanizing', have led to an increasing demand for a return to 'natural childbirth'. Health authorities in many countries have responded with newer policies which encourage minimal medical intervention in normal births, rooming-in of mothers with babies, breastfeeding, community midwifery, and so on. This is an area in which anthropological evidence (some of it ill-substantiated, such as the frequent claim that childbirth is 'easier' in traditional societies) has often been cited to support the case for changes in social policy.

black. This term came into prominence in the United States during the 1960s when it was adopted by Civil Rights and BLACK POWER movements and quickly spread into popular usage. Black political and civil rights activists rejected the labels 'coloured' or 'negro', deliberately adopting the term 'black', which had previously been considered an insult, and stressing the importance of positively identifying with 'black pride'. In the United Kingdom, the term has also been widely adopted to refer to people of African and Caribbean descent. (See RACE.)

black economy. The growth of Third World cities, coupled with the fact that the modern industrial sector has been unable to provide employment for most of the incoming migrants, has meant that a majority of urban households have, in order to survive at all, had to resort to a range of different kinds of economic activity: hawking, street-trading, small-scale production, reciprocal kin-based exchange and servicing. This sector has been called the black, underground, marginal, or, most commonly, the informal economy, since it operates outside formal market structures and outside fiscal control (national accounts and tax registers) as well as employing those who are not part of the statistically-defined labour force. Considerable attention has been paid by anthropologists, economists and governments to the operations of this sector, and it has proved remarkably difficult to quantify. The emphasis has recently shifted in work on this topic from regarding it as separate from, and parasitic upon, the formal economy, to seeing it as an integral part of the capitalist market. As the world recession has hit the First World, so too it is increasingly recognized that the informal economy exists there as well and it is not just a Thirld World phenomenon.

Black Power. An influential movement of social transformation in the USA, and one which has provided models for many other movements of protest and 'consciousness raising'. Black Power grew out of the Civil Rights movement of the 1960s, from which it differed in its emphasis on the independent development of political organization and ethnic pride among blacks. In their anthropological study of the movement, L.P. Gerlach and V.H. Hine (1973) characterize it as a 'grass roots' organization rather than a more centralized revolutionary movement, and typify it as segmentary, decentralized and 'reticulate' (forming unbounded and loose networks between local cells, each of which crystallizes around a charismatic leader). They conclude that these features are adaptive in implementing social change, because they make the movement hard to suppress, encourage innovativeness, and maximize recruitment from different socio-economic strata.

blood feud. A type of FEUD distinguished by the prevalence of homicide and revenge killing. (*See* WARFARE.)

blood relations. *See* CONSANGUINITY.

Boas, Franz (1858–1942). Franz Boas was born and received his education as a geographer in Germany. He was led to take up anthropology as a result of his experiences living among the Eskimos of Northern Canada, and he became the dominant figure in US professional anthropology. He criticized the tendency in anthropology towards premature generalization and SPECULATIVE HISTORY, and argued in favour of meticulous collection (aiming at 'total recovery') of ethnographic data before generalization could be attempted. Unlike earlier evolutionary theorists who had emphasized overall cultural similarities, Boas stressed the differences and particularity of each culture as a result of its specific and divergent historical development. Thus his approach has been termed 'historical particularism', which is characterized by its rejection of the comparative method of the UNILINEAR EVOLUTIONISTS (1911). He also developed an interest in the psychological aspects of culture(e.g. 1940). His holistic approach to fieldwork and the breadth of his research interests – which spanned linguistics, physical anthropology, archaeology as well as cultural manifestations – was inherited by many of his students. The Boasian school established CULTURE as the key concept in US anthropology, and has been criticized both for its CULTURAL DETERMINISM and its CULTURAL RELATIVISM.

body, anthropology of the. The anthropology of the human body has been most fully developed in the study of bodily decoration, which is seen as a way in which the natural human body is transformed into a cultural manifestation. The ways in which this process is carried out include temporary changes (dress, ornament, hair style, body paint etc.) and permanent ones such as tattooing, scarification, and what might be considered by Western standards as 'deformations'. While in modern society bodily decoration may be regarded as an expression of FASHION in simple societies it often involves sacred and social symbolism. Bodily decoration symbolizes group membership, status and role change, often by referring to animal characteristics or by stressing sexual features (*see* TOTEMISM; INITIATION). Structural analyses of the use of the human body in social symbolism have shown how natural differences are accentuated and used as a language to talk about sociocultural differences and processes. An area of body anthropology which is little developed is the comparative study of bodily attitudes, movements, and so on, though there have been some significant contributions both from PSYCHOLOGICAL ANTHROPOLOGY and the anthropology of DANCE in this field. The human body need not simply be the instrument of symbolic expression, as in bodily decoration, dance or movement, but can also become the symbolic model: as for instance when the community, the house, or the social unit is conceived of as being like a human body, or human bodily processes provide the model for religious symbolism.

borrowing. Most of the countries of Latin America and Africa are in a situation of chronic indebtedness to First World financial institutions. With the world recession that began in the late 1970s, the situation has become acute. Borrowing orginally occurred to finance a specific Western model of DEVELOPMENT which stressed modern heavy industrialization. This was to lead to increased foreign exchange earnings through growth in the export trade and was therefore to generate more than enough to pay for the substantial import (from the West) that was involved in such a programme. During the 1970s borrowing was heavy (increasing among non-OPEC developing countries over four times between 1970 and 1978), world trade doubled, interest rates were relatively low and money easy to borrow. However, with the beginning of the world recession at the end of the 1970s, the situation changed. Interest rates increased dramatically through the 1980s, world trade shrank, and the anti-inflation policies pursued by many First World countries meant a substantial drop in exports from the Third World. In addition, one of the other sources of foreign exchange, the remittance from migrant workers, with unemployment hitting the First World. The debtor countries found themselves unable to pay the interest on their loans and found that banking institutions were no longer willing to loan more, and were demanding repayment within much shorter time periods than was the norm in the 1970s. Living standards in many of the debtor countries have fallen significantly and are continuing to fall. The situation is extremely serious.

boundaries. In anthropological studies of SYMBOLISM, considerable attention has been paid to boundaries as inherently dangerous or powerful areas (*see* LIMINALITY; RITES OF PASSAGE). The theories of TURNER, for example, and those of M. Douglas (1966), on the relationship between symbolism and social structure, postulate that boundary areas are inherently dangerous and powerful because they are outside the formal and controlled structure of CLASSIFICATION. While it is true that everywhere boundaries tend to be marked by anomalies, it does not necessarily follow that they are regarded as particularly dangerous or powerful, and the cross-cultural generalizations assumed by various authors who have developed the concept of liminality need more careful examination.

bourgeois democracy. This concept refers to the fact that under capitalist economic regimes, even though the formal apparatus of democracy exists, power structures are secured and protected in the hands of the bourgeoisie no matter how votes are cast. In a people's democracy, however (with or without elections) power is controlled by the representatives of the people or the working class.

bourgeois economics. A Marxist term for economic theory which treats EXCHANGE and EXCHANGE VALUE as the fundamental economic facts, and views the laws of the MARKET as natural rather than historically specific phenomena. Such economic theory is thus not scientific but pseudo-scientific, its true function being ideological.

bourgeoisie. Under CAPITALISM, the owners of property, who as a class replaced the ARISTOCRACY as power holders when capitalism replaced feudalism. In Marxist theory the modern State is held to represent the bourgeoisie as a class. The distinction between *petite* and *haute bourgeoisie* (small and large property owners) is important historically: the latter progressively forced out the former and caused them to become part of the proletariat.

breast feeding. In societies without effective contraceptives, population size is frequently controlled through long periods of breast feeding, which reduces the risk of pregnancy, as well as through *post partum* taboos on sexual intercourse. It is increasingly recognized that breast feeding is also extremely important in terms of infant mortality rates, since breast milk contains a range of essential immunities which bottled milk does not. There is concern acout the increasing popularity in the Third World of what is successfully represented as the modern and progressive way to feed your children: bottle feeding. (*See also* CONTRACEPTION AND ABORTION.)

bricolage. An analogy employed by LEVI-STRAUSS in his discussion of mythic thought (1969). The *bricoleur* is a kind of professional do-it-yourselfer or Jack of all trades, who uses a set of whatever tools and materials are at hand to construct his projects. Mythical thought, Levi-Strauss claims, similarly uses elements or signs which are 'half way between percepts and concepts'. In a process of 'continual reconstruction from the same materials, it is always earlier ends which are called upon to play the part of means: the signified changes into the signifying and vice versa'. Thus mythical thought uses events (or the odds and ends left over from them) to create new structures; while scientific activity uses structures in order to create events.

bride capture. The capture of women of the enemy group may be a feature of raiding and warfare among groups who are traditionally warlike (a well-known example would be the Yanomamo, an Amazonian group studied by N. Chagnon (1968)). According to the theory of primitive marriage expounded by McLennan, the earliest form of marriage was bride-capture, since early man practised female infanticide and was thus obliged to seek his mate in war.

brideprice, bridewealth. See MARRIAGE PAYMENTS.

brideservice. The services rendered by a man to those from whom he has received a wife. Such services are usually rendered to his father-in-law, but he may also be required to perform some services for his mother-in-law, brothers-in-law or other affines whether as individuals or as a group. Such services are imposed on him in return for the granting of a woman in MARRIAGE. The custom of brideservice often involves a period of UXORILOCAL residence which may be more or less extended. The duration of the period of brideservice may be subject to negotiation between the parties concerned, or it may be a permanent obligation of the wife receiver, conceived of as a permanent debt. The control exercised by the wife-givers over the wife receiver may form an important part of the system of political relationships in societies where brideservice obligations are considerable. Brideservice is a custom associated mainly with HUNTING AND GATHERING or horticultural societies: for example, it is common throughout the native groups of Amazonia.

brokerage. ACTION THEORY in anthropology has brought to the forefront the study of brokers and their importance in sociopolitical networks. E. Wolf's studies of brokers in peasant society (1966), and C. Geertz's work on 'cultural brokers' (1960) focused on the role of brokers who mediate between local and national levels, and their role in the changing local, regional and national political economy. Brokers are typically located in marginal or frontier areas of economic expansion. They may be missionaries, traders, patrons, teachers or any other kind of 'middleman'. The 'broker model' of social interaction has been elaborated most fully by F.G. Bailey (1969). An example of a study of brokerage is that of N. Long (1975), who analyses the circumstances under which different types of broker emerge in rural Peru to occupy strategic positions in local, regional and national economies.

bureaucracy. Rule by administrative offices. Used in general to describe systems of formal, hierarchically organized authority characteristic of large areas of modern society. Bureaucratic organizations, which may be civil, religious or military, are distinguished by their ability to organize large numbers of people in terms of impersonal or RATIONAL goals, and by the existence of sets of explicit rules of procedure which regulate the actions of their members. We tend to associate bureaucracies with modern industrial societies where they have their fullest development, but there are of course many examples of pre-industrial and even pre-literate bureaucracies (for example, in the ancient Inca empire in Peru) which provide interesting comparative material. A key element in WEBER's theory of the progressive RATIONALIZATION of behaviour and authority systems in the modern world is his analysis of bureaucracy, which he takes to be the ideal type of rational-legal AUTHORITY. According to Weber, bureaucratic organizations geared to the rational attainment of goals and to centralized, impersonal and ROUTINIZED authority would eventually transcend the opposition between capitalism and socialism and become the dominant mode of organization. A key issue for investigation by the social sciences related to bureaucracy is the link between its political and administrative aspects, and it is questionable to what extent we may accurately refer to 'rule' by administrators. If bureaucracies are the ideal type of organization for the rational attainment of goals, then we must examine at what level these goals or policies are determined, how they are communicated to, reinterpreted and executed by the bureaucracy, and to what extent the bureaucratic organization itself may generate unacknowledged or contradictory goals as a product of its internal organization. The political control over bureaucracies and the extent to which these are themselves politicized are crucial issues in the study of their organization and functioning. Many of the ills attributed to bureaucracy itself are in fact the intended or unintended products of political decisions, or of the contradictions between central policy and administrative norms, structure and resources. Thus the bureaucrat, administrator or clerk often acts as a buffer between a public which has a certain expectation of service, and a central government or other organization which does not place him in a position to meet this expectation – an expectation which may itself have been created by explicit central policy. In this situation, the administrator takes refuge in the rules and regulations in order to refuse or delay service, but the real problem lies not in the bureaucracy itself but in the lack of political will to implement stated policy. The bureaucracy, rather than serving as a mechanism for the attainment of goals, thus becomes the apparent obstacle to their attainment, but this apparent obstacle only serves to disguise the real problem of a central government or organization which cannot or does not wish to implement its stated policies. The proliferation of bureaucracy in developing countries may be understood better in this light than if we employ a model of the bureaucracy as a 'rational' organization. Third World bureaucracies, as well as providing employment for a large proportion of the middle class in economies characterized by massive unemployment and underemployment, are also the mechanism by which governments are able to display at the level of law and policy an impressive array of institutions, projects, services etc. which they do not have the resources or the political will to implement. The necessarily inefficient bureaucracy serves to delay, dilute or effectively strangle the implementation of these policies and services. The anthropological study of bureaucracies in developed and developing countries has been a somewhat neglected area of research, and this is unfortunate since they are an important element in the study of national and international power structures.

burial. *See* MORTUARY RITES.

C

cannibalism. The practice of cannibalism or anthropophagy seems to date from the Paleolithic era, according to the archaeological evidence, and reports of it in modern times are scattered throughout the ethnographic record, concentrated mainly in New Guinea and Amazonia but occurring occasionally in other areas. There are two distinct forms of cannibalism. One, associated with MORTUARY RITES, is the eating of the flesh of dead kinsmen or group members. This is referred to as 'endo-cannibalism'. The second, associated with WARFARE, is the eating of enemies, referred to as 'exocannibalism'. The two types of cannibalism are not usually found together in one society. It has been suggested that cannibalism may relate to protein shortages in the diet, but most anthropological interpretations have focused on the symbolic nature of the cannibalistic act, representing as it does the 'incorporation' (literally) of the dead kinsman, or the dead enemy, into the person or the group who eats his flesh. W. Arens (1979) has argued that the evidence for cannibalism has been exaggerated, that accounts of this practice are nearly always at second hand, and that it is always a practice attributed to neighbouring peoples but never to one's own. He concludes that it is in fact a 'myth' relating to stereotypes of savage behaviour among others, and that the actual evidence for its ever having been practised is slim. However there are several well-documented accounts of cannibalism which are not so easy to dismiss: for example, among the Kuru of New Guinea, consumption of the remains of the dead by their kinswomen was shown to be responsible for the transmission of a rare and fatal viral infection. Similarly in other areas of the world accounts of both endo- and exocannibalism occur with sufficient frequency and are sufficiently well-documented to call into question Arens' thesis.

cantometrics. A system developed by Alan LOMAX which aims to describe musical style objectively (in a similar fashion to CHOREO-METRICS in the anthropology of DANCE) and to relate it to other aspects of culture. Lomax attempts to establish correlations between the organization of musical performance and more generalized sociocultural beliefs and values such as individualism, co-operativeness, democracy, authoritarianism, and so on. (*See* ETHNOMUSICOLOGY.)

capital. Capital is one of the three factors of production (the others are land and labour). As a factor of production, capital is defined as that part of the produced goods which is put into the system to stimulate further production. In a narrower sense it can also be used as a term for financial assets. (*See* HUMAN CAPITAL.)

capital accumulation. The build up of capital stock through investment. This is difficult to achieve in underdeveloped countries because of the low income levels of the vast majority of their population and because capital is diverted from these countries to the developed nations or to the transnational corporations.

capital intensity. The ratio of capital to labour in production. The historical development of capitalism is towards greater capital intensity made possible by techno-logical advances, but this model is in many cases inapplicable to Third World countries where capital is scarce but labour is plentiful. (*See* APPROPRIATE TECHNOLOGY.)

capitalism. A socioeconomic system or formation in which the MEANS OF PRODUC-TION are controlled by the BOURGEOISIE and in which SURPLUS VALUE is extracted from the labour of the PROLETARIAT or working class. The latter, because they do not control

30

the means of production, must sell their labour and are thus obliged to participate in an alienated labour process in which they are exploited by the dominant class. According to Marxist theory, capitalism is the stage which succeeds FEUDALISM in the evolution of human society, and will itself be succeeded by SOCIALISM and COMMUNISM. The process of transformation from capitalism to socialism, or the proletarian REVOLUTION, will be brought about as a culmination of the basic contradiction in capitalism between the socialized nature of work and the privatized nature of ownership.

Theories of the historical development of capitalism vary greatly, reflecting the political and ideological stance of different social scientists. WEBER, for example, strongly disagreed with Marx's contention that the final cause of the emergence of capitalism must be located in the development of the FORCES OF PRODUCTION (the materialist hypothesis). Weber claimed that under certain circumstances changes in belief systems could produce changes in the social order, and he developed his theory of the PROTESTANT ETHIC and the rise of capitalism as a demonstration of this argument. There are similarly varying views regarding the existence and nature of primitive or pre-industrial capitalism. Some anthropologists have examined capitalist-type behaviour in tribal societies or peasant communities, but many social scientists would argue that these small-scale 'capitalist' strategies should be distinguished clearly from capitalism as a SOCIOECONOMIC FORMATION. Thus the first truly capitalist productive system in history is considered to be the mercantile capitalism of 17th-century Europe, which developed into industrial capitalism at the time of the industrial revolution. The characteristic form of capitalism in the 20th century is monopoly capitalism, which is a product of the historical tendency for wealth to concentrate in fewer and fewer hands and for the scale of capitalist enterprises to increase. This latter phenomenon is related to the tendency for increasing CAPITAL INTENSITY in industry, as the capitalist class invests in progressively more advanced machinery in order to increase productivity. MULTINATIONAL AND TRANSNATIONAL CORPORATIONS are a special development of monopoly capitalism.

Intrinsic to the historical development of the capitalist system of production is the tendency to expand frontiers of economic activity in order to amass surplus value. Historically, capitalism is thus an expansive or predatory system, constantly in search of new fields of operation. Thus the phenomena of IMPERIALISM, COLONIALISM and NEO-COLONIALISM may all be interpreted not only as phases in the development of a capitalist productive system, but also as expansions which are necessary to sustain the capitalist system in developed countries. Thus prosperity at home, giving the means to satisfy increasing consumer and welfare demands of the proletariat, is acheived at the expense of colonialist and neo-colonialist strategies of exploitation abroad. (*See* WORLD SYSTEMS; DEPENDENCY; INDUSTRIALIZATION.)

cargo cult. This term is applied to a number of characteristic MILLENARIAN movements occurring in Melanesia in the first part of the 20th century. In these movements, which were products of the early years of European colonization, charismatic CULT leaders emerged among the native population, claiming that European trade goods (cargo) would arrive in the near future and be delivered to the natives in large quantities, heralding the dawn of a new era of plenty in which the 'cargo' would be controlled by the natives and not by the white man. Accompanying beliefs included, for example, that the first page of the Bible, explaining that Christ was black and that all the trade goods were made by God for the natives, had been removed by the white man at the same time as he had diverted the cargo from its rightful owners. P. Lawrence (1964) suggests that cargo cults arose because of a combination of pre-existing Melanesian religious beliefs about the supernatural origins of material culture and the new situation of relative deprivation brought about by the colonization process. Since in traditional Melanesian culture there was no distinction between work and the accompanying ritual, and wealth was believed to be a product of supernatural forces, it was thought that the white man's goods too came from his God or from Jesus, and that they could be obtained by the natives if they found the correct ritual formula. This gave rise to various recommendations: in some cases, to emulate certain distinctive features of the white man's conduct, dress etc.; in others to destroy previous possessions and crops in order to bring about the millenium, and so on. Over time, and as the native population acquires more accurate and extensive information as to the real nature of the dominant society and the origins of 'cargo', these cults tend to transform themselves into political movements drawing support from the lower socioeconomic categories.

cargo system. In Central and South American peasant communities, a series of ranked religious or civil-religious offices through which individuals pass as temporary office holders. In some communities, the cargos are purely concerned with the realization of religious duties and celebrations, while in others both civil and religious offices are integrated into a single system. These cargos involve heavy expenditure in the realization of religious FESTIVALS and have been interpreted as mechanisms whereby the office-holder is obliged to spend any surplus wealth, thus militating against CAPITAL ACCUMULATION and acting as LEVELLING MECHANISMS which prevent the emergence of significant wealth differences among members of the community. For example, in Zinacantan, a Maya community described by F. Cancian (1965), the cost of holding one of the higher offices in the cargo hierarchy involves the incumbent in heavy indebtedness and it may take years of saving and work to build up sufficient resources to occupy another cargo. Since the cargos themselves have political importance and prestige value, they should perhaps be regarded as the exchange of short-term economic surplus for long-term political advantage, rather than as purely 'ceremonial' in function. Additionally, it is probable that the expense involved in the cargo is not always sufficient to 'recycle' the individual back down the economic ladder, as suggested in many studies of the cargo system. This misconception is part of a general tendency to underestimate the differences in wealth within PEASANT communities, partly due to the fact that within many of these communities such differences

are extremely well-hidden, though at the same time highly significant.

carrying capacity. This concept is used in ecology and is linked to the notion of population pressure. In studies of human ecology and CULTURAL ECOLOGY, the term is generally employed with reference to the potential of soils for the production of food crops, giving a limit to population density for a given area. However the concept has often been used somewhat carelessly and without scientific substantiation, and it is important to bear in mind that it is related to a number of variables such as the level of technological development of the population, their preferred subsistence strategy, and a series of decisions regarding the amount and type of labour to be devoted to crop raising.

case study. A detailed record of the experience of an individual or a series of events occurring within a given framework (such as, for example, the history of a dispute in legal anthropology, the history of a patient and his complaint in medical anthropology, the account of a life-cycle or ritual etc.). The case study method has perhaps been most systematically employed in the field of the ANTHROPOLOGY OF LAW.

cash. *See* MONEY.

cash crops. Crops which are grown for sale in the market rather than those devoted to SUBSISTENCE or REDISTRIBUTION. Cash crops in the Third World often occupy the best land and are the only ones eligible for government support or subsidies to agriculture. Nevertheless the prices of these crops are dependent on world markets and on the transnational companies who control their worldwide commercialization, and the return to the smallscale producer or agricultural labourer is often extremely low. (*See* AGRIBUSINESS.)

caste. Castes are corporate social units which are ranked and generally defined by descent, marriage and occupation. Castes need never meet as wholes in one place but members of one caste share a concern for its rank and morality. The general characteristics of caste systems can be compared with other systems of STRATIFICATION such as those based on class or race. Undeveloped forms of caste exist in many parts of the world but caste organization and ideology are elaborated to such an extent in Hindu societies that some scholars have considered caste a uniquely Hindu phenomenon. In Hindu society caste rank is hereditary and linked to occupational pursuits. Castes also tend to be ENDOGAMOUS and the boundaries and differences in rank between castes are expressed and maintained by restrictions on commensal relations and intermarriage. These restrictions create the illusion that caste systems are rigid and that individual mobility is impossible. In fact individuals can improve their social standing and prestige and castes can, sometimes over long periods of time, move to higher positions in the rank order. The term caste derives from *casta* meaning species, lineage, race or clan, and was used by Portuguese traders to describe the people they met on the West coast of India when they arrived there in the 16th and 17th centuries. In many Indian languages the word for caste is *jati*, which can also mean a genus, a distinct sex, a tribe, a family, a lineage or clan, a population or a nation. Hindus classify all living beings into genera and each genus (caste) is thought to share substances (such as for example blood, bones or flesh). These substances have embodied in them particular codes for conduct which govern the exchanges between one caste and another, and also maintain its morality. Through procreation the bodily substances from both parents are mixed to make a child who will share characteristics particular to the nature of his or her caste. Correct moral actions maintain these shared characteristics, but acts which mix wrong bodily substances such as improper procreation or commensal relations change the shared morality of a caste and its offspring. The code for conduct of each caste and its rank with respect to other castes is therefore concerned with regulating marriage (*see* HYPERGAMY), with regulating the consumption of food and with regulating service relationships between castes (*see* JAJMANI).

Early European observers attempted to explain the origin of caste systems. Abbé Dubois saw castes as a result of rational legislation instituted by a past authority in order to maintain order and civilization. The differences in the racial characteristics between castes was noted by H.H. Risley, and explanations of castes as the result of repeated invasions and conquests by Indo-Europeans from Central Asia have also been popular. J.H. Hutton (1946) saw castes as the result of a historical accident, in which a number of distinct factors combined. In the first half of the 20th century the explanations started to show a greater understanding of Hindu society as an integrated whole and a better appreciation of the role of religion. Celestin Bougle (1971) postulated a set of three underlying characteristics – hierarchy, economic interdependence and separation – based on an opposition between the pure and the impure. These ideas were later to form the starting point for the work of L. Dumont (1970). A.M. Hocart saw castes in Vedic times as organizations for the carrying out of sacrifice, and in modern India for worship. He emphasized the religious and political role of the king. The consolidation of religious and political processes in caste systems has posed a major problem for sociological theory since 1945. Srinivas has proposed two concepts in order to illuminate the relationship between religion and politics: 'dominant caste' and 'sanskritization'. Other theorists, such as McKim Marriott (1976), R.B. Inden (1976) and S. Barnett (1932) have increased our understanding of castes as moral systems. They have concentrated particularly on what may be said to constitute a Hindu person, and the interaction between persons against the background of the conceptual order. L. Dumont also considers caste systems as moral systems of relations, though his point of departure is the whole rather than individual castes or persons. By introducing the idea of structure Dumont attempts to reduce all relationships between castes to their essence. Underlying Bougle's three principles of hierarchy, separation and interdependence is a structure of opposition between purity and pollution which derives from the polluting nature of bodily substances and organic processes. Purity and its opposition, pollution, underlie hierarchy because the pure is superior to the impure; they underlie separation because the pure and the impure must be kept separate and they underlie interdependence because the continuation of superiority depends on inferiors removing pollution from superiors. The opposition is the foundation of all levels of segmentation in caste systems, but this hierarchy is not a linear one; instead, lower levels are subsumed and encompassed by higher ones. The theory of *varnas* serves as an illustration of this. The conception that society contained *varnas* (genera, but sometimes also referred to as colours) developed in Vedic society and reached its most elaborate form in the classical code book *Dharma-sastra* (c 200 BC–200 AD). In late Vedic society four *varnas* were defined. Three of them – the Brahmana, the Ksatriyas and the Vaisya – twice-born because they became divinized by a ritual second birth. The other was defined as Sudras, once-born. Untouchables were outside this division. The Sudras were opposed to the twice-born. The twice-born were divided into a further two genera: the Vaisyas opposed to the Ksatriyas and the Brahmanas who were also divided into two parts. The moral order of Vedic society was upheld through sacrifice, from which all *varnas* benefited and to which they all contributed in different ways. The Sudra offered his labour and services. The Vaisyas were the farmers and grazers of cattle and provided the wealth offered in sacrifice to the Gods. The Ksatriyas had royal power, superior wealth, and could also command and protect the Vaisyas. The Brahmanas possessed godly power and were the only ones who could perform sacrifices for the Ksatriyas and Vaisyas, for which they received gifts from them. In modern Hindu society sacrifice has generally been replaced by image worship, but the Vedic theory continues to provide a conceptual model for the system of proliferating castes and subcastes at the local level. Dumont saw in the *varna* model a unique separation between the role of the priest and that of the king. The opposition between the pure and the impure presupposes this separation because the priest alone is pure enough to mediate between men and Gods. In this way an ideal type of hierarchy emerged in which status is superior to power and religion encompasses everything.

This Dumontian scheme has dominated social anthropological work on caste systems for the last few decades. Increasingly, however, the secondary and encompassed nature of political and economic processes is being questioned. More attention has been recently directed towards the 'Hindu kingdom' and the religious as well as political role of the king in rituals. In conjunction with scholars working on Indian history, social anthropologists are beginning to reappraise such aspects as agrarian relations, land tenure and economic differentiation. This work, which is still in its infancy, should bring a better understanding of local variations in the order of castes, of changes occurring in caste relationships and of the way caste systems have responded to the impact of colonialism, industrialization and independence.

catastrophe theory. Originally a mathematical theory developed by René Thom concerning transitions from one configuration to another, this has also been applied to the study of social change. Catastrophe theory concerns laws of development and structure which apply up to a certain point but which then bring about the collapse of existing structures and the advent of new laws.

category. This term has two main uses in anthropology. Firstly, it is contrasted to the term GROUP. A social category is an observer's construct, based on the classification of persons according to a characteristic or characteristics selected by that observer. A social group, however, is characterized by some common identity or group consciousness as well as by the criterion of face-to-face interaction. The second use of the term relates to the anthropological study of systems of CLASSIFICATION, where it is common to refer to 'conceptual categories' or 'cultural categories', which are sets of entities, events or phenomena classed together by informants within a given context.

cattle culture. See PASTORAL NOMADS.

caudillismo. A Latin American term for a political system dominated by violence and by the periodic emergence of *caudillos* or leaders who gain their position through their success in warfare and raiding.

ceremony. This term is sometimes used as a loose equivalent of RITUAL. It is useful, however, to retain a distinction between the two terms. A ceremony is a formalized or stylized performance, often public and always involving more than one participant and/or observer, characteristic of a particular cultural tradition. The study of ceremony is thus the study of these stylized performances and their cultural, social and ritual context. The study of ritual itself is broader than the study of the ceremony which may accompany it, and includes the study of its magico-religious and symbolic aspects. There are many ceremonies which do not have a strong ritual component, in the sense that they have little or no religious significance or symbolic ramification (the presentation of a diploma or degree in modern society is, for instance, without doubt a ceremony, but there is little to be gained by studying it as a ritual) and by the same token there are many ritual acts which are not ceremonies, in that they may be informal, private or 'unceremonious' but still be classed as ritual because of their magico-religious and symbolic importance.

change. Changes in culture and in society are one of the major theoretical preoccupations of anthropology, and one of the areas where theoretical differences manifest themselves most clearly. HISTORICAL PARTICULARISM versus EVOLUTIONISM, FUNCTIONALISM versus CONFLICT theory, different schools of MARXIST ANTHROPOLOGY, and so on all present different interpretations of the phenomena of change, instability and development in sociocultural systems. In functionalist social science, the tendency is to regard change as a negative or pathological manifestation, since it is assumed that the natural tendency of social systems is towards equilibrium. Thus the study of 'social change' or 'cultural change' in functionalist-oriented anthropology in Britain and the USA has tended to constitute a separate field focusing on particularly rapid processes of change brought about typically by situations of contact, conquest or COLONIALISM, and often resting on the implied premise that apart from contact situations normal social systems do not change. In Marxist-oriented social science, however, change is regarded as built into in the social order, since every historical stage of society's development holds within itself the germs of the contradiction which will eventually lead to its destruction. Another major area of dispute

is the relationship which holds between changes in environment, technology, social organization and cultural systems, or between the INFRASTRUCTURE and the SUPER-STRUCTURE of Marxist terminology. Different theories of change, which are nothing more or less than different theories of HISTORY, imply different philosophical and political positions, and in many cases we cannot speak of 'debate' between different positions, since they do not even possess a common vocabulary to discuss the phenomena concerned.

Marxist theory holds that 'in the last instance', changes in the material base of society will determine changes in the superstructure, and the driving force in human social evolution according to this theory is the development of the contradiction between the FORCES OF PRODUCTION and the RELATIONS OF PRODUCTION. Since the productive forces are never static, but always evolve, the social relations of production become obsolete and instead of allowing the development of the productive forces they become obstacles to this development. This contradiction between forces and relations culminates in the overthrow of the latter and their replacement by new social relations better suited to the development of the productive forces. In pre-class societies, this qualitative leap (or REVOLUTION) in the relations of production expresses itself through the release of technological potential and the establishment of new and more complex social forms. CHILDE has described the Neolithic Revolution and the Urban Revolution in prehistory in this way. In class-based societies, the revolution takes the form of the replacement of one social class by another as controllers of the MEANS OF PRODUCTION. Interpretations differ as to the application of Marxist theory to traditional or pre-industrial society, particularly to the status of pre-class societies in the general Marxist theory of history. There is also considerable debate as to the meaning of the 'last-instance' determinism of the economic order in social organization, and its implications for those societies where the dominant idiom of social relations is provided not by the economy but by the kinship system or by religion.

In non-Marxist theory of social and cultural change, the notion of material determinism is maintained, for example, by ecologically-oriented anthropologists who view cultures as adaptive systems with relation to the environment, and who argue that cultures change as a result of the cumulative effects of their interaction with the ecosystem (*see* CULTURAL MATERIALISM; CULTURAL ECOLOGY). The tradition of ACCULTURATION or culture contact studies, on the other hand, has developed an elaborate typology of culture change in which 'superstructural' elements are given priority, and in which change is seen as the result of the interaction and mutual transformation of cultural configurations, and of the cumulative effect of INNOVATION, DIFFUSION and SYNCRETISM.

charisma. One of the three types of AUTHORITY described by WEBER is charismatic authority, which is based on the personal characteristics of a leader. This type of leadership emerges especially in times of social crisis. Charisma means literally 'gift of grace', and examples of charismatic leaders are prophets, military heroes and revolutionary leaders. As an ideal type, charismatic authority is diametrically opposed to the rational authority which finds its expression in BUREAUCRACY. Charismatic leadership is however inherently unstable, and after the initial phase of social crisis there generally follows a stage of ROUTINIZATION of charisma whereby bureaucratic institutions take over the leadership role.

charter. The set of rules and justificatory principles of an ASSOCIATION or INSTITUTION, rules which may be formalized as a written code or which may be informal and implicit rather than overtly expressed.

charter, social. MALINOWSKI, in his theory of MYTH, claims that it acts as a 'social charter': that is to say, it justifies the manner in which things are done in present day society by reference to a mythical or sacred past. This theory has been influential in the study of myth, though critics were quick to point out that in many myths antisocial or forbidden acts are committed and go unpunished, and that the mythic universe goes beyond the bounds of the social order. The theory receives a sophisticated revival in C. Levi-Strauss' 'The Story of Asdiwal' (1967), where he argues that the mythic variations in marriage types serve to demonstrate that none of the possible permutations is viable except that which is currently practised.

chiefdom. In the evolutionary scheme often used to classify different social types, and popularized especially in US anthropology by E.R. Service (1975), the chiefdom is the LEVEL OF SOCIOCULTURAL INTEGRATION which succeeds that of the TRIBE. The chiefdom is characterized by greater specialization in the DIVISION OF LABOUR, the emergence of SOCIAL CLASSES or at least incipient social classes, and by an economic system based on REDISTRIBUTION. Unlike the ACEPHALOUS political systems of the tribal level of evolution, the chiefdom has a centralized authority uniting a number of local communities, but unlike the STATE, the chiefdom has no formal apparatus of repression or of military power. Under the chiefdom system, there is an expansion of craftwork and agricultural technology and productivity, creating and maintaining fulltime specialization in these fields. There is also often a development of ceremonial/religious cults with specialized priesthoods, as well as of a noble class associated with the chiefs and their families or kinsmen. Some chiefdoms are characterized by the development of SLAVERY (for example, in the Northwest Coast area of North America). Some examples of the chiefdom level of social development are the Circum–Caribbean chiefdoms of pre-Hispanic America, and the traditional chiefdoms of Polynesia.

Childe, V.G. (1892–1957). An anthropologist and archaeologist who had a considerable influence on evolutionary and ecological perspectives in the USA. Childe's works interpret prehistory and the development of complex societies according to the Marxist scheme of evolution of socioeconomic formations (e.g 1942). His view of archaeology as a social science and his synthetic view of prehistory and history were pioneering developments.

childhood. *See* AGE, ANTHROPOLOGY OF.

choice. *See* DECISION.

choreometrics. A system devised by Alan

LOMAX for the objective cross-cultural measurement of DANCE performance.

church. A set of religious institutions, usually with a full-time professional priesthood, to which individual believers or followers are affiliated. The term is generally restricted to the divisions within the Christian religion, where it may be applied also to voluntary associations of believers more correctly termed SECTS or CULTS.

circuit. In CYBERNETICS, any path along which a message may travel. Analysis of such circuits may lead the anthropologist to disregard conventional divisions between organisms, tools and environment, to consider instead the systems of communication which link all these phenomena.

circumcision, female. The removal of the genital labia of a woman, performed as part of female INITIATION rites in some African and other societies.

circumcision, male. The removal of the foreskin, performed as part of INITIATION rites in societies widely distributed around the world. The circumcision of boys is a common practice also in modern industrial societies, among Jewish and other communities. Various psychoanalytically-oriented theories have been advanced to explain the significance of male initiation rites accompanied by circumcision, by subincision (cutting the lower part of the penis), by supercision (cutting the upper part of the penis) or by other genital mutilations. (*See* RITUAL SEXUAL SYMMETRY.)

city, anthropology of the. The comparative study of cities raises important questions in anthropology, particularly about the universality or specificity of aspects of the rural/urban contrast so often taken for granted in anthropological studies. Different types of city – the pre-industrial city, the Western and non-Western industrial city, the colonial and the post-colonial city – have been described and compared. Generalizations prevalent in sociology which were based on evidence from Western cities have thus been called into question. The idea that kinship networks must inevitably decline in cities, for example, is manifestly inaccurate when

cases of pre-industrial and Third World cities are considered. G. Sjoberg (1960) has sketched an ideal model of the pre-industrial city, and has argued that it was principally a centre of government and religion and only secondarily of commerce. Within the city the extended family household, grouped together with others in ethnic enclaves, was the dominant mode of social organization. Sjoberg believes that power was held by a hereditary elite, and expressed itself mainly in political and religious spheres, merchants being of lower status. His ideal type has been criticized as being too generalized, and it has been suggested that he fails to take into account the variations in type among pre-industrial cities in different parts of the world. Postcolonial cities, with their large marginal or squatter populations and their colonial heritage of social and cultural forms, provide interesting cases for study, as do cities such as the Japanese which have developed largely in isolation from the Western model.

In anthropology, cities have usually been regarded as special environments with distinctive psycho-social characteristics, an idea advanced by DURKHEIM in his *Division of Labour in Society* (1893) and which influenced both the Chicago school of urban anthropology and REDFIELD's model of the FOLK-URBAN CONTINUUM. However, as Blanton (1976) has pointed out, the problem of defining a 'city' and its relation to the phenomenon of URBANISM is not a simple one. Sjoberg defined the city by the presence of a literate elite, while P. Wheatley advances a functional definition of the 'ethnocity' as a 'node of concentration' of population and social activities of any kind. The city itself (or the town, which is distinguished only by an arbitrary criterion of size) is a product of increasing role specialization and the centralization of social institutions. Thus the city as a centre for social, economic and political integration in a specific region must be studied not in isolation but in relation to its regional context.

In modern urban anthropology studies have focused on interethnic relations within the city (*see* ETHNICITY), on the sociocultural characteristics of marginal or slum districts (*see* SHANTY TOWNS), on processes of rural-urban MIGRATION and on the mechanisms of sociogeographical separation and integration which act to perpetuate the distinctive profile of each urban centre. (*See* CIVILIZATION; INDUSTRIALIZATION.)

civilization. A relatively complex society with a state-type political organization. It is linked to the process of URBANIZATION, and the increasing DIVISION OF LABOUR into limited and specialized functions. The term also implies that there is an increasing complexity in the cultural tradition, which is generally accompanied by the emergence of LITERACY and the flowering of artistic, religious or ceremonial life. In referring to 'a civilization', the anthropologist is envisaging two distinct historical and political phenomena: the emergence of a state-controlled society, and the parallel growth of the artistic and cultural traditions with which it is associated. In the evolutionary schemes popular in anthropology in the 19th century, 'civilization' was seen as the highest category to succeed BARBARISM.

civil society. In political theory, this refers to the society formed by the SOCIAL CONT-RACT, as opposed to the institutionalized framework of the STATE.

clan. This term has been used rather differently in British and US anthropology. US anthropologists, following MORGAN, have generally reserved the term for a unilineal descent group recruited through the female line, while a unilineal descent group recruited through the male line is called the GENS. In Morgan's earlier work these two groupings are also termed *matriclan* and *patriclan*. In British social anthropology, however, the definition established in LINE-AGE THEORY is that of a descent group who trace their ancestry to a common apical ancestor or ancestress, but do not know the precise links to that ancestor. The use of the term 'clan' in this sense thus includes several distinct types of lineage. They may all be generally defined, however, as being composed of unilineal descent groups, which are united by known links to a common ancestor. MURDOCK suggested that the term SIB could be used to designate the group referred to in British anthropology as the clan. The word is derived from the Gaelic word *clann*, which was in fact a bilineal KINDRED group.

class, social. Class systems or class societies are characterized by the horizontal division of society into strata. In Marxist terms such classes are defined by their differential access to the MEANS OF PRODUCTION. The dominant class appropriates the SURPLUS produced by other classes through its control of the means of production, and thus exploits their labour. The relationship between classes is fundamentally antagonistic, and class conflict is inevitable in class systems.

In anthropological theories of the evolution of human societies, the emergence of social classes is usually attributed to the CHIEFDOM level of social integration, where the increasing specialization in the division of labour results in the differentiation of nobles, craftsmen, soldiers, priests, agricultural producers and in some cases slaves. Such groups are regarded as potentially constituting social classes, which will become further differentiated with the rise of URBANISM and the STATE. Sociological studies of class have tended to follow WEBER and considerable attention has been paid to power and STATUS as well as economic position as markers of social class. Recent work on class has extended its frame of reference; one strand of feminist theory argues that the basic class relationship is between women and men and some Marxist anthropologists have argued that in lineage societies the elders exploit the labour of young men and women and thus constitute a class. (*See* STRATIFICATION.)

class consciousness. Class consciousness, or the phenomenon of 'class for itself', as opposed to merely 'class in itself', is a central element in Marxist political and social theory. A class becomes a class for itself when, through CLASS STRUGGLE it comes to recognize its common interests and objectives. According to Marxist theory, social classes under capitalism become increasingly polarized, and this is accompanied by increasing class consciousness and politicization of the working class, a process which will culminate in REVOLUTION. The commitment of Marxist social science to class based political party activism rests on the notion that class consciousness is essential to the revolutionary process, since historical 'laws' of social development express themselves not in spite of or regardless of man's will but by means of his will.

classification. Systems of social and cultural classification have been an important element of study in many areas of anthropological theory, and STRUCTURAL and COGNITIVE ANTHROPOLOGY, as well as a variety of perspectives within SYMBOLIC ANTHROPOLOGY have approached the subject rather differently. A pioneering early study, and one which was extremely influential in British STRUCTURAL FUNCTIONALISM, was DURKHEIM and MAUSS' *Primitive Classification*. In this work, the authors argued that society is the elemental model for logical classification and the first logical classes were thus classes of men. Logical classifications have therefore been seen as extensions of social ones, such as for example Australian MOIETIES and section systems, where the basic social division is extended throughout all of nature (*see* TOTEMISM). This primitive system of classification, they argued, then evolved into more complex philosophical or scientific forms which are detached from the social order. RADCLIFFE-BROWN and subsequent structural functionalist anthropologists developed this approach to classificatory systems to a considerable extent. They saw the systems as a reflection of features of the social order, particularly in their studies of kinship, and of religious and RITUAL systems in tribal societies. (*See* LINEAGE THEORY; RELIGION.)

LEVI-STRAUSS (1949) takes as his starting point the element of Durkheim's sociology which has to do with the theory of COLLECTIVE REPRESENTATIONS and his proposed 'social psychology', which was to be a study of the independent existence or life of collective representations and the manner in which they combine and recombine, attract, repel, or transform each other. Like other theorists of social classification, Levi-Strauss is greatly influenced in his approach by linguistic models. He was inspired by the advances made in phonology, where the model of BINARY OPPOSITIONS or contrasts had been used to impose an order on the sound system. In the same manner, he sought in his studies of kinship and of symbolic and mythic systems to elucidate the binary logic behind cultural and social classifications. In *The Elementary Structures of Kinship* this theory of classification is closely linked to theories of EXCHANGE and RECIPROCITY. So close is this link, indeed, that changes in principles of classification are seen as the correlatives of evolutionary development in systems of marriage exchange and social relationships. In his later work, however, such as his *Mythologiques*, Levi-Strauss moves towards a theory of SUPERSTRUCTURES alone. He sees them as constituting a vast network of transformations, and variations on cultural themes which are both regional and universal (*see* MYTH).

The British anthropologist R. Needham (1973) has developed Levi-Strauss' approach to systems of classification and furthered the study of how pervasive the principle of opposition is in the construction of symbolic systems. Needham has also contributed to the anthropological definition of some principles of classification: he distinguishes, for example, between 'monothetic' classes and 'polythetic' ones. In the former, all members are linked by one or more common characteristics, while in the latter members are linked by chain or serial resemblances. He suggests that the latter may be an important and somewhat neglected principle of classification in anthropological studies. Similarly, he distinguishes classes according to their internal organization, which may be hierarchical (nested) or non-hierarchical, ordered by the principle of analogy.

Cognitive anthropology represents a different approach to systems of classification, and focuses on linguistic categories and on TAXONOMY as a key to cultural knowledge. As well as taxonomies, cognitive anthropology has also paid considerable attention to the analysis and development of classificatory principles and typologies of categories, and has laid stress on careful recording of communicative behaviour as a guide to cognitive and cultural systems.

classificatory/descriptive kinship terminology. This distinction was made originally by MORGAN. Classificatory kin terms subsume various biological kin types: specifically, they place lineal and COLLATERAL kin in the same category, while descriptive terms refer only to one specified biological kin type, and distinguish lineal from collateral relatives.

Morgan argued that the most primitive kinship terminologies were classificatory and the more advanced ones descriptive by nature. Tylor and Frazer both suggested that the origin of the classificatory system is in DUAL ORGANIZATION. For Frazer, 'the classificatory system of relationship flows directly from the organization of society into two exogamous classes'. Levi-Strauss develops this suggestion in his discussion of dual organization and the elementary structures of kinship. Modern kinship studies however have moved away from the wholesale classification of terminologies as either 'classificatory' or 'descriptive', since it has been observed that all systems have some elements of both types. Instead, they have examined the criteria by which classes of kin are distinguished and differentiated, and the degrees of EXTENSION OF KINSHIP TERMS, as well as the different contexts in which native speakers may choose in referring to a particular person to employ a more specific or a more general term.

class struggle. This concept is central to the Marxist theory of history, since once social classes emerge in the evolution of human society the struggle between them becomes the driving force of history. The transition from one MODE OF PRODUCTION and one socioeconomic formation to another (e.g. from feudalism to capitalism, from capitalism to socialism etc.) is marked by the taking over of control of the MEANS OF PRODUCTION by a different social class. The overturning of the status quo by a rising social class constitutes a REVOLUTION in Marxist terms.

client. In anthropology, a client is the subordinate partner in a relationship of PATRONAGE or a similar relationship – such as brokerage or sponsorship – in either the political or the economic domain, or in both. In political anthropology ACTION THEORY has paid especial attention to the relationships between patrons, brokers or FACTION leaders and their clients. In theory, clientship is at least at first a voluntary tie entered into by the client because of the services, protection or favours he expects to receive from his patron or broker. However there are instances in which the voluntary side of the relationship is more apparent than actual, and in most cases it is limited to the client's ability to choose between one patron and another, but not to dispense with having one altogether. In many systems of political and economic patronage, as the relationship between client and patron develops over time, it also becomes increasingly difficult for the client to extricate himself due to his indebtedness. The institution of clientship may then become one of DEBT SLAVERY or of obligatory political allegiance. One of the structural features of clientship in terms of political and economic organization is that it tends to divide less powerful sectors of society vertically along the lines of their individual allegiances to particular patrons or leaders, thus militating against the development of horizontal divisions between the more powerful and the less powerful, and discouraging the development of collective or communal strategies of seeking access to power or wealth.

cline. The gradual variation in distribution of a given characteristic of population, language or culture may be expressed in terms of the technique of geographically mapping this variation in a manner similar to the use of contour lines in physical geography. These linguistic or cultural 'contours' are called clines, and may be used to study the geographical patterning of genetic traits in physical anthropology, of dialects in linguistics, and so on.

clique. A relatively informal and overtly unacknowledged interest group which may form at any level of social interaction or within any institution, and which exists to further the interests of its members, or to protect their access to scarce resources. The study of NETWORKS and network formation in POLITICAL ANTHROPOLOGY and in ACTION THEORY includes the study of such covert interest groups and their functioning.

clitorectomy. The removal of the clitoris, performed as part of female INITIATION rites among some African groups and occasionally in other parts of the world. Female initiation rites are generally associated with horticultural societies, but the reason for their accompaniment by clitorectomy is unclear. It is probable that their operation is part of a generalized ideology of male dominance or sex antagonism.

closed corporate community. A term coined by E. Wolf to describe PEASANT communities in Mesoamerica, and which has been applied to other parts of the world where small peasant villages predominate. The peasant community is described as a CORPORATE group because its unity or integrity depends fundamentally on its corporate ownership of land or other resources, and on its relative economic independence from outside markets. In addition, the community is 'closed' by virtue of its self-contained and inward-looking social and cultural organization. This inward-looking tendency is in part a result of the desire to protect the community's resources from outside encroachment. Such communities are regarded as naturally conservative and traditional, resisting innovation and change. Their ideologies are defined as egalitarian, and reinforced by mechanisms which inhibit conspicuous displays of personal wealth (*see* EVIL EYE) and tend to redistribute surplus wealth (*see* CARGO SYSTEM).

The concept of the closed corporate community has been considerably criticized in modern studies of peasant sociocultural organization, particularly by those authors who emphasize the links between the peasant community and the wider society, and by those who contest the image of peasant conservatism.

coalition. A temporary political alliance or 'patching up of differences' by political parties, factions or groups who maintain their separate identities but join together for the performance of a specific task. Coalitions are among the phenomena which have been studied within the ACTION THEORY approach in POLITICAL ANTHROPOLOGY.

code. Refers in one usage to a set of regulatory rules, as in the 'code of etiquette' or the 'legal code'. In COMMUNICATION studies, it is more usually a communicatory device containing a set of rules for the transcription of one domain, or one set of semantic parameters, to another.

code switching. In SOCIOLINGUISTICS and in anthropological studies of linguistic behaviour, this concept has been used to refer to the changing over from one linguistic code or type of discourse to another. The phenomenon of code switching allows us to perceive what the norms are which govern the appropriateness of different kinds of speech in different social contexts.

cognate. Kinsman related to EGO through CONSANGUINEAL links to either sex.

cognatic. This term has been used in two senses. 'Cognatic kinship' has been used as a synonym for BILATERAL or CONSANGUINEAL kinship. In the second more restricted sense, 'cognatic descent' refers to descent from an APICAL ANCESTOR/ANCESTRESS through any combination of male or female links. (*See* KINDRED.)

cognitive anthropology. The subfield of CULTURAL ANTHROPOLOGY which concerns itself with relationships among language, culture and cognition. Its development was influenced by cognitive psychology and structural linguistics, as well as by structural anthropology, although it differs from the latter in a number of its central preoccupations. Cognitive anthropology is based on the notion of CULTURE as an ideational system – that is, a system of knowledge and concepts – in contrast to the materialist interpretation of culture as an adaptive system or a set of observable behaviours. Cognitive anthropologists devote considerable attention to the accurate description of ethnographic reality, particularly to the recording of what people communicate, which can be used as a guide to what they know. Frake, for example, claims that a record of communication will provide a record of the cognitive system a people employ in order to organize their everyday activities. When approaching the subject in this way, the words people use for significant objects and phenomena must be carefully recorded as well as alternative meanings to words (or polysemy), variations in meaning according to the context of communication, and so on. The ethnographic technique of cognitive anthropology or the 'New Ethnography' of the 1950s and 1960s was marked by the attempt to avoid ethnocentric bias and to meticulously record the 'view from inside' another culture. An early emphasis on the relativity of cultural and cognitive categories, however, later gave way to a greater concern for the establishment of universal cognitive schemes, the most famous example being perhaps Berlin and Kay's study of COLOUR TERMS, which showed that the progression from simpler to more complex systems of colour classification follows the same course in all peoples.

In the 1960s, many studies within cognitive anthropology focused on the classification of the natural world in other cultures, and on other systems of botanical or zoological knowledge. This approach was termed ETHNOSCIENCE, and generated a flow of folk TAXONOMY studies which continues to be of major anthropological importance, and which has been applied not only to studies of knowledge of the natural world but also to those of kinship terms, subsistence techniques, and social organization. This broadening of interest to embrace all areas of folk knowledge and meaning was pioneered mainly by the anthropologists W.H. Goodenough, C.O. Frake, and H.C. Conklin, and has been termed ETHNOSEMANTICS or ETHNOGRAPHIC SEMANTICS. The influence of linguistics on cognitive anthropology is evident not only in the emphasis placed on the recording and study of linguistic categories, but also in the borrowing of linguistic models and paradigms to account for cultural phemomena. However it should be remembered that not all cognitive schemata are linguistic, and the indiscriminate borrowing of linguistic models may not always be appropriate to the study of either cognition or culture.

Another difficulty arises in defining the relationship between individual cognition and culture conceived as a system of shared meanings. Since knowledge, ideas and values will vary in different members of society, a cognitive model from psychology cannot be applied to a culture as a whole. There are sometimes also a number of alternative formal models to account for a cognitive system, and the ensuing debates as to which model is more psychologically 'real' are perhaps more relevant as accounts of the method being employed than of the phenomenon under study (see FORMAL ANALYSIS; COMPONENTIAL ANALYSIS).

Cognitive anthropology and parallel areas of study such as the ethnography of speaking share with structural anthropology a concern for conceptual universals, but differ in their modes of analysis of communication and of systems of classification.

cohesion. A term used in two rather different senses. 'Social cohesion' is used to refer to the phenomenon of social SOLIDARITY, or the sense of group unity. It may also be used to refer to the phenomenon of social INTEGRATION, or the way in which the institutions of a society function together as a co-ordinated whole.

collateral. In KINSHIP studies, consanguineal relatives; that is, those 'of the same side' not in a line of descent but related 'horizontally', such as brothers or cousins.

collective consciousness. *See* CONSCIENCE COLLECTIVE.

collective representation. In the sociology of DURKHEIM, *representations collectives* are states of the CONSCIENCE COLLECTIVE, as distinct from states of individual consciousness. These representations are expressions of the way in which the group conceives of itself and its relations with the world, and for Durkheim the essential task of sociology is to study how these representations form and combine. S. Lukes (1973) points out that Durkheim's development of this concept entails two important ambiguities. Firstly, he fails to distinguish modes of thought or cognition from the thing which is thought or perceived: thus both concepts and typical forms of thought on the one hand, and specific examples of beliefs, myths, legends and so forth on the other hand, are called 'collective representations'. Secondly, a definition of such representations as 'collective' is not only a description of their generation or creation – which is social – but also of what they refer to since they are about society. Durkheim considered collective representations to be SOCIAL FACTS, and thus to have an 'independent reality' irreducible to that of individual states of consciousness. He proposed that the discipline of 'social psychology' should study the life of these collective representations and the manner in which they combine, recombine and transform one another.

colonialism. A specific form of IMPERIALISM in which territories annexed by a dominant power are clearly defined as subordinate in status. Local political and governmental authorities and institutions are either replaced by colonial authorities (direct rule) or incorporated into the colonial power structure (indirect rule). Colonialism is a product of the need for territorial expansion, a need generated by economic pressures at home which triggers a search for new markets, new resources, profit and surplus VALUE. The history of colonialism is thus inseparable from that of the growth and development of an economic WORLD SYSTEM. European colonialism began in the 15th and 16th centuries, with the exportation of FEUDAL types of socioeconomic systems to conquered territories – the Spanish and Portuguese domination of South America is typical – and has continued into the 19th and 20th centuries. It has been the major force in the creation of the THIRD WORLD, and has been accompanied consistently by ideologies of RACISM which are attempts to justify the white man's dominance over the conquered races. The persistence of relations of domination and DEPENDENCY along colonial lines after the formal granting of independence is termed NEO-COLONIALISM.

In the 19th and early part of the 20th century, anthropology and ethnography were very much influenced, and even shaped, by what has been called the 'colonial encounter' (Asad (1973)). Anthropological research itself was financed by government or private vested interests. In the United States the concentration was on the Amerindian population, while in Britain the focus was on the colonial territories. The Royal Anthropological Institute of Great Britain supported the establishment of a teaching centre for colonial officials, arguing that the anthropological perspective might avoid misunderstandings which would otherwise lead later to costly military intervention. During the period in which STRUCTURAL FUNCTIONALIST theory was being developed in Great Britain, the majority of anthropologists were employed by the Foreign and Colonial Office. Most ethnographers did not see their research as primarily for government use, but believed it could smooth the task of colonial administration. While the actual influence of anthropology on policy development was slight, the uncritical attitude of anthropologists towards colonial and neo-colonial power structures led to a movement of CRITICAL ANTHROPOLOGY arising in the 1970s which culminated in a call for the 'decolonization' of the profession. These critiques focused not only on the historical importance of colonialism in the development of anthropology but also on the claim that many anthropologists continue to play a covert role in the maintenance of neo-colonialist or imperialist power structures. Also, they pointed out that the 'primitive' world studied by anthropologists, which was often conceived of as if it were a pre-colonial 'traditional' reality, was in fact a system radically transformed and in many ways created by colonialism. Naturally anthropologists have defended themselves against the charge of being merely an epiphenomenon of colonialism, arguing that the relationship between anthropology and administration was never a simple one, and pointing to the pre-colonial philosophical and scientific roots of the discipline. This defence does not however entirely obviate the need for anthropology to evaluate critically its attitude towards the international power structure and the effect this has on apparently 'pure' research. Groups which are committed to the documentation and the critique of the advance of world CAPITALISM and the colonial/imperial encounter include the International Working Group for Indigenous Affairs, Cultural Survival, the Anthropological Resource Centre and Survival International.

colonialism, internal. The reproduction of colonial type social, economic and political relationships within a single national territory, a phenomenon of special interest and concern for anthropology. The internal colony is a subordinate population within the state, usually an ethnic minority and often an indigenous population which has been largely displaced by a dominant and non-native national group. This minority internal colony is maintained at the margin of national political power structures, in much the same manner as former colonial elites marginalized the entire national population, and is employed to provide labour, raw materials or other services for the dominant group. In cases such as that of the native population of Amazonia, the indigenous groups are regarded mainly as an obstacle to the development of the region and the extraction of its resources, and the resulting GENOCIDE and ETHNOCIDE there has attracted worldwide attention due to the massive scale of the destruction of indigenous ethnic groups and their rainforest environment. In cases such as these the phenomenon of internal colonialism must be considered in conjunction with that of NEO-COLONIALISM, to which it appears, here as in other cases, as an additional ramification. Internal colonialism is thus usually studied as an aspect of neo-colonialism, in which a national elite perpetuates the exploitation of minority and majority populations in favour of international or transnational economic interests. However the concept of internal colonialism has been applied to a wide range of cases, including some where a considerable degree of interpenetration of the 'colony' and the 'colonizers' can be observed: the situation of American Blacks and other ethnic minorities, for example, in relation to the dominant white group. The relationships between dominant and subordinate ethnic groups within national territories have also of course been approached from other angles, such as the study of RACE relations, or employing the concept of the PLURAL SOCIETY.

colour terms. An important landmark in the development of COGNITIVE ANTHROPOLOGY was the comparative study of colour classification by Berlin and Kay. The study suggested that human beings make the same discrimination of primary colours regardless of cultural experience or definition, and that the pathway towards more refined and complex colour classifications is a similar one for all peoples (that is to say, colour classification schemes all evolve in a similar way). The method of hierarchical analysis of classificatory schemes employed in Berlin's and Kay's study has been applied to other types of classification (of natural objects, technological inventories, kinship terms etc.). This method offered a means of developing a general theory of knowledge based on the exploration of cognitive systems. It also stood in opposition to Sapir's and Whorf's hypothesis about the nature of

language and thought, which had postulated that it was the structure of language which imposed form on experience rather than the other way around, and that areas like colour classification were relative to each language and the distinctive view of reality it governed.

commensality. The state or act of eating together, one of the fundamental acts of social SOLIDARITY. Different relations of commensality, which are prescribed and proscribed by social and cultural convention, are an important guide to the study of social relationships and cultural categories as far as SHARING, common substance and IDENTITY are concerned. Often the DOMESTIC GROUP is the commensal unit, and the criterion of commensality is frequently taken as part of the definition of such a group. However there is considerable cross-cultural variation in this respect, and the situations in which the commensal unit is expanded or is typically constituted by larger groups are particularly interesting for anthropological analysis. (*See* FOOD.)

commerce. *See* TRADE.

commodity. Commodities are goods and services which have both use VALUE and exchange value within an economy. The concept of commodity is thus closely linked to that of the MARKET, in which commodity exchange creates a relationship between things, as opposed to GIFT exchange which creates a relationship between people.

commodity fetishism. In Marx's economic theory, the tendency whereby the social nature of the production of commodities is disguised or hidden in the market economy. Thus in the market, each commodity appears to possess an intrinsic exchange value, disguising the fact that value is created by the process of human labour.

communes. Contemporary communes in Europe and the United States are generally associated with COUNTER-CULTURAL movements, and express varying degrees of rejection of the wider society's prevailing value system and social relationships. These communes are examples of the cultivation of what TURNER termed *comunitas*, or solidary and egalitarian personal relationships. They are characterized by the common ownership and use of property and resources, and by a breaking down of the normal barriers in the division of labour between domestic units and families. The history of communes may be traced back to a variety of groups, including socialists, utopians and others who have sought to establish small communities according to a range of different ideologies and value sets.

communication. Communication, or the sending and receiving of messages, is essential to all social life and cultural systems, so much so that it is often taken in anthropological theory to be the paradigm of all culture and of all social organization. Communication can take several different forms: it may be verbal or linguistic, paralinguistic, or non-linguistic. Models derived or adapted from LINGUISTICS have been extremely influential in the formation of anthropological models of cultural and social organization. Paralinguistic communication, which accompanies language and provides extra messages about it (*see* METACOMMUNICATION), has also been a focus of interest in anthropological linguistics and in the ETHNOGRAPHY of speaking. The study of nonverbal or non-linguistic communication has been pursued in various areas of anthropological enquiry, among them SYMBOLIC ANTHROPOLOGY and the fields of kinesics and PROXEMICS.

Communication among animal species is characterized mainly by the use of SIGNS and signals, while human communication is distinguished by its extensive use of SYMBOLS, which allows the communicative system a far greater complexity and independence. The evolution of human linguistic and symbolizing ability is functionally linked to the evolution of cultural and social systems dependent on constant and complex communicative acts. LEVI-STRAUSS, in his theory of the elementary structures of KINSHIP, links the idea of communication by the word with the basic structures of RECIPROCITY and EXCHANGE which are central to human society. He thus examines systems of exchange and circulation of goods or PRESTATIONS, and of women, as systems of communication between social groups.

Another approach to the study of communication in society focuses on the relationship between communication and IDEOLOGY, and the manner in which communicative acts convey ideological messages. The issue of who controls the means of communication in society therefore becomes an important one. J. Goody, in his studies of LITERACY and the evolution from 'primitive' to 'advanced' societies, has emphasized the role played by changes in the technology and means of communication.

communism. A socioeconomic formation in which the MEANS OF PRODUCTION are owned and controlled communally, that is to say by the producers themselves or their representatives. Thus private property in the means of production does not exist, and private ownership is limited to personal property for the immediate use of the consumer. In this type of economic system, according to Marxist theory, use value would replace exchange value with the elimination of COMMODITY FETISHISM and of the domination of the MARKET and market forces. The term also refers to political ideologies which advocate this type of social system, and to political movements designed to bring about a change in capitalist society towards the establishment of such a system. There is some degree of confusion regarding the distinction to be made between communism and SOCIALISM. The term communism was initially used to distinguish Marxist political and social theory from earlier Utopian socialist movements. Later, some Marxist theorists came to use the terms almost interchangeably, while others distinguish between socialism as a first phase in the establishment of communism. Thus it is sometimes said that Soviet society is 'socialist', that is to say is in a phase of transition from capitalism to communism (*see* STATE SOCIALISM).

The SCIENTIFIC SOCIALISM of MARX and ENGELS is characterized by an insistence on the linkage between political and social theory and political and social action (*see* PRAXIS). Thus according to Marxist theory the study and analysis of society is inevitably linked to political party action designed to bring about the social REVOLUTION which is a necessary condition for the transition from capitalist to communist society. The revolutionary nature and political party commitment of communism thus distinguishes it from other types of reformist movements, sometimes referred to as socialist, but not necessarily committed to revolutionary change.

communism, primitive. In Marxist theory, a stage of the evolution of human society in which the forces of production were little developed: more specifically, to the period of human history in which HUNTING AND GATHERING or primitive agricultural technology predominated. The primitive communist MODE OF PRODUCTION is characterized by the common ownership and control of the MEANS OF PRODUCTION and the absence of EXPLOITATION and social CLASSES. Anthropologists have questioned the use of this term, and have argued that the means of production in less advanced societies are not always held by the community as a whole: they may be controlled by kin groups (hence E. Terray's concept of the 'lineage mode of production') or by domestic groups (*see* DOMESTIC MODE OF PRODUCTION). R. Keesing has suggested the term 'tribal communal mode of production'. Recent debate has also centred on whether in these so-called primitive communist systems incipient forms of exploitation (for example, of junior men by elders, of women by men) and therefore incipient forms of social class exist.

community. This term has a range of meanings in anthropology and sociology. In its broadest sense, it may refer to any group of persons united by a 'community of interests'. In this sense a professional group, a residential unit, such as a village or town, a sector within such a unit, or a club or voluntary ASSOCIATION may all be referred to as communities. The term is also much employed in phrases such as 'community action', 'community medicine', 'community participation', 'community projects', and so on, where it designates a commitment to the interests and welfare of majority or popular sectors of society, and in consequence to policies and strategies of 'grass roots' involvement in the planning and execution of individual projects or more general programmes. This approach is often linked to calls for APPROPRIATE TECHNOLOGY in DEVELOPMENT programmes and for the decentralization of political structures. The emergence of the concept of community as an important element in modern political ideologies owes a great deal to the influence of the social sciences and to sociological and anthropological perspectives.

In its more limited anthropological and sociological senses, the term is restricted to mean a local community, generally fairly small-scale and often described as 'traditional' or 'closed' (*see* CLOSED CORPORATE COMMUNITY). In this sense it is mainly used to describe PEASANT communities or traditional isolated or semi-isolated groups which persist within modern industrial societies, especially those which are united by a common occupational category such as fishing, mining and small-scale farming. In this sociological and anthropological usage community is implicitly or explicitly contrasted with SOCIETY or ASSOCIATION (*see* GEMEINSCHAFT/GESELLSCHAFT; FOLK-URBAN CONTINUUM). 'Community' is thus in this instance taken to mean face-to-face personal relations in a small-scale social network or residential settlement, as opposed to the more impersonal or contractual relationships characteristic of modern industrial and urban society.

community study. The community study has been the dominant mode of anthropological analysis in studies of PEASANT society in Mesoamerica, South America, Europe, and Asia. The method has also been applied to the study of other types of COMMUNITY; to sectors of urban society, for example. The community study focuses on a relatively small and independent local settlement, and emphasizes the practical interrelation of social institutions and cultural patterns within such a community. It aims accordingly at a holistic and complete description of patterns of social relationships, values and institutions in the community, and the manner in which it maintains and reproduces its social structure and cultural system over time. The functionalist orientation of community studies has provoked considerable criticism, and has the tendency to concentrate on intra-community dynamics to the neglect of wider social and political power structures affecting the community and its relationship to regional and national systems.

compadrazgo. A Spanish term which may be translated as 'co-parenthood'. In Spain and the Spanish-speaking New World, it refers to the relationship between the parents and godparents of a child, a relationship often more important or more visible than that between godparents and their godchildren. Also referred to as RITUAL KINSHIP, *compadrazgo* has been interpreted as an example of the DYADIC CONTRACT; that is, an example of the various means by which the individual may extend his personal network by extending kin-like relationships to non-kin. *Compadrazgo* relationships may be classified according to the social status of the partners in the relationship. They may be established with social and economic equals for the purpose of mutual support, or with persons of superior status (*see* PATRONAGE) in order to obtain benefits or access to extra-community power sources. Bloch and Gugenheim in their survey of the topic (1981) point to two main trends: an analysis from a sociological point of view of the links formed by the *compadrazgo* arrangement within a network of social relations, and the analysis of the symbolism of *compadrazgo* and the opposition between spiritual and natural kinship. Sociologically *compadrazgo* as an institution takes a wide variety of forms and performs a wide variety of functions, and several anthropologists have explored its historical and geographical variability: the inter- and intra-class aspects of *compadrazgo*, its use to create or to solidify social relations, and so on. Many writers have conceived of *compadrazgo* as a form of ritualized personal relationship which is always underpinned by some form of instrumentality. Others, however, have explored its symbolic or ideological basis, which consistently underlies its historical and cross-cultural variability. J. Pitt-Rivers (1971), for example, relates it to baptism, and to the name and social identity conferred upon an individual by ritual kinship. S. Gudeman relates it to the notion of man's dual nature as spiritual and natural being, and the superiority of the spiritual parents over the natural ones. *Compadrazgo*, according to these views, thus creates the social or juridic person out of the natural one. Bloch and Guggenheim relate the ideology of *compadrazgo* to the symbolism of GENDER relationships and of ritual rebirth in general, which they argue serve to devalue the natural (female) BIRTH and substitute for it

ritual rebirth controlled by men. (*See* RITUAL SEXUAL SYMMETRY.)

comparative method. This should not be confused with CROSS-CULTURAL COMPARISON. It refers to the 19th-century practice of equating existing simple societies with extinct groups ('living fossils'), in order to substantiate theories of EVOLUTION.

competence and performance. In LINGUISTICS, a distinction is made between linguistic competence, or the speaker's mainly unconscious knowledge of language, which he draws upon in order to speak or understand speech, and linguistic performance, which is actual observable speech behaviour. This distinction, important in structural linguistics, can be made in a parallel fashion for culture: 'cultural competence' would in this case refer to the system of knowledge or cultural models of an individual, and 'cultural performance' to his observable behaviour.

competition. Competitive behaviour and competitive social relationships involve the use of strategies designed to gain access to scarce resources and at the same time to exclude others from such access. Competitiveness, like co-operativeness, is part of the range of tendencies or attitudes which occur universally among human beings, but it is Western society and culture in particular which channels such competitive or co-operative tendencies into certain standardized behaviours and relations. Competitiveness thus may be encouraged in one domain of social life, while co-operativeness is favoured in others. Competition is closely related to CONFLICT, from which it is however sometimes distinguished, in that competition is governed by a set of shared rules and norms, while conflict involves divergences of norms and values. However this distinction is not a hard and fast one, since competition will generally tend to create a degree of value divergence.

complementary filiation. A term coined by FORTES in his study of unilineal descent systems, to refer to the rights, obligations and relationships channelled through the maternal line in patrilineal systems or the paternal line in matrilineal ones. Fortes suggested that complementary filiation provided counterbalancing elements in the lineage system, complementing the formal, jural relationships of unilineal descent with the more informal affective ties of the non-descent relationships. Subsequent critics of his hypothesis have argued that it is an artefact of the LINEAGE THEORY itself, which has to invent a special category to account for relationships which are in reality expressions of DOUBLE UNILINEAL DESCENT, BILATERAL kinship, or AFFINAL ties. (*See* KINSHIP; ALLIANCE THEORY.)

complex society. This term is sometimes used, with or without its implied contrast, the 'simple society', to distinguish modern industrial from traditional or pre-industrial societies. Like any simple dichotomy, this classification raises many problems when the appropriateness of its application to the diversity and range of human societies is examined. The so-called simple societies may be extremely complex in certain aspects of their social and cultural structures. The criterion of simplicity or complexity is generally taken to be the nature of their social networks (predominantly small-scale and face-to-face in the simple society, predominantly large scale and 'open' in the complex society) and/or the level of technological development. It is immediately apparent, however, that the term cannot be used with any precision, nor can a definite border be drawn between the simple and the complex.

complex structure. In LEVI-STRAUSS' theory of kinship complex structures are opposed to ELEMENTARY STRUCTURES. Complex structures are those in which marriage rules are expressed negatively: that is to say, there are categories of kin who are prohibited partners for marriage, but the system does not prescribe marriage with a given category of kin. (*See* PRESCRIPTION.)

componential analysis. A technique which has been employed in kinship studies and other areas of anthropological enquiry, componential analysis belongs to the group of techniques of FORMAL ANALYSIS developed within COGNITIVE ANTHROPOLOGY for the examination of data. R. Brown describes componential analysis as defining 'all of some set of words in terms of the same semantic dimensions or components. The meaning of each word in the set appears as a unique bundle of values on the common dimensions.' In the study of KINSHIP TERMINOLOGY, for example, a componential analysis would proceed first by defining the universe of kin terms (denotata) and by attempting to discover their meanings (significata). Each term is mapped on to its designata (biological kinship types; e.g. MB, MZH, FB, FZ etc.). After the 'core term' or 'kernel' for each of the ranges has been decided, all of the terms are defined by isolating in each case the smallest number of distinctive features which put an individual term apart from the rest of the set. These features, or criteria, are 'components' which distinguish each kin term from every other and which, when 'bundled together' in an individual definition, identify each term and define its place on the domain. There may be more than one way of doing this, and the choice of components to be used depends on the analyst's preference and his intuitive understanding of the informants' cognitive map. Componential analysis can only endow a very limited meaning on a kinship term, and does not include all culturally and linguistically relevant dimensions or connotations. Like other types of formal analysis of kinship systems, it gives an account of a closed system within a deductive framework, and to avoid a sterile formalism this closed deductive model must be related in some way to the open-ended system of attitudes, and cultural, social and linguistic contexts within which kinship is embedded.

computers in sociocultural anthropology. The development and spread of computers has had a major impact on sociocultural anthropology. Mainframe computers in academic centres have been used for over two decades to evaluate anthropological models and analyse data, and personal computers are increasingly employed in field situations.

When anthropologists first gained access to computers in the 1960s, many articles on programming discussed how computer simulations could be used to construct and test anthropological models. Since that time anthropologists have devised numerous ingenious computer programs simulating demographic processes and resource use. However, simulation efforts have often foundered because of unrealistic assumptions, programming problems, and time constraints.

While only a small minority of anthropologists have attempted simulation, the use of computers in data analysis is widespread. Easily learned 'canned' programs such as the SPSS (Statistical Package for the Social Sciences) allow complex data manipulations which were previously prohibitively time-consuming. The increasingly sophisticated use of STATISTICS by anthropologists can be largely attributed to the availability of these programs. The ease of use of statistical packages, however, has often caused problems when anthropologists with limited expertise have tried to use analytic methods which they understand incompletely. Anthropologists have also sometimes been insufficiently critical of the quality of data analysed.

The development of battery operated machinery has stimulated the use of personal computers even in the most remote field sites. Word processing programs and printers are great aids in the writing, storage, revision, reproduction and cross-referencing of field notes. Statistical packages allow preliminary data analysis in the course of fieldwork. The only major drawback of computers in remote settings is the difficulty of obtaining supplies and maintaining and repairing equipment.

Comte, Auguste (1798–1857). This French philosopher and sociologist worked closely with SAINT-SIMON. Comte coined the term SOCIOLOGY, and divided the discipline into two parts, the study of social statics and that of social dynamics. He advocated the scientific study of society and history according to the methods of 'positive philosophy' (e.g. 1877). This was linked to his evolutionary scheme of social forms, in which three basic types of society – the military, the legalistic and the industrial – were accompanied by three types of thought, the theological, the metaphysical and the positive or scientific.

conception. There has been considerable debate in anthropological circles where certain beliefs about conception and paternity (or maternity) are concerned. The most well-known example is that of the Trobriand islanders, who in common with some Aust-ralian aboriginal peoples deny that pregnancy is a result of copulation between the mother and her husband or lover. In the Trobriand islands, pregnancy is said to result when a woman's matrilineal ancestors, at the request of her matrikin, send her a 'spirit child'. Much debate has centred on whether this is to be interpreted as a literal statement of what the Trobriand islanders believe, or as a dogmatic or symbolic assertion which they actually know to be false. It has been pointed out that the Trobriand islanders are in constant contact with other peoples who are perfectly aware of the role of the father in conception, and that they themselves apply to animal breeding this knowledge, and thus it has been argued that the 'belief' in question should be regarded rather as a dogma: sexual intercourse is a necessary condition for pregnancy, but not a sufficient one, since the spiritual element is regarded as essential to the animation of the potential child. The Trobriand denial of physiological paternity is merely an extreme example of a wide range of beliefs about respective contributions of father and mother to the spiritual and/or physical development of the child. At the other extreme, there are peoples who deny the role of the mother in the creation of the child, asserting that she is merely a container for the growth of the baby which is deposited in her by the man. The Lakher of Burma, for example, assert that two children of the same mother but different fathers are not related. Such beliefs or dogmas should be considered in relation to the ideology of kinship and affinity in the society concerned. The denial of physiological maternity or paternity may be regarded as a logical extension of the principle of separation of kin and AFFINAL ties: if the mother is regarded as an affine, for example, in a system where kin relationships are conceived of as transmitted through males, then it is a logical extension of this to deny the mother's part in forming the child and to conceive of the relationship between mother and child as an affinal one. Similarly, where kinship is regarded as transmitted through females, the denial of physiological paternity amounts to the assertion that where there is affinity, there is no kinship. Other societies have less drastic resolutions of the problem of reconciling kin and affinal relations, but which also reflect their ideology of relationships. In some groups the mother is thus considered to contribute 'blood' or 'flesh' and the father 'bone' to the child, and these substances are in turn endowed with symbolic properties which link it to a particular kind of social relationship.

concubinage. A permitted sexual relationship between a man and a woman, or women, to whom he is not legitimately married (*see* MARRIAGE). The children born of such women do not have claims on the father's status or property, and this is one of the key distinctions between concubinage and POLYGYNY. Whereas polygyny is consistent with 'open' kin groups where people are regarded as an asset, the emergence of concubinage is consistent with 'closed' kin groups which desire to restrict inheritance of property to a limited range of persons. Concubinage might thus be viewed as a kind of compromise between MONOGAMY and polygyny, and also as a form of expressing high status and prestige for a dominant elite in those societies where concubinage is restricted to the wealthy or politically powerful strata.

conditioning. In BEHAVIOURIST psychology, this is a central concept and is held to account for most if not all learning and behaviour patterns. Two types of conditioning are distinguished: the 'classical conditioning' described by I. Pavlov and the 'operant conditioning' described by B.F. Skinner. In classical or Pavlovian conditioning, the association of a normally neutral stimulus with another stimulus which evokes an automatic response leads to the association of the previously neutral stimulus with the response. Thus, in a typical example of Pavlovian conditioning, a dog may salivate at the sight of his food dish, a previously neutral stimulus, because he has come to associate the dish with food by the repeated presentation of the two stimuli simultaneously. In operant conditioning, the subject is exposed to a punishment or reward (positive or negative 'reinforcement') following a random act. By repeated trial and error, the subject comes to associate the act with the reinforcement and thereby learns to repeat or avoid the behaviour. By using operant conditioning techniques, animals can be trained to perform a variety of mechanical operations and even to replace human labour in certain routine industrial work. The limitations of the conditioning model as a comprehensive account of human learning and behaviour have been pointed out by cognitive and developmental psychologists who emphasize the importance of the organization of knowledge into hierarchical schemata by the individual, who takes an active and dynamic part in the process of learning.

Condorcet, Marie Jean Antoine Nicolas Caritat, Marquis de (1743–94). One of the main figures in the French ENLIGHTENMENT, this philosopher, mathematician and social scientist saw history (and progress) as the result of the development and perfection of the human intellect. For Condorcet, the purpose of the study of history was to discover and apply the laws of human progress, which he divided into ten stages of development towards more rational government and society. Condorcet's views influenced COMTE, among other social scientists.

configurationalism. Also called GESTALT THEORY, this is a psychological theory of perception and thought which stresses the importance of the consistency and 'wholeness' of mental configurations. Its emphasis on the integration of thought and perception influenced the development of CULTURE AND PERSONALITY theory. An influential figure in the development of this theory was SAPIR, who was closely associated with BENEDICT, widely regarded as the leading exponent of this approach in anthropology. The concept of CULTURAL PATTERN is closely related to that of configuration, though KLUCKHOHN distinguished between the two in that he reserved the term 'pattern' for overt manifestations of a culture's underlying configuration.

conflict. A broad term, including phenomena which may be classified under a number of different headings. Thus the ANTHROPOLOGY OF LAW, the anthropology of WAR, POLITICAL ANTHROPOLOGY and the study of social and cultural CHANGE all have as a central concern the phenomenon of conflict between individuals, groups or social classes. Approaches to conflict in anthropology and in the social sciences in general vary considerably according to the theoretical significance attached to the disputative relationships. The tradition of studies of deviance and SOCIAL CONTROL established by DURKHEIM and developed by FUNCTIONALIST and STRUCTURAL FUNCTIONALIST anthropology and sociology has frequently been criticized for failing to take into account fundamental conflicts of interest between different groups or sectors in society, conflicts not accounted for by a model of functional equilibrium and systems maintenance. In MARXIST ANTHROPOLOGY, on the other hand, conflict is regarded as built into the social system, and is seen as productive or positive, inasmuch as it is the expression of underlying contradictions which will culminate in the transformation of society itself. In the anthropology of law, too, there are a number of approaches to the study of conflict and dispute settlement, which depend on whether the anthropologist and legal institutions view mechanisms for resolving disputes as necessary elements in the maintenance of social cohesion and a common moral order (see CONSCIENCE COLLECTIVE) or rather as coercive instruments serving the interests of a dominant class.

Conflict is a primary source or stimulus for social change, for, when it cannot be handled by institutionalized mechanisms of dispute settlement, the opposing parties will be forced to create new strategies either to resolve the conflict or avoid the situation which produces it. The organization of social groups for the purposes of conflict or in order to cope with its consequences is also a major force for social integration: conflicts at one level (for instance, between local communities) may thus promote cohesion at another (within the local community). By the same token, real conflicts of interest within a given group or community may be disguised by the strategy of focusing on more or less artificially created conflicts with other groups, as in the time-honoured political strategy of declaring war on a neighbour in order to distract attention from troubles at home. In the anthropological study of conflict we must thus carefully distinguish between levels of analysis: the levels at which conflicts occur and are managed, as well as the levels of social cohesion or integration which come into play in the creation and management of conflict.

Conflict is sometimes distinguished from COMPETITION, in that the latter is governed by a set of shared goals or values, while the former is characterized by divergent goals and values between the parties involved. But this is rather a difference of degree than kind, since competitive social relations and situations will inevitably generate some degree of conflict or value divergence. BATESON in his theory of SCHISM argues that communication itself generates increasing tensions and conflicts culminating in the fission of social groups.

When referring to conflict, we use the term in two rather different senses, which it is useful to distinguish. One is that of a 'conflict situation', which might also be called an overt or expressed conflict, and the other is a 'conflict of interests' or implicit conflict. The distinction is helpful, for the two do not always coincide, and the relationship between underlying or implicit conflicts of interest and the overt expressions of conflict in a society is an interesting field of anthropological enquiry. Fundamental conflicts of interest in society may be diverted to find their expression in conflict situations unconnected with their real underlying causes via mechanisms of both an ideological and a social psychological nature.

conjugal. Having to do with the MARRIAGE relationship.

connubium. In Roman civil law, the condition of marriageability. In anthropology, the term has been used, following DURKHEIM, MAUSS and LEVI-STRAUSS, to refer to the right and obligation of men of a certain group or category to marry members of another group or category. The connubium is thus said to exist between such groups or categories. (See PRESCRIPTION.)

consanguinity. 'Blood' or kinship relations based on biological ties. Consanguineal relatives are thus persons related through parental and/or sibling ties. There is considerable debate in the anthropological study of KINSHIP about the correspondence between consanguinity or the 'biological facts' and the system of kin classification. On the one hand it is recognized that our intuitive definition of kinship is that it has something to do with biological relationships, and it is sometimes argued that the core meanings of all kinship terms are biological kin types (*see* EXTENSION OF KINSHIP TERMS). On the other, it is pointed out that there is great cross-cultural variation in the definition and interpretation of 'biological' kinship (*see* CONCEPTION), and it has been shown that the analysis of kinship terms as CATEGORY terms, without reference to biological core meanings, is also a productive approach.

conscience collective. This term, coined by DURKHEIM, is defined by him as 'the set of beliefs and sentiments common to the average members of a single society [which] forms a determinate system that has its own life'. The inclusion of both 'beliefs' and 'sentiments', that is to say, both cognitive and emotional, moral or religious elements in the *conscience collective* introduces an important ambiguity in English, where it is possible to translate this term either as 'collective unconscious' or 'collective conscience'. The concept is important in his work *The Division of Labour*, where it is particularly linked to less advanced societies characterized by MECHANICAL SOLIDARITY. In his later works, however, Durkheim moved away from his original concept towards the more detailed analysis of COLLECTIVE REPRESENTATIONS, which are specific states of the *conscience collective*, occurring in advanced as well as simple societies.

consciousness, altered states of. *See* ALTERED STATES OF CONSCIOUSNESS.

consensual union. In societies where a formal or legal MARRIAGE ceremony exists, a consensual union is one between a couple who maintain a common residence without having gone through this ceremony. The high incidence of this type of union in certain social groups (for example in black families in the Caribbean and the USA) has generated debate as to whether this is a pathological phenomenon (that is, an index of social disorganization) or a normal feature of such social groups. It has been pointed out in this respect, that the legal marriage is often regarded as the ideal, although consensual unions are the norm at certain stages of the domestic cycle, or due to economic reasons. (*See* MATRIFOCALITY.)

consensus. The converging of opinion, or the process of forming a common decision or judgment in a group. The role of consensus in social and political life is of considerable importance in all societies as an expression of, and an essential condition for, social solidarity and cohesion. The repeated or continuous breakdown of consensus (or the formation of dissensus) is, by the same token, expressive of, and a key factor in, situations of social CONFLICT or disintegration. The process by which a consensus is arrived at in a group may include a number of formal and informal devices for minimizing conflict or its overt expression, and may also involve a complex series of political manoeuvres designed to influence the opinions and actions of others. This process of consensus forming may be studied from the point of view of POLITICAL ANTHROPOLOGY, where it is important to distinguish the structural value of consensus in the society under study. In many non-state political systems, particularly those where the leader is conceived of as a *primus inter pares* with limited formal authority, political decisions and strategies at the level of the group or the community emerge essentially from group consensus, and the power of a leader to go against such a consensus is limited (*see* CONSENT). The ideological system of a society is closely connected to the process of consensus formation, and constitutes a common set of beliefs and values subscribed to by all members of society while at the same time justifying the dominant position of one group or class. In pre-class societies, such ideologies may maintain the dominant position of elders versus juniors, of men versus women, and so on, while in class-based societies they serve to generalize throughout society the values and beliefs espoused by the dominant class. By means of such ideological systems, a general consensus may be assured which includes even those groups or classes who are objectively being subordinated or exploited. However there is no general agreement among anthropologists as to the degree of value and norm consensus which is necessary for the functioning of society, since recent studies have increasingly tended to demonstrate the diversity of individual viewpoints, and the extent to which consensus is a pragmatic rather than a normative process.

Consensus formation may also be studied from the point of view of COMMUNICATION, or the study of linguistic and paralinguistic mechanisms involved in the creation of a group opinion or judgment. The ethnography of speaking, with its emphasis on how we create social and cultural systems as products of our communication and interaction, has made important contributions in this field. BATESON, in his development of the concept of SCHISM, pioneered the analysis of the opposite phenomenon, whereby communicative acts generate a build-up of opposed or contrary values and concepts, culminating in the breaking up of a social group.

FUNCTIONALIST and STRUCTURAL FUNCTIONALIST theories of society have sometimes been termed 'consensus theories' because they emphasize (and many would argue overemphasize) the degree of consensus of values and beliefs in society. 'Conflict theories', on the other hand, have shown that such consensus is not a necessary feature of social organization, which may rely instead on pragmatic acceptance of POWER structures.

consent. In POLITICAL ANTHROPOLOGY, a distinction is sometimes made between political systems based on consent and those based on coercion. Consent, which may be implicit or explicit, has differing structural significance in different types of political system. Consent of most of the population most of the time is essential to the maintenance and continuation of any political and social system, but in STATE societies such consent is backed up by the organized coercive force of military, legal and other potentially repressive institutions. In pre-state political formations, however, such coercive apparatus does not exist, and the structural role of consent is therefore a primary one.

conservatism. The preference and maintenance of traditional ways of acting, forms of social institutions and cultural patterns. Extreme conservatism has often been cited as a feature of both 'primitive' and PEASANT societies studied by anthropologists. It is often argued that pre-literate societies, where the ORAL TRADITION is the dominant way of transmitting knowledge and values, are inherently resistant to INNOVATION and CHANGE. Although this assumption is common, it needs more careful examination, and in particular we need to distinguish between different kinds or levels of innovation and change. LEVI-STRAUSS, for example, has shown in his studies of MYTHOLOGY how mythic systems can be innovative in the sense that they constantly combine and recombine elements in new configurations, and at the same time deeply conservative in that they preserve a common underlying structure which always tends towards the preservation of equilibrium and the 'suppression of (historical) time'. We need far more careful investigation into the sense of HISTORY of pre-literate peoples before we can categorize whole cultures as 'conservative' or otherwise. Similarly, the broad assumption of peasant conservatism has been challenged considerably both by those writers who emphasize conflict and change in peasant societies and by those who argue that the supposedly 'irrational' conservative tendencies of peasant communities are in fact a perfectly reasonable reaction to the uncertainties of their relationship with the wider regional and national society. In fact pre-literate and peasant peoples from different geographical areas and types of community do diverge widely in degrees of conservatism and of social and cultural stability.

conspicuous consumption. Coined by Thorstein Veblen in his *Theory of the Leisure Class* (1899), this term refers to the wasteful consumption of luxury goods which serves to indicate membership of the leisure class in capitalist society. The term has been applied in anthropological studies of pre-capitalist societies, to refer to the display of consumption of goods for prestige purposes.

contagious magic. FRAZER divided MAGIC into two broad categories or types: contagious magic, which operates on the principle that two substances or objects which have once been in contact may continue to influence one another in the future, and sympathetic magic, which relies on the principle that like affects like.

contraception and abortion. Contraception is the prevention of conception, while abortion is the termination of an existing pregnancy. In addition to contraceptive and abortive practices, INFANTICIDE and cultural restrictions on sexual intercourse are the other two available means of limiting population and fertility. In the case of restrictions on sexual intercourse, the limitations may relate to taboos on male or female sexual activities at certain stages of the life cycle or during the performance of specific activities, or to moral values regarding sexual 'purity'. The reduction of fertility may thus be an unintended consequence in this instance, whereas in the cases of contraception, abortion and infanticide the limitation of family size is the direct and intended consequence. That there is little detailed ethnographic evidence regarding contraceptive and abortive practices in the majority of technologically simple societies is largely due to the intimate nature of the information involved, and it is thus generally impossible to assess the efficacy of contraceptive methods within folk medicine. In HUNTING AND GATHERING societies there is as a rule a strict control of population density, achieved in many cases by the practice of infanticide, but influenced too by a complex combination of factors including the effects of diet on fertility, prolonged lactation (which delays ovulation and thus inhibits fertility), and so on. The need for birth spacing in hunting and gathering societies is directly related to the nomadic lifestyle and the burden placed on a woman by the caring, feeding and carrying of small children while at the same time going about her daily subsistence routine. In sedentary populations, there tends to be an increase in fertility, due at least in part to the fact that in agricultural communities children are valuable additions to the domestic workforce and thus become assets rather than liabilities. With the shift in domestic group organization from a productive to a consuming unit in industrial society, there tends to be once more a drop in fertility, facilitated by the advent of more efficient contraceptive methods.

contract. A voluntary agreement between two or more persons, which creates and specifies the terms of a legal obligation or relationship between the parties concerned.

Contract has often been taken as one of the key features of modern industrial society, and contrasted with simple societies governed by STATUS (MAINE) or COMMUNITY (*see* GEMEINSCHAFT/GESELLSCHAFT). The notion of the contract, or voluntary assumption of rights and obligations by rationally acting individuals, is an important one in many theories of political and social organization. (*See* SOCIAL CONTRACT.)

contradiction. In logic, a contradiction is the conjunction of a proposition and its negation. The term is used very broadly to refer both to inconsistencies in thought, beliefs or values and also to refer to institutional contradictions or CONFLICT. (*See* DIALECTIC; MARXIST ANTHROPOLOGY.)

control, social. *See* SOCIAL CONTROL.

conversation analysis. *See* ETHNOMETHODO-LOGY.

conversion, religious. Religious conversion has attracted the attention both of anthropology and social psychology, which have studied the forms and functions of conversionist CULTS or SECTS. Such sects rely on the experience of personal conversion in order to recruit their members. They have often been linked to situations of social stress or social change, and particularly appeal to migrant or marginal sectors in urban environments. Such sects may in time become progressively more respectable and institutionalized, becoming religious DENOMINATIONS associated with certain sectors of the community. This process of denominalization is linked to that of social mobility and stabilization of migrant groups.

co-operatives. Economic entities owned by their members. In the case of productive co-operatives, which may be agricultural or industrial, the members are the producers or workers. There are also a variety of other types of co-operative organization: co-operative marketing organizations, for example, and consumers' and savings and credit co-operatives, etc. These co-operative organizations, when they exist within the framework of a dominant capitalist economy, may come to resemble more or less the private concerns with which they compete. In socialist states, the co-operative has greater potential for development and centralized support, though there are within socialist programmes ambiguities in the distinction and delimitation of generalized collective ownership, controlled by the state, and true co-operative organization where a paramount role is played by the membership as direct owners and managers of the concern.

In Third World countries faced with the failure of capitalist free enterprise to achieve the DEVELOPMENT and growth of the economy as a whole, co-operative organizations have sometimes appeared to hold much promise, attempting to build on traditional patterns of communal organization. Yet the resemblance between a traditional communal economy and a modern co-operative organization is largely illusory, and in any case does not resolve the structural, economic, and political problems in the wider national environment. Many co-operative experiments in developing countries have therefore failed due to lack of organized centralized support and to their relegation to the less profitable areas of economic activity which do not attract international capital investment or participation.

corporate group. A social GROUP which owns and controls significant property or resources. Thus, following MAINE, the corporate group is defined as an aggregate of persons who share rights over property or an 'estate' which has continuity over time. WEBER, however, saw corporateness as a function of the distribution and relationship to AUTHORITY within the group. In legal and administrative terms, a corporate group is one which is considered as a single individual as far as the rights, responsibilities and functions relating to its corporate property are concerned. A corporate kin group is thus a kin group which has economic and property holding functions, and a corporate DESCENT group is one which in addition transmits these rights and functions throughout a period of time in accordance with a rule of descent. In anthropology, groups are defined as 'corporate' not only in connection with forms of property such as land or economic goods, but also in relation to property of a ritual, religious or political nature (names, ritual procedures and pre-

rogatives, offices etc.). STRUCTURAL FUNCTIONALIST anthropology and LINEAGE THEORY place great emphasis on corporate kin groups, seeing them as the basis of jural order and of sociopolitical organization in the majority of pre-state societies. ACTION THEORY in POLITICAL ANTHROPOLOGY moved away from this emphasis on corporate groups, and modern kinship studies have also done so to some extent, as other types of group and relationship have been shown to be significant factors in social organization.

corvée. A kind of labour which is exacted by a political authority as a form of tribute or in lieu of taxation. The term was originally used to refer to the system in which a FEUDAL lord in Europe could compel his peons to work for a period of time on his lands. The term has also been extended to other types of labour tax in feudal or feudal-type states, including that directed towards the realization of public works, as in the Inca empire of pre-conquest Peru, and that required by COLONIAL authorities of the local population.

cosmogony. A theory or explanation of the origin of the universe or cosmos. In anthropology the study of indigenous cosmogonies forms part of the analysis of RELIGION, MYTH and BELIEF systems.

cosmology. A theory of, or set of beliefs concerning, the nature of the universe or cosmos. These beliefs may include postulates of the structure, organization and functioning of the supernatural, natural and social worlds. In some contexts the ethnographer finds cosmological systems which are coherent and complex, while in others they may be incoherent, contradictory or apparently incomplete. (*See* RELIGION; MYTH; BELIEF.)

cotradition. A term coined by LINTON (1955) in an attempt to refine the concept of CULTURE AREAS by specifying their historical depth. The concept of culture areas refers to geographical continuities in culture types, and that of cotradition to historical continuities. Thus an 'area cotradition' is a culture configuration which has both historical and geographical continuity.

counter-culture. A phenomenon which develops in defiance of traditional or majority norms and values, and relates to the norms and values of an 'alternative' society or social group. The counter-culture is thus distinguished from the SUBCULTURE, which is simply a variant of the dominant culture but not necessarily in explicit opposition to it. The term has been applied to 'youth cultures' in industrial society, and may also be related to certain types of deviance.

court. The original sense of this term was a king's or lord's palace, subsequently extended to refer to certain institutions, specifically legal ones, related to the functions of political authority. In the ANTHROPOLOGY OF LAW the study of the functioning of different kinds of courts, and the manner in which these bring power or authority structures to bear on the resolution of CONFLICT or the transgression of norms, is an important area of enquiry. Normally the term 'court' is restricted to formal legal institutions, where there is an appointed authority empowered to judge, and backed up by a system of coercive means to enforce the decision, generally the police or miltary. However there are many other institutions or settings for the settlement of disputes, from a formal legal institution where judges and lawyers are legal specialists, to a more informal 'community court' or 'moot', where cases are decided between neighbours and kinsmen. In pre-state societies the function of courts is not usually specialized, and judicial authority thus overlaps with kinship, ritual and political authority. FORDE, for example, described the 'priestly council' of the Yako village in the 1930s as an institution based on ritual and moral authority which served to resolve disputes and punish offenders. The council also served as a forum for the discussion and deliberation of political matters and issues of common concern. However it was not backed up by any specific coercive force. In the centralized Tswana chiefdoms described by Schapera (1955), however, there existed an elaborate traditional court system including legal specialists and a complex legal code at its highest level.

cousin marriage. Marriage between cousins has attracted considerable attention in the study of KINSHIP and ALLIANCE in anthropology. In PRESCRIPTIVE marriage systems (those with a positive marriage rule) the prescribed category of spouse is very commonly typified or represented by a particular category of cousin. We have, therefore, the categories of PARALLEL COUSIN MARRIAGE and CROSS-COUSIN MARRIAGE, depending on whether the marriageable cousin is a child of the parent's same sex or opposite sex sibling. In addition there are distinct categories of MATRILATERAL, PATRILATERAL and BILATERAL cousin marriage. There has been considerable anthropological debate as to the significance of these prescriptive marriage categories, with particular reference to opposing interpretations of cousin marriage, either as a relationship primarily between individual kinsmen, or as a relationship principally between alliance categories, which are simply typified by the actual cousin (see KINSHIP TERMINOLOGY). In alliance theory it has thus been argued that the concept of cousin marriage itself is an erroneous one, since the marriageable categories are to be conceived of as alliance categories, not kinship relationships. The different kinds of alliance pattern are thus better described by terms such as ASYMMETRIC/SYMMETRIC ALLIANCE.

cousin terms. *See* KINSHIP TERMINOLOGY.

creativity. The ability to form new patterns or structures, to perform new actions, and to solve new problems. In linguistics, the term is used to describe the individual's ability not only to reproduce accurately utterances which he or she has heard, but to generate a potentially infinite number of new utterances employing the linguistic structures which he or she has mastered. Cultural creativity is the ability of a group as a whole to incorporate INNOVATIONS into its cultural repertoire. At the level of individual behaviour, creativity is manifested constantly in the individual's ability to adapt to changing personal and social conditions, generating new behaviour patterns accordingly, as well as in those domains which are culturally defined as proper outlets for creativity of a more deliberate or artistic kind. The phenomenon of human creativity is important in the evolution of our species: creative behaviour like PLAY, enables humans to adapt better to a wide variety of environments and to elaborate and complex cultural traditions. Human creativity also lies at the root of the universal phenomenon of CHANGE in culture and society.

credit. There is an important distinction to be made between types of credit or delayed RECIPROCITY where the repayment is identical to or equivalent to the original loan (food for food, labour for labour, money for money) and those where repayment takes a different form (labour for goods, goods for money). Similarly, there is a vital difference between systems of credit without interest and those where the principle of interest applies. Credit relationships are a basic principle of operation of a pre-money economy, whether they be the generalized relationships of credit which obtain between kinsmen and neighbours, or the more formalized continuing obligations of trading partners. However these credit relationships are not of the same kind as the relationships of financial credit in a capitalist economy, or the credit given by a patron to his client, which permit capital accumulation and encourage economic differentiation. (*See* ECONOMIC ANTHROPOLOGY.)

creole. A creole language is a mixed language – that is to say, an amalgam of two languages which results from a contact between two peoples. Typically a creole language develops from a PIDGIN. The two may be distinguished by their levels of complexity; while a pidgin is a simplified means of communication between groups who do not share a common tongue, the creole is a first language in its own right. The term creole is also used in Latin America and the Caribbean to refer to local born descendants of European families. In colonial Spanish America there was a rigid division into social groups according to origin: between Spaniards, *criollos*, *mestizos* and Indians, each of which had specified rights and obligations within the sociopolitical hierarchy. In parts of the United States, the term refers to descendants of French families.

crime. A violation of law which attracts a sanction. It differs from other kinds of transgression of NORMS or violation of CUSTOM, in that there exists a formal social process for handling and penalizing the criminal (*See* COURT). The definition of what constitutes a crime is a political one, since it rests with the political authority, via its legal institutions. Two broad categories of crime may be distinguished: those in which one member of society commits an offence against another (crimes of property or offences against the person), and those in which there is no specific victim. These may be crimes against public morals or custom, or crimes of a political nature in which the 'victim' is the state or the dominant political authority. The social and political processes and pressures which cause these different kinds of crime and create different types of criminal have been the subject of considerable sociological study in the fields of law and deviance, but have as yet attracted little attention from the comparative and cross-cultural perspective of anthropology. (*See* LAW, ANTHROPOLOGY OF.)

crisis. A moment in the development or functioning of a system in which the contradictions generated internally within itself and/or between it and its environment, reach a point at which they place intolerable strain on the system itself. The ensuing crisis will precipitate either the destruction of the system or radical structural changes. The concept of crisis resolution has broad applicability in the study of social CHANGE and REVOLUTION.

crisis of capitalism. This term is used in two rather different though overlapping senses within Marxist interpretations of CAPITALISM. In one sense, it is used to refer to the social conflicts and tensions generated within capitalist society as a result of the contradictions inherent in the capitalist system. In another sense, it refers to the specific historical moment, predicted by Marxist theory, when the productive forces of capitalism will outgrow its productive relations, precipitating the collapse of the capitalist productive system. (*See* REVOLUTION.)

critical anthropology. An amalgamated discipline, in which scholars of diverse theoretical positions have combined analyses of a given people's mode of life and the effects on it of the political-economic activity of nation states and other 'control systems'. A loosely-knit field of anthropological expertise and concern, it draws from MARXISM, literary criticism, and post-structuralist philosophy as well as anthropology and welds aspects of such schools of thought to certain traditional anthropological specialities. The features that are common to critical anthropology include the ethnography of a given people carried on through time; continued analysis and monitoring of the nation state and WORLD SYSTEM as they impinge on a given people; a knowledge of world ethnology and an ability to confront ethnological generalizations continuously with fresh ethnographic data; and a willingness to enter various literary and political arenas on behalf of given peoples caught up in struggles for autonomy, or more satisfactory ecological, economic, political, social or cultural circumstances.

Critical anthropology accepts, admires and seeks to illuminate the inner integrity of a cultural system – the structure – without assuming that such a system is homogenous, functional, a retention of the past, the result of marginality or the creation of a dominant system. It rejects the use of terminology that implies racist, sexist or other unequal status ('primitive culture,' 'primitive society,' 'savages') and maintains continuing sensitivity to the outlooks and opinions of ethnic minorities. For example, it recognizes tendencies to generalize about 'Indians have tribal culture,' 'Primitives are superstitious,' 'Paranoia is a cultural trait of the Bongo-bongo,' and so on, and tries to demonstrate the ways in which anthropology can inadvertently project to its lay readers an image of a world of savages waning in the face of 'superior civilization'. It is directed as much inwardly, toward disciplinary concerns, as outwardly, toward human concerns.

Critical anthropology accepts cultural, ETHNIC and individual variation as basic to human nature. It regards centralized control over either cultural variety or cultural homogenization as a potential infringement on human freedom which requires constant monitoring. It accepts that there is a place for cultural adaptation, albeit without accommodative or assimilationist tendencies, and for cultural PLURALISM, but without

centralized imposition of segmental order (for example, racist APARTHEID in South Africa). It also assumes that cultural transformations may occur at any level of any system at any time, and that the need for clarity about what constitutes CHANGE and what constitutes continuity is inevitably problematic. It regards inconsistency, irony, paradox, contradiction and antinomy as part of the human condition, not as evidence of the dissolution or disorganization of a society or culture.

Critical anthropology seeks to raise novel questions about society and culture and to answer them in a way that will promote understanding of the world's diverse peoples, to contribute to a revitalized and transformed humanistic and scientific field of cultural anthropology, to attack injustices and stereotypes extant in nation states, industry, and other dominating political-economic formations, and to maintain total integrity in preserving the dignity of the host cultures that are the subjects of its research.

This sort of anthropology, because of its stress on holistic ethnography, may be antagonistic toward both general social criticism and standard ethnography. It is not prominent in the United States; its development has come more from Latin America, with a number of European contributions. It should not be confused with romantic travelogues that plead for greater understanding, nor quests for indigenous support for political ends. Whatever its alliances, critical anthropology maintains a healthy respect for sectors of ethnological and social anthropological theory and method, and sees them as a means of penetrating critically the relationships of dominance and the versatility and integrity of a given people and the relationships of dominance which impose a structure upon them.

critical theory. This broad school of thought is associated principally today with the German philosopher J. Habermas. Critical theory developed in the 1930s and 1940s in the Frankfurt Institute for Social Research from the work of a number of scholars who drew elements from both Marxist and Freudian theory. Among the leading exponents of critical theory were M. Horkheimer, T.W. Adorno, H. Marcuse and E. Fromm. There is a considerable diversity of perspectives within what has been labelled critical theory, but it may be broadly characterized by its emphasis on the early Hegelian Marx and the primacy of the interpretation of consciousness. Critical theory is distinguished by its opposition both to positivist philosophies of science and society on the one hand and to economic determinism within Marxism on the other. Its exponents have developed the tools for the analysis of false consciousness, ALIENATION and IDEOLOGY, emphasizing the primacy of the interpretation of SUPERSTRUCTURES for the understanding of society. In this respect they stand in opposition to crude material or economic determinism. On the other hand, they also oppose the positivist ideal of a 'value-free' social science, and view the function of the social sciences as that of undertaking a critical and committed analysis of society and ideology.

cross-cousin. A cousin related to Ego by a cross-sex link: that is, the child of Ego's mother's brother (actual or CLASSIFICATORY) or of Ego's actual or classificatory father's sister. (*See* KINSHIP TERMINOLOGY; ALLIANCE THEORY.)

cross-cousin marriage. The practice of cross-cousin marriage occurs in most ethnographic areas of the world, with the exception of Europe. In ALLIANCE THEORY this type of marriage PRESCRIPTION is interpreted as a relationship between alliance categories rather than between kinsmen. The prescribed marriage category, according to alliance theory, is thus not 'child of parent's opposite sex sibling', but 'child of parent's affine'. In other words, what creates the marriageable relationship or CONNUBIUM is not the kinship relationship (cross-cousin) which exists between potential spouses, but rather the alliance relationship which they inherit or perpetuate from the previous generation. (*See* ELEMENTARY STRUCTURES.)

cross-cultural comparison. This method was widely used by cultural evolutionists in order to develop and demonstrate their theories, using data from classical and historical as well as proto-ethnographic sources. TYLOR, in a pioneering attempt to create a methodology for the explanation of sociocultural

phenomena, collected information from 350 societies around the world. He applied statistical methods in order to determine whether relations among social institutions (in this case, kinship and marriage patterns) recurred consistently in such a way as to indicate the orderly and lawful progress of cultural evolution. He concluded that there had been a 'maternal' stage of culture, which had evolved through a transitional mixed stage to the 'paternal' type. In this kind of study, the units of analysis, or variables, in statistical terminology are culture traits. As well as Tylor's original application to the study of cultural evolution, the method may be used to test a variety of hypotheses which seek to explain regularities in culture. Problems with the method of worldwide cross-cultural comparison include that of defining or isolating variables (traits), and that of adequately interpreting statistical results. The problem raised by Galton in a critique of Tylor's model is one which has continued to haunt this type of study: that is, the difficulty in defining what is to be considered an independent or a representative sampling unit for the collection or comparison of traits. The failure to adequately define units of comparison, which is linked to the whole problem of delimiting 'cultures' or CULTURE AREAS, must cast doubt on the validity of subsequent statistical analysis. The tremendous scholarly contributions of MURDOCK (1967) and WHITE to cross-cultural comparison are similarly plagued by this problem of judging what may be taken as the unit of analysis, a judgement which cannot be other than impressionistic. The assessment of correlations which could be expected to occur by chance, an essential element in the statistical method, also raises a series of problems about the relationship between sampling units and the similarities which could be expected to occur due to common heritage, INVENTION or DIFFUSION. More sophisticated analysis using computers allows larger data sets to be employed in order to explore patterns of regional correlation and of functional interrelations of traits, as well as questions of invention and diffusion. However the method of comparison which considers constellations of traits without regard to their historical context has limited explanatory value: it gives timeless correlations among variables which tell us nothing about their historical development. World-wide cross-cultural analysis has often been used in order to test hypotheses concerning cultural universals or the regular recurrence of functionally related features. But it should be remembered that causal inferences derived from statistical correlations may be questionable, and that while such data may provide evidence about a causal hypothesis it cannot be taken as proof. This is because certain assumptions are fed into the model before the analysis begins: assumptions which relate to anthropological theories (Freudian, functionalist, evolutionist etc.), and which therefore predetermine the variables which will be taken into account.

A related method, known as continuous area cross-cultural analysis, was pioneered by BOAS (1911) in his comparative study of mythology in a continuous area sample of North American Indian groups. This type of analysis samples available data within a specified region, enabling controls to be exercised for geographical, linguistic, and environmental relations. Early studies of this kind by KROEBER and his students took societies as the units of analysis, and compared inventories of traits in order to elaborate 'cultural similarity matrices'. This type of study also suffers from limitations determined by the assumptions which the investigator builds into his model, and from the problems involved in making historical inferences from synchronic data. However the greater possibility of controlling linguistic, environmental and other relationships between sampling units makes this arguably a more manageable type of study than the world-wide cross-cultural survey.

A major advance in cross-cultural analysis came when Driver (1967) joined together the two types of statistical analysis employed: one using cultural traits as the units of analysis, and the other using societies or 'tribes'. His reanalysis of the *Ethnographic Atlas* compiled by Murdock seeks to derive inductively culture area schemes or 'sets of strata' by this more statistically sophisticated method. New statistical approaches have been used in a similar way to analyse the relationship between language and culture on a cross-cultural basis, as well as to evaluate a variety of hypotheses concerning the relationships between cultural and environmental factors. Jorgensen (1974), in a review of this topic, points to the need not only to refine statistical methods but also to carry out extensive ethnographic research in order to generate hypotheses for testing by these methods. Perhaps the major limitation of this type of study is still the fact that as yet there is no statistical method for testing hypotheses about diachronic data sets: in other words, for the incorporation of the historical context into the statistical model.

cross-cutting relationships. The principle of cross-cutting relationships or allegiances is often invoked in anthropological analysis, particularly within FUNCTIONALIST interpretations of social organization, as a factor conducive to social cohesion. It is argued that cross-cutting ties (for example, COMPLEMENTARY FILIATION in lineage systems, common ties of ethnic or regional origin which cut across class boundaries in multi-ethnic societies, kinship ties which cut across political divisions, and so on) act in favour of overall social cohesion because they bind different groups and factions into one social and cultural system, thus preventing fission. However it should not be forgotten that such cross-cutting ties may also produce conflicts of interest and situations of stress and conflicting loyalties for the individual and the group, and thus produce CONFLICT as well as cohesion.

Crow. This term, like other tribal names (OMAHA, IROQUOIS etc.) has passed into general anthropological usage as the definition of a type of KINSHIP TERMINOLOGY found among this group, which is similar in its structural features to terminologies widely distributed among other peoples. The Crow type of kinship terminology is a variant of the BIFURCATE merging type: that is to say, it distinguishes paternal from maternal kinsmen but merges siblings with COLLATERALS. In addition, the Crow-type terminology SKEWS the terms for cross-cousins, assigning them to different generations. Thus while PARALLEL COUSINS are merged with siblings, cross-cousins are classed as relatives of the first ascending generation, in the case of the father's sister's children, and of the first descending generation, in the case of mother's brother's children. The Crow-type terminology thus gives the following equations:

FZS   =   F
FZD   =   FZ
MBS   =   S
MBD   =   D

This type of kinship terminology was often linked by anthropologists to systems of MATRILINEAL descent, and it was argued that since in these systems Ego inherited his mother's brother's property or position, it was logical that he should also class his mother's brother's children as his children. However later studies have shown that Crow-type kinship terminology is not always associated with matrilineal descent, and it has been argued by ALLIANCE theorists that it should be related rather to alliance patterns and specifically to MATRILATERAL CROSS-COUSIN MARRIAGE or ASYMMETRIC ALLIANCE.

cult. A type of religious organization or movement which deviates from the dominant or orthodox religious tradition of the community. The use of the term is not always clearly distinguished from that of the term SECT, though the latter is generally reserved for more organized, authoritarian and closed groups adhering to a minority religious code. The cult, on the other hand, tends to be a more spontaneous and open movement, often crystallizing around a particular religious leader, and lacking specific formal authority structures and membership requirements. Cults may be of a politico-religious nature, such as Melanesian CARGO CULTS or MILLENARIAN movements in many parts of the world, or they may be persistent traditions associated with healing practices, and with the complexes of folk belief which coexist in many areas with an orthodox world religious tradition. Such is the case of *umbanda* and other SYNCRETISTIC healing and magical cults of Brazil, for example, which combine elements of Catholic, African and Amerindian origin. These cults have special appeal to marginal or impoverished sectors of the community. I.M. Lewis (1971) has interpreted these healing cults as compensatory activities which endow members of society who are in structurally weak or marginal positions (for example, women in male-dominated Islam communities) with a certain degree of magical or spiritual power or influence.

The term cult is also applied to regional cults within the Catholic religion, which may be linked to the existence of regional SHRINES, to PILGRIMAGES, or to annual festivals in honour of local patron saints.

cultivation. *See* AGRICULTURE.

cultural anthropology. Generally regarded as the dominant tradition in US anthropology, cultural anthropology comprises both ETHNOGRAPHY or the study and recording of specific cultures, and ETHNOLOGY or the comparative and historical analysis of cultures. The term 'cultural anthropology' has both a broad and a narrow sense. In the broad sense, it includes prehistoric ARCHAEOLOGY and anthropological LINGUISTICS as well as the comparative study of human cultures and societies. In the narrow sense, the term is restricted to the study of human cultures and societies only. In British anthropology this field has usually been labelled SOCIAL ANTHROPOLOGY in accordance with the traditional British emphasis on SOCIAL STRUCTURE which contrasts with the US emphasis on the concept of CULTURE. Cultural anthropology is generally regarded as a separate discipline from PHYSICAL ANTHROPOLOGY, and in practice there is considerable separation of these two fields of enquiry, though recent developments have brought them together in certain areas, as can be seen for example in new developments in archaeology which draw from both physical and cultural anthropology.

cultural baseline. In studies of ACCULTURATION or culture contact, the cultural baseline is taken to be the description of two cultures as they were before the came into contact with each other. This baseline is important in order to assess the impact that the contact has had. It is, however, too static a concept, as it leads us to assume that there is a traditional and unchanging pre-contact culture which may be regarded as a fixed and stable system before it came into contact with another culture. In reality, the phenomena of contact between cultures and the resulting transformations are so common and constant that it would be impossible to conceive of any meaningful cultural baseline in most ethnographic areas of the world. Instead, the anthropologist must undertake a continuous historical and ethnohistorical study of the influences that different human groups have had upon each other, without assuming that at any time there were separate and bounded cultures which were self-contained and had no outside contact.

cultural determinism. This term has been applied to the CULTURAL RELATIVIST position associated especially with students and followers of BOAS in North American cultural anthropology. It implies that the concept of CULTURE is invoked by these anthropologists as an explanatory principle which can account for all differences and forms of behaviour in human groups. For example, the CULTURE AND PERSONALITY theory interprets the personality types found in different human groups as components of typical or 'model' personality configurations produced by cultural patterns. The dominance of the culture concept in North American anthropology has often led to the neglect of the analysis of social, political and economic structures and processes. For example, studies of culture contact and change have often attributed to cultural differences problems which are clearly the result of conflicting political and economic interests or contradictions between different social classes or groups. Thus to analyse the relationship between a colonial power and a local subject population in terms of the contact between two cultures is in a sense to ignore the fundamental fact that it is not cultures which interact, but groups of people who have specific power relationships and specific interests. (*See* CRITICAL ANTHROPOLOGY.)

cultural ecology. An area of anthropological enquiry, also called ecological anthropology, which focuses on the relationship between human populations and their environment, and attempts to provide a materialist explanation of human society and culture as products of ADAPTATION to given environmental conditions. Orlove, in a review of this topic (1980), indicates that the central concerns of cultural ecology are the study of the relationships which pertain between environment, population dynamics or DEMOGRAPHY and human culture and social organization. Such studies may be diachronic or synchronic, and may focus either on a single group or a comparison of different

groups and different environments. Ecological anthropologists all share a common view of human cultures as adaptive systems, a view which has been influenced by ARCHAEOLOGICAL research as well as by diverse developments.

In the modern school of cultural anthropology the contributions of P. Vayda, R. Rappaport and M. Harris have been particularly distinguished. Harris' theory of CULTURAL MATERIALISM (1979) is influenced by Marxism in its division of infrastructure, structure and superstructure as levels of analysis, but his theoretical position is not Marxism but environmental determinism, and he has devoted his attention to elaborating on materialist, or environmental, explanations of superstructural phenomena. Vayda and Rappaport have focused on systems functioning and the flow of energy, borrowing components both from CYBERNETICS and from biological ecology. All of these writers, and those influenced by them, stress that population pressure is a principal mechanism of change in the adaptation of human populations to their environment, and use the idea of CARRYING CAPACITY in order to determine the potential population density in an environment with a given level of technological development. It has been observed in criticism of these theories that not all populations do in fact retain equilibrium with their environment; some exceed their carrying capacity and change their environment, with varying historical consequences. There is, in other words, no automatic equilibrium mechanism built into human culture. Another common charge is that of ecological determinism or vulgar materialism: opponents have argued that cultures and societies have their own logic and their own principles of organization, and cannot be reduced to a series of adaptations to environmental conditions. Other criticisms mentioned by Orlove include the difficulty of defining what is to be regarded as a population unit, and the failure to establish the manner in which the ecological factors relate to or determine human motivations and decisions. It is frequently argued as a result that to demonstrate unintended ecological consequences of social institutions is not to explain them.

Orlove mentions new 'processual' approaches in cultural ecology which overcome some of these difficulties. By eliminating functionalist models and the assumption of equilibrium maintenance, these new approaches have been able to examine critically such areas as the relationship between productive systems and demography and the response of populations to environmental stress. New models of cultural ecology incorporate the notions of ADAPTIVE STRATEGY and decision-making in order to integrate the level of individual behaviour into the overall theory. They also recognize that not all goals or behaviours are shared by entire populations, and that there may be conflict and competition within population units. The concept of the population unit itself is refined too, and both the smaller units of groups and persons and the larger ones such as regions form part of the analysis. The basic problem of reconciling ecological systems theory with the study of cognitive systems and the inner logic of culture has however yet to be resolved.

cultural materialism. This approach has been developed by the North American anthropologist Marvin Harris (1979), who advocates cultural materialism as a research strategy which links ecological and sociocultural branches of anthropology. Harris bases his theory on a materialist explanation of social reality derived from MARXIST ANTHROPOLOGY, but unlike Marxism Harris' theory is not dialectical. In addition, his theory rests on the central importance of reproductive or population pressure and ecological pressure in determining sociocultural systems. Thus, he argues, the biopsychological constants of human nature (the need for food, for sexual relations, for affective stimuli etc.) create four universal components or levels of human organization. These levels are: (*a*) the infrastructure or the domain of production and reproduction; (*b*) the structure or the domain of domestic and political economy; (*c*) the behavioural superstructure of social relations; and (*d*) the mental or EMIC superstructure of goals, values, beliefs etc.
These levels are also orders of determination: that is to say, the first level determines the second, which in turn determines the third, which in turn determines the fourth. However, the way determination operates

between levels, and their internal coherence, need further explication.
In practice, Harris' theory is usually interpreted as a variant of ecological determinism, and he has devoted his energies in his work to seeking ecological explanations for such seemingly bizarre and/or irrational practices as food prohibitions, TABOOS, and CANNIBALISM, which have traditionally been interpreted in anthropology as symbolic or religious expressions.

cultural pattern. The concept of pattern has been used in several rather different ways by anthropologists. CONFIGURATIONALISTS used the term to refer to the constellations of formal features (or 'styles') which characterize particular cultures. Thus BENEDICT, in *Patterns of Culture* (1934) classifies different cultures according to their dominant orientation (Dionysian, Apollonian etc.). The term may also be used to refer to culturally standardized behaviour patterns such as rituals, ceremonies, or simply customary or typical sequences of activity. Yet another use of the term is in Parson's (1963) concept of pattern variables or sets of alternative orientations towards social action.

cultural relativism. An approach or theory in anthropology associated with students and followers of BOAS in North America, also termed CULTURAL DETERMINISM. Cultural relativism continues to be an influential force in anthropology, in spite of increasing doubt about the concept in modern anthropological theory. In the works of Boas and of many of his students, there was a reaction against 19th-century evolutionist theory or 'speculative history' in favour of a HISTORICAL PARTICULARIST approach, which stressed the need for careful and holistic study of each culture's unique features as an antidote to premature evolutionary generalizations. The growth of the anthropological fieldwork tradition, which was also nourished by the contributions of MALINOWSKI and the emerging STRUCTURAL FUNCTIONALIST school in British anthropology, led to an increasing emphasis on the systemic nature of other cultures and other societies, and the need for the anthropologist as ethnographer to penetrate the inner logic and inner reality of that world view and social system. Anthropologists on both sides of the Atlantic thus assumed the defence of indigenous and peasant peoples against the ETHNOCENTRIC and RACIST assumptions of much 19th-century anthropology, and assumed it under the banner of cultural relativism, arguing that each culture or each society possessed its own rationality and coherence in terms of which its customs and beliefs were to be interpreted.

However, the concept of cultural relativism has more recently come under increasing attack, on the grounds both of its philosophical underpinnings and its ultimate conseqences for anthropologists' commitment to the societies they study. For example, COGNITIVE ANTHROPOLOGY, which was characterized in its initial stages of development by a general commitment to the notion of cultural relativism, has moved increasingly towards the search for universal principles of classification. In the study of the relationship between language and culture, the theory of LINGUISTIC RELATIVISM put forward by Sapir and Whorf, which argued that linguistic categories determine and limit our perception of reality, was closely linked to the cultural relativist hypothesis in anthropology. However the notion of linguistic relativity has been broadly rejected as a result of modern investigations in STRUCTURAL LINGUISTICS and cognitive anthropology. One of the major problems in the concept of cultural relativism when held dogmatically is that it leaves the anthropologist without a theoretical basis for comparative generalizations regarding human societies or cultures. The cultural relativist position is that we should understand ethnographic material in terms of informants' or EMIC models. But if we accept that etic models, which transcend the boundaries of one particular culture in order to construct comparisons and generalizations will become a necessary part of the enquiry, then hypotheses or theoretical constructs must be employed which are not dependent on a particular ethnographic context. Some anthropologists hold that such 'scientific' generalizations are impossible, and that the most anthropology can hope to achieve is a task of description and translation of culture. Others, however, believe that it is possible to discover regularities or laws of structure or of historical process in social systems. Many anthropologists share the view that cultural relativism is also an ethically unacceptable position since, taken to its logical extreme, it would imply the impossibility of any form of moral judgement or ethical standpoint on behaviour, including the ethical standpoint of the anthropologist who analyses the situation of subordinate or exploited peoples.

Another important feature of cultural relativism is its tendency to presuppose that cultures or societies are closed and self-contained systems within which a separate reality is created, a reality which does not confront that of other such units. In fact it has been amply demonstrated by studies within MARXIST ANTHROPOLOGY, CRITICAL ANTHROPOLOGY, DEPENDENCY theory, and other historically oriented approaches that self-contained and bounded sociocultural systems, unchanging through time, have never existed. The ethnographic world is in fact made up of communities and cultures in constant contact and change, where models of reality are not perfect and coherent, but provisional and transitory. Once we accept that human beings and human groups are engaged in a constant process of confrontation between models, values and reality and that cultural systems themselves are subject to constant transformation, the issue of cultural relativism evaporates.

cultural revolution. A REVOLUTION in consciousness which often accompanies a socio-economic revolution. The term is most frequently employed to describe the process which took place in China in 1967–8, and which aimed to bring about the ideological and subjective transformations which are necessary for the growth of a socialist society. The notion of the cultural revolution provides an interesting challenge to Marxist theory and the basic tenet that it is the INFRASTRUCTURE which determines the SUPERSTRUCTURE and not vice versa. (*See* HEGEMONY; CRITICAL THEORY.)

cultural selection. Employing by analogy the principle of natural selection, in which species with strong adaptive traits are seen as more successful and therefore tend to survive and increase in a given environment, it is sometimes argued that there is a process of cultural selection. This process may be conceived of in two different ways. The first is a natural selection of cultures or of cultural traits, so that in the process of cultural EVOLUTION more adaptive cultures or more adaptive cultural traits survive and spread while less adaptive ones die out. The second is the process in which the cultural environment controls the selection of individual personality traits, behaviours or tendencies. Thus physical anthropologists and SOCIOBIOLOGISTS have argued that cultural environments have shaped man's genetic evolution, selecting for certain traits and eliminating others.

cultural themes. This concept, developed by OPLER (1967), is related to the CONFIGURATIONALIST approach to culture, from which it differs in that while configurationalists seek an overall dominant cultural pattern, Opler postulates that cultures can be studied as distinct sets of dominant themes. These themes, which may be mutually inconsistent or contradictory, help us to understand the manner in which a people structure their behaviour, their attitudes and values, and their belief systems. The approach thus recognizes that cultural systems are not fully consistent or coherent, and provides a model for dealing with internal contradictions.

cultural traits. Cultural elements which may be material or non-material. In the CULTURE AREA approach and in theories of DIFFUSION and CROSS-CULTURAL COMPARISON the concept of the culture trait has been of central importance. Traits are conceived of as isolatable elements not necessarily linked to one another, though many theories of diffusion and culture pattern do in fact postulate functional interrelationships between such traits.

culture. The classic definition of culture is generally taken to be that of TYLOR, considered by many to be the founder of modern cultural anthropology. Tylor, in *Primitive Culture* (1871), said: 'Culture or civilisation, taken in its wide ethnographic sense, is that complex whole which includes knowledge, belief, art, morals, law, custom, and any other capabilities and habits acquired by man as a member of society'. Since this statement, however, the concept of culture has been defined and employed in a great variety of different ways, and there is no

overall consensus as to its precise meaning. Thus KROEBER and KLUCKHOHN (1952) are able to list and survey nearly 300 different definitions of the term. They conclude that it should not be used as Tylor uses it, to describe a set of manners or traits, but should refer to a form or pattern which is abstracted from observed behaviour. They consider it, therefore, to be an analytical, not a descriptive term, but its use in this way raises a series of problems about whether we are dealing with ideal types, with normative values or with statistical means when we speak of culture as an 'abstraction' from observable series of events and behaviours.

Much of the debate regarding the concept, and especially regarding the SUPERORGANIC view of culture, is couched in philosophical terms, but as Kaplan (1965) points out in a review of this topic this metaphysical debate obscures the fact that there is a large degree of practical consensus about the kind of things anthropologists consider under the rubric of culture. This common universe of discourse is based on a view of culture as 'a class of phenomena, conceptualized for the purpose of serving their methodological and scientific needs'. Kaplan argues that the basis of this common conception is the consensus that culture is composed of patterned and interrelated traditions, which are transmitted over time and space by non-biological mechanisms based on man's uniquely developed linguistic and non-linguistic symbolizing capability.

Given this general consensus, the term 'culture' is used in a variety of ways. Sometimes we refer to 'a culture' (as we might refer to 'a society'), meaning an autonomous population unit defined by distinctive cultural characteristics or shared tradition. This sense of the term is often imprecise, since it is often extremely difficult to define the boundaries of such population units, and an arbitrary division may divert the anthropologist from investigating important relationships which cross-cut such boundaries. It may also refer to a system of values, ideas and behaviours which may be associated with one or more than one social or national group (e.g. 'black American culture', 'Western culture', and so on). The term SUB-CULTURE is used to refer to minority cultures within a larger dominant culture. We may also speak of the 'personal culture' of a single individual. In these usages the term identifies not a population unit but a system of ideas, beliefs and behaviours which the anthropologist isolates for the purposes of his study.

culture and personality. Studies of the relationship between culture and personality type were pioneered by BENEDICT, who based her typology of cultures on psychological types. Following Nietzsche, she contrasted the 'Dionysian' and 'Apollonian' temperaments which she claimed could be held to characterize whole cultures as well as individuals. She argued that integrated cultures were the result of historical selection of customs and VALUES in accordance with the dominant character type. In *Patterns of Culture* (1934) she says, 'a culture, like an individual, is a more or less consistent pattern of thought and action. Within each culture there come into being characteristic purposes...and...the heterogeneous items of behavior take more and more congruous shape...The form that these acts take we can understand only by understanding first the emotional and intellectual mainsprings of that society.' Thus Benedict, like Margaret MEAD who followed her in developing this approach, Benedict saw culture as 'personality writ large', and this school has consequently incurred a considerable current of criticism of its psychological reductionism. In studies which had considerable influence on American public opinion, Mead argued that the natural variation in basic temperamental dispositions was universally the same, but that each culture selected and shaped certain limited forms and moulds from these natural possibilities. Thus sex roles, for example, were held to be culturally and not naturally determined, and therefore potentially variable from the model which had traditionally been present in American society.

Benedict's emphasis on CULTURAL PATTERN or the stylistic profile of each culture was also influenced by Gestalt theory or CONFIGURATIONALISM, which supplied the analogy of wholeness and integration in psychological and thus in cultural systems. SAPIR, who later went on to formulate with Whorf his hypothesis of the unique language-thought configuration of each cul-

ture, was an influential associate of Benedict.

Another strand in the interpretation of the relationship between culture and personality has been supplied by Freudian and other psychoanalytical theories in PSYCHOLOGICAL ANTHROPOLOGY. In the United States the psychiatrist Kardiner developed an influential theory in culture and personality studies by arguing that the BASIC PERSONALITY acted as a mediator between the primary and secondary institutions of a society. Characteristics of the basic personality, formed by socialization and subsistence patterns, were thus projected onto the secondary institutions such as religion, politics etc. LINTON (1945) and DUBOIS both adopted this theory, and DuBois coined the term MODAL PERSONALITY to refer to the statistical behavioural manifestations of the basic personality.

The influence of psychoanalytical theory is clearly manifested in the National Character Studies undertaken by anthropologists, which were stimulated in large part by the desire to obtain a strategic advantage by understanding the motivations and attitudes of allies and enemies during World War II. Other well-known instances are Benedict's study of Japanese national character, *The Chrysanthemum and the Sword* (1967), or the works of the British anthropologist Geoffrey Gorer.

Culture and personality studies became unpopular in the 1960s and 1970s, largely due to the criticisms of psychological reductionism levelled at the work which had been carried out in the previous three decades. It was pointed out by the critics of this approach that there is is fact no general uniformity of personality type within a culture, and that since culture itself is reconstructed or abstracted from a series of individual behaviours, values and attitudes it was then meaningless to claim that culture determines personality. Moreover, the notion of individuals 'internalizing' their culture gave rise to the view of each culture as a historically unique and self-contained system, determining the nature of the personality types within its boundaries (*see* CULTURAL DETERMINISM; CULTURAL RELATIVISM).

More sophisticated recent approaches to the problem of the relationship between culture and personality recognize both the complexity of the individual personality and its development, and the need for a scientific methodology for cross-cultural measurement of personality types. Most psychological anthropologists would accept that individual personality is a result of a complex combination of our species-specific potential, our individual temperamental disposition, and our social and cultural experience. However there is some disagreement about the extent to which the basic structure of human personality is universally or biologically programmed and the extent to which it is culturally determined or learned.

Modern approaches also recognize the fact that the individual does not reproduce a model of his culture in his personality, but rather that there is considerable diversity in personality types within a culture. The influential psychological anthropologist A.F.C. Wallace (1970) suggests that we should regard culture as a mechanism by which individual variability is organized and structured according to the characteristics of the social system. Wallace has also pioneered the approach to certain culturally standardized types of mental illness as products of biochemical imbalances due to diet, and so on. (*See* PSYCHOLOGICAL ANTHROPOLOGY.)

culture area. This concept developed out of the CULTURE HISTORY approach of BOAS and his followers, and in the USA is associated principally with the works of MURDOCK, and with the Human Relations Area Files and the Ethnographic Atlas, both of which he directed (1967; 1972). A culture area is defined on the basis of the distribution of CULTURE TRAITS, and is a geographic area where the population shares many common characteristics such as related languages, common artistic traditions, similar features of social organization, and so on. The culture area concept has usually been linked to theories of the relationship between ecology and sociocultural systems, and culture areas are generally considered to coincide with variations in ecological conditions. However ecological limitations do not determine the variability and historical development of culture: instead, culture and environment co-exist in a reciprocal and DIALECTICAL relationship. Through their

culture humans interpret and transform their environment, and the environment in turn exercises a modifying influence on culture and society. There may, therefore, be cultural and social links of a historical or contemporaneous nature which transcend the limits of ecological variation.

Culture areas themselves, like individual societies or cultures, may be difficult to define and are in any case not rigidly bounded units. The definition of a culture area must be arbitrary to a certain extent, since in reality there are no fixed limits to intercultural contact, influence and communication. Culture area theorists have accordingly tended to emphasize ecological boundaries which give the concept greater concreteness. In addition, the culture area approach is based on the premise that ecological conditions and the material responses of human groups to them are primary determining factors in the organization and development of sociocultural systems.

Perhaps the principal problem for the culture area approach is that of dealing with the relationship between historical and geographical variation. Since both historical and contemporary ethnographic data are used in reconstructing culture areas, it is easy to fall into the trap of constructing a 'timeless' ethnographic area which does not take into account the historical process of development and change among the peoples concerned. LINTON's concept of COTRADITION attempts to compensate for this deficiency. In any case, the culture area concept must be complemented by a mechanism for dealing with and analysing the history of regional social systems and interethnic and intercultural contacts. (*See* CROSS-CULTURAL COMPARISON.)

culture bearer. This concept is frequently used in US anthropology, especially when considering processes of MIGRATION and the emergence of new cultural types. The individual or group is seen as the bearer of certain cultural traits or trait-complexes which they may transport to other regions as they migrate.

culture contact. *See* ACCULTURATION.

culture core. In the works of STEWARD and other anthropologists influenced by his evolutionary theory, the culture core is the area of human culture which is most directly related to adaptations to the environment. (*See* CULTURAL ECOLOGY; EVOLUTION.)

culture hero. In the study of MYTH and FOLKLORE the culture hero is a common type of character, and represents the members of a social or ethnic group. In myths and legends he is responsible for establishing certain characteristics of the group and its way of life: he may pass through ordeals, undergo competitions or battles with gods and spirits, or he may win or achieve certain objects or privileges for the group. The culture hero functions as a sort of intermediary between the supernatural and mythic past and the everyday world of human society.

culture history. This is a perspective developed in the United States by BOAS (1940) and his followers, and in Europe by the KULTURKREIS school and other anthropologists whose common concern is the inference of historical relationships from the observed spatial distribution of CULTURE TRAITS. Boas argued against the 'speculative history' of the evolutionary anthropologists and in favour of the historical method, in which the history of each people would be reconstructed by means of detailed comparison with neighbouring peoples. Followers of Boas such as LOWIE and HERSKOVITS continued the approach, attempting to reconstruct culture history according to the distribution of traits, but in the USA a united school of culture historicists did not emerge. The concept of CULTURE did become central to US anthropology, but the principle of historical analysis did not. In Germany the culture historical approach was developed by Frobenius, Graebner and other members of the *Kulturkreis* school. One modern anthropologist who has been considerably influenced by the culture historical method is LEVI-STRAUSS, who credits Boas with the first clear formulation of the problem of the relationship between cultural structure and variation. (*See* CULTURE AREA.)

culture morphology. A school which was associated with the German scholars Frobenius, Spengler and Jensen, and which

converged with developments in US CULTURE HISTORY which stressed the concepts of cultural integration through VALUES and WORLD VIEW. Jensen, for example, contrasted the world views of archaic hunters with those of cultivators. He argued that elements of these ancient world views were transmitted by migration and diffusion, succeeding one another as intellectual culture strata. This theory represented the application of German philosophical romantic idealism to the theory of society, since it focused on man's imaginative understanding of nature as the basic culture forming experience.

culture of poverty. A theory of the life of peasant peoples in urban contexts developed by LEWIS (1961; 1966), which may be compared to FOSTER's concept of the LIMITED GOOD in rural areas. Lewis claimed that POVERTY was not simply a question of economic deprivation and social disorganization, but generated a way of life with its own features of strategy and order. The 'culture of poverty' was particularly developed in situations of rapid social change, urbanization, conquest and colonization, but once in existence it acquired a considerable stability as it was passed on by families from generation to generation. The culture of poverty is composed of a mixture of economic, social and social-psychological factors. Some of the principal features that Lewis identified are the lack of participation of the poor in major social institutions, their distinctive patterns of family life, sexual relations and childrearing practices, and a series of apathetic or resigned attitudes towards their situation and future possibilities. Lewis' formulation of the concept is somewhat confused, due to his failure to distinguish features which are to be regarded as positively valued norms and organizational factors from those which are to be viewed as negative or disorganizational factors. His descriptions of family and community life among the poor continue to be valued in anthropology, but the theory of the culture of poverty has come under considerable attack, especially by those who contend that it has unacceptable political implications in its suggestion that poverty is self-perpetuating and is due to attitudes rather than to politico-economic structures.

culture shock. An individual or group psychological response to exposure to a new and unfamiliar cultural environment, whether it is a result of migration, invasion, colonization, or some other social or political upheaval. In situations of culture contact this culture shock may be a mutual one. The components of culture shock are both emotive and cognitive. The term is in fact a label for a wide variety of different possible responses to this particular kind of stress, which may include disorientation, depression, apathy, irrational or inappropriate responses, and so on.

culturology. A term coined by WHITE to refer to the scientific study of culture, but which has not passed into general usage.

custom. Cultural TRADITIONS or habitual forms of behaviour within a given social group. The concept of custom implies not only the statistical occurrence of a given behaviour but also a prescriptive dimension: customary behaviour is that which is required or expected of the members of society under any given circumstance. To behave contrary to custom may attract sanctions ranging from social disapproval to ostracism or other forms of punishment. In the ANTHROPOLOGY OF LAW it sometimes argued that custom in stateless societies performs the functions of social control attributed to law in state systems. The concept of custom has declined in importance in anthropology and is no longer emphasized, as it was by writers such as SUMNER (1906) and later by both MALINOWSKI (1926) and FORTES, as a central focus of anthropological enquiry. Instead, modern anthropology has tended to move away from the notion of a static or timeless tradition implied by the concept of custom, towards analysis of the act of creating cultural systems through the process of social interaction.

cybernetics. A form of systems theory which was originally developed to discuss engineering but has been widely applied to both the natural and social sciences. The central focus of cybernetics is the study of information processing systems and their control, and of feedback mechanisms. The concept of feedback is the most widely known contribution of cybernetics to modern scientific theory, and refers to the process in which an information output from a system is fed back into the system as information input. Feedback mechanisms are thus employed in engineering to create self-regulating systems which automatically maintain a given steady state. One of the major applications of cybernetics has been the development of computers and artificial intelligence, but cybernetic theory has also been influential in the study of COMMUNICATION in general, as well as in the study of ecology and biological systems. In anthropology, a leading exponent of the cybernetic approach was BATESON, who argued persuasively for the interdisciplinary potential of cybernetics (1972).

Cybernetics transcends traditional disciplinary boundaries in favour of the study of total systems of communication and interaction: human beings, their actions and their environment are thus all interpreted as a single system. It is important to note that when cybernetic theory is applied to anthropology it does not necessarily imply a simplistic FUNCTIONALIST presupposition that social systems are harmonious self-regulating wholes. In systems of communication and control, feedback does not always have the effect of 'negative feedback', which regulates or stabilizes the system. There is also 'positive feedback', which has the effect of throwing the system into disequilibrium. A cybernetic approach which focuses on the totality of human behaviour and environment requires no assumptions that any specific social system is a separable unit or organism striving to maintain equilibrium. Instead, it encourages us to seek interconnections or circuits of information within total systems of humans-in-environment.

D

dance. Little systematic attention has been paid by anthropologists to the study of dance, though it has important links with the study of RITUAL and the anthropology of ART. Early DIFFUSIONISTS studied dance data along with other traits in order to test their hypotheses, but it was perhaps in the work of BOAS that dance was first analysed as a cultural phenomenon in its own right. Boas argued that dance, like art, should be assessed through categories which would vary from culture to culture, and not as part of a universal language of artistic communication, which has been the usual approach of Western art and dance theorists. For Boas, each culture possessed a unique configuration of which its dance forms were a part. G.Kurath (1960), often regarded as the founder of modern dance ETHNOLOGY, has coined the term 'choreology' to refer to the anthropology of dance. She has collaborated with anthropologists in dance analysis, and has suggested to ethnographers a technique for recording forms of dancing in the field. Her method involves observation and recording of dance in its cultural context, and the analysis of cultural symbolism as reflected in choreographic patterns.

In the 1960s Alan LOMAX initiated a cross-cultural survey of 'choreometry', claiming that 'danced movement is patterned reinforcement of the habitual movement patterns of each culture', and that 'dance style varies (with)...the level of complexity and the type of subsistence activity of the culture which supports it', but there is insufficient data to test these hypotheses satisfactorily. During the same period, some analysts began to use models derived from structural linguistics and structural anthropology to analyse dance. For example, Kaeppler (1978) analysed Tonga dance in terms of 'kinemes' (units of movement) which combine into 'morphokinemes', while Williams attempted to develop a transformational grammar of dance 'language' in his study of the 'deep structure of dance'.

Kaeppler suggests that we should not limit ourselves to our own category of 'dance', which if ethnocentrically defined could obscure significant features of what she calls 'human movement systems' in other cultures. For example, there are important differences between participatory dances and performing ones, between ritual dances and other forms of stylized movement which might or might not be considered 'dance' by Western standards. She also draws attention to the fact that while dance has often been analysed as a 'reflection of culture', less attention has been paid to dance as part of different activity systems: in other words, to the dance as action rather than simply as passive vehicle of social or artistic symbolism.

death. Like BIRTH and other LIFE CRISES, every human group possesses a social organization of the experience of death: both as a personal and family crisis and as a crisis of social structure and role replacement. The immediate crisis is met by the MORTUARY RITES and practices of each society, while the long-term problem of transmission of property and position is met by the rules of INHERITANCE and SUCCESSION. Death itself may be regarded in some societies as a RITE OF PASSAGE in which the dying person becomes an ANCESTOR who will continue to have a social personality, while in other societies the dead are completely removed from the sphere of social life among the living. Often the recently dead may be seen as continuing to influence or manifest themselves in the world of the living, as there may be a period of transition in which they are not fully separated from it. Beliefs about the dead are generally a mixture of conceptual opposition to and projections of the world of the living: on the one hand, for example, the dead are set apart by certain characteristics which oppose them to the living, while on the other they also share or reflect certain features of the social and cultural organization of the living. The analysis of beliefs and conceptual schemata about death and the dead may therefore reveal features of the sociocultural system both directly, as a projection of the world of the living, and by opposition or indirectly, as a transformation of the world of the living. Death itself is also often employed as a symbol in the domains of myth and ritual. In rites of passage a symbolic death is a common feature of the transition from one status to another. In SACRIFICE and ritual killing the symbolism of death is employed more literally. We can analyse two distinct dimensions of the social and cultural organization of death: first, the manner in which the crisis of death itself is managed within the group, and secondly, the wider symbolic significance of death within conceptual, ritual and social systems.

debt. *See* CREDIT; GIFT.

debt slavery. A relationship within a system of economic PATRONAGE in which the CLIENT is indebted to his patron to the point where it is impossible for him to pay off his debt and he is obliged to work indefinitely without payment. This situation is likely to arise in contexts where the client population is socially and politically subordinate to the patron class or group, and where the value of the clients' labour or produce is fixed at prices much lower than the goods or services supplied by the patron.

decedence. In KINSHIP, a principle whereby relatives linked to Ego through living persons are distinguished from those linked through dead persons.

decision. Decisions or choices between alternative strategies or courses of action may be analysed through a study of their cognitive dimension or the processing of information and KNOWLEDGE involved in decision making, as well as from the point of view of the political factors involved. In COGNITIVE ANTHROPOLOGY, in discussions of RATIONALITY and in GAME THEORY,

decisions are considered as products of information processing or of the interaction between a purposive decision maker and the environment. In POLITICAL ANTHROPOLOGY and the study of POWER an analysis of decision making is often helpful in locating where power lies.

deep and surface structure. The concept of deep and surface structures of language was developed by the linguist N. Chomsky (1965). According to Chomsky's theory of language, which has deeply influenced the development of STRUCTURALISM in anthropology and other disciplines besides linguistics, it is not enough to study language solely on the basis of generalizations about observed behaviour. It is necessary, rather, to postulate underlying rules or models which make sense of the behaviour we observe. Chomsky distinguishes the surface structure of language, or its series of 'morphemes' as they are arranged in acceptable utterances from the deep structure. The deep structure of language is created by a set of rules ('phrase structure' or 'base rules') and contains the necessary information for a speaker to generate and understand the meanings of an utterance. A series of transformation rules operate in order to convert deep structures into surface structures or actual utterances. In anthropology, structuralist theorists led by LEVI-STRAUSS attempted to apply an analogous methodology to the study of culture, distinguishing the surface structure of observable behaviour or events from the deep or generative structure underlying them.

deme. The term deme originates from the Greek root 'people', that is, a group of human beings who are considered in some ways as one. The vagueness of the term is explained by the fact that at various times in ancient Greece it referred to a group of people united through descent from a common ancestor, and at others to a group of people living in a given ancestral territory who intermarried among themselves. It is this combination of DESCENT, locality and preferential ENDOGAMY which has made the term useful. It was reintroduced into modern anthropology by MURDOCK in his *Social Structure* (1949) where it was defined as an aspect of an evolutionary scheme of kinship which is little favoured these days. It has however been used by a number of anthropologists working in Southeast Asia and Madagascar to define groups in which the ideas of locality, descent and inmarriage are so merged that it could be misleading to privilege any one aspect.

democracy. A term with a broad range of meaning, including both the sense of participation and that of representation. We speak of democratic procedures or democratic styles of management when we wish to refer to the participation of persons affected by a decision in the taking of that decision. On the other hand, we also speak of democratic political systems as being those where representatives are elected by free voting procedures to take decisions on behalf of the persons affected, in which case those persons do not participate in the decision making process and their representatives may be more or less accountable to the voters. Some schools of Marxism distinguish between BOURGEOIS DEMOCRACY where elected governments act in the interests of a capitalist ruling class and people's democracy where the government, whether or not elected by free votes, is held to represent the interests of the working class. (*See* POLITICAL ANTHROPOLOGY.)

demography. The study of human populations, mainly in quantitative or numerical terms. Demographers are concerned with the size of populations and their breakdown by sex, age and social category as well as their density and geographical distribution. Demographic studies may be synchronic, examining population structures or characteristics at a given moment, or diachronic, as when they study processes of change in population composition and distribution over time. Demography establishes reliable estimates of total population numbers and composition, and of rates of fertility and mortality, as well as the interrelationships which exist between different variables such as age, sex, social class, ethnic origin, migrant status and vital rates. Studies of this kind must be adapted to the kind of data available within given historical and geographical contexts, which gives rise to a number of sub-specialities within the discipline. Paleodemography, for example, is the study of prehistoric populations, and borrows heavily from the methods of ARCHAEOLOGY in order to reconstruct the demographic structures of early populations and to study the processes of population growth and redistribution which accompanied, for instance, the evolution of AGRICULTURE or of urban life. Historical demography, working with historical materials such as census data, parish records and legal and administrative documents, attempts to rediscover the demographic structures and processes of past populations and critically assess and reformulate theories of the relationship between, for example, population size, family structure and INDUSTRIALIZATION. The broad area of social demography is concerned in general with the relationships between population and social process, and has links both with ecology and with sociological and anthropological theories concerning population and social structure.

It is generally true to say that in anthropology insufficient attention has been paid to substantiating hypotheses about population scientifically using the demographic methods available. This is partly due to the difficulties, especially in the field of anthropological enquiry, of obtaining reliable demographic data. Sociologists and demographers of modern industrial society possess a wide range of data and survey methods, with a considerable time depth, upon which to base their studies. But the anthropologist or anthropological demographer is not likely to have comparable sources: he may have to rely on poorly executed or incomplete surveys or censuses in Third World countries, and may in addition be dealing with numerically small populations and/or areas where there is little historical information. Since a sizeable population unit and a time depth of perhaps 150 years or so are needed in order to be able to establish a demographic trend, this may effectively limit the ability of the anthropologist to substantiate his hypotheses. In order to overcome these limitations some use has been made of computer simulations. These have been employed where reliable data is not available to simulate population data in order to test hypotheses regarding KINSHIP and MARRIAGE as well as theories of fertility, population growth and genetic change.

Anthropological demographers have concerned themselves particularly with the relationships between environment, population, social systems and social evolution, and demographic studies in anthropology have had particular importance in EVOLUTIONARY and ecological theories. The concept of population pressure has often been invoked in theories of CULTURAL ECOLOGY as part of an explanation of culture as an adaptive system within a given environment. One of the first theorists to draw attention to the relationship between population pressure and social process was MALTHUS, who argued that human populations tend to outgrow their resource base until curbed by the resulting poverty and hunger. Modern demographic theory of course recognizes that there are many more complex variables involved in the relationship between environment, fertility and society (*see* CONTRACEPTION AND ABORTION). There have for example been several studies of the physiological and cultural mechanisms limiting population size in HUNTING AND GATHERING societies. In the tradition established by STEWARD and developed by R. Carneiro and others there has been increasing refinement of theories of the relationship between population pressure and sociocultural evolution.

demystification. A term which has been employed in Marxist theory and related areas such as CRITICAL THEORY to refer to the process of critical analysis of IDEOLOGY, demystification reveals the objective social realities which are concealed by ideological elements.

dependency. Dependency theory, associated mainly with the works of A.G. Frank (1967; 1969), argues against conventional theories of economic DEVELOPMENT and contends that it is not internal factors which impede the development of Third World nations but their relations of dependence on Western powers. Dependency theorists point out that historically the development of Western CAPITALISM has not been an independent process but one which has depended upon COLONIALIST exploitation and the consequent impoverishment of Third World nations. Thus, while conventional economic development theory tends to view underdeveloped or developing nations as those

which have not yet undergone the process of industrialization and economic growth, dependency theory views them as nations which have become underdeveloped as an integral part of the process in which the Western industrial nations became 'developed'. Frank analyses world economic relations in terms of the concept of METROPOLIS-SATELLITE links, and argues that Third World development is only possible by means of a radical break with the world capitalist system. P. Baran (1957), whose theories were precursors of Frank's, argued against the traditional Marxist notion that capitalism is universally a progressive phenomenon, since in colonial and NEO-COLONIAL contexts the consequence of overseas capitalist domination has been the prevention, rather than the encouragement, of domestic economic development.

Dependency theory has links both with the WORLD SYSTEMS approach and with Marxist theory, though it is not fully identified with the Marxist perspective and has also been adapted to bourgeois nationalist ideologies.

desacralization. The process of passing from a SACRED to a less sacred or PROFANE condition. (*See* RITES OF PASSAGE.)

descent. Descent has conventionally been defined in anthropology as a principle of transmission of group membership: descent rules are the rules which in a given society assign membership in a kin group, which is thus referred to as a descent group. It is this definition of descent upon which descent or LINEAGE THEORY is based. Descent is thus conventionally distinguished in anthropology both from INHERITANCE, which is the transmission of property from one generation to another, and from SUCCESSION, which is the process of transmission of social position or OFFICE. By this definition, descent is not a universal feature of all human societies, but is only present in those which possess kin groups recruited according to lineal principles. However this original definition formulated by RIVERS in his *Social Organization* (1924) is not consistently maintained in modern anthropology, where the term is sometimes used simply to refer to a privileged principle of the FILIATION of children and does not imply the existence of CORPORATE descent groups.

There may be several principles of descent or descent rules. An initial distinction can be made between UNILINEAL and NON-UNILINEAL DESCENT. Unilineal descent systems utilize links through one sex only: through males (PATRILINEAL descent), or through females (MATRILINEAL descent). A special case is that of DOUBLE UNILINEAL DESCENT, where matrilineages and patrilineages co-exist in the same society. In non-unilineal descent systems links through both sexes are recognized: these systems are called BILATERAL, COGNATIC, undifferentiated or BILINEAL. Some authors have made a distinction between these terms, but there is no generally-agreed terminology which can be applied to non-unilineal descent systems. Many authors now reserve the term 'cognatic' for descent groups tracing their ancestry from a common or APICAL ANCESTOR or ancestress through links which take no account of sex. The term 'bilateral' can be applied to EGO-focused kinship reckoning in which an individual traces relationships outwards from himself by links which are regardless of sex. Some authors similarly employ the term 'bilineal' only with reference to the section systems found in Australia, where there is a special kind of intersection between matrilineal and patrilineal principles of descent. But others use 'bilineal' as a synonym for double unilineal descent, while still others prefer 'bilineal', rather than 'cognatic', to refer to ancestor focused descent groups tracing their descent through male and female links. Where a choice is made between either male or female ascendants but not both we may speak of 'utrolateral filiation'. Another special type is constituted by those systems where females trace their descent through female links only and males trace their descent through male links only, thus producing a sex-specific double unilineal descent system which is referred to as PARALLEL DESCENT. In part the proliferation of terminology for classifying descent systems is due to the great variety of possible variations in the type and combination of relationships which may be singled out or privileged within a given system. There are also many terms which have been applied in a range of ways by different authors to describe the component parts of a descent system, or the descent groups which are produced by the application of specific descent principles; some of the more common terms employed are LINEAGES, CLANS, PHRATRIES, SIBS, RAMAGES, and KINDREDS. Because there is no overall consensus on the use of these terms, one should be careful in anthropological writing to specify which sense of a term one is using.

Further distinctions have been made (by Goodenough, for example) between descent groups which are 'restrictive' (including only some descendants) and 'unrestrictive' (including all descendants). FIRTH distinguishes 'definitive' descent groups, which are bounded and non-overlapping, from 'optative' descent groups where membership is not fixed but the individual may opt to belong to one or other of a number of overlapping descent groups. In the case of such overlapping kin groups as those generated by cognatic descent reckoning other principles may come into play – for example, marriage or residence criteria – which determine the emergence of bounded and non-overlapping corporate groups. As the study of non-unilineal descent has amply demonstrated, it is always necessary to consider the interaction of descent principles with other features of the system of KINSHIP and ALLIANCE.

The study of unilineal descent has had great importance in anthropology, and the so-called descent or lineage theory dominated kinship studies until comparatively recently, though it has come under increasing critical scrutiny from the 1960s onwards as anthropologists have directed their attention both to the study of non-unilineal descent and to the importance of principles other than descent (especially marriage rules) in the study of kinship and of social systems.

descriptive kinship terminology. *See* CLASSIFICATORY/DESCRIPTIVE KINSHIP TERMINOLOGY.

despotism. A form of rule in which power is concentrated in the hands of a single person, party or group. Despotic systems are thus characterized by their highly centralized power, and occur under special conditions: when a centralized STATE controls a key element of the means of production, for

example (*see* ASIATIC MODE OF PRODUC-
TION; ORIENTAL DESPOTISM), or in times of
WARFARE. The term 'dictatorship' is sometimes used as a synonym of despotism, but is
usually used in a more general sense to refer
to governments which are not democrati-
cally elected.

determinism. A term applied to a number of
theories in the social sciences which attempt
to demonstrate that social and historical
phenomena obey discoverable laws which
may be related to one principal or determining factor: thus we have theories of
ecological determinism, or of economic or
material determinism. (*See* MARXIST
ANTHROPOLOGY; MATERIALISM; DIALECTI-
CAL MATERIALISM.)

detribalization. A term which was applied
especially to African nations in a process of
social CHANGE, in which it was supposed
that tribal identities were being lost in new
urban and national contexts. The critical
reappraisal of the concept of TRIBE, which
suggests that it is largely a creation of the
colonization process, casts doubt on any
simplistic notion of detribalization, and the
concept has been largely abandoned in
favour of a more careful examination of
ETHNICITY and changes in ethnic identity.

development. The notion of development,
which in its broadest sense includes both
economic development and the social and
cultural changes which accompany it, is
closely linked to certain ideologies or theories of international relations and of world
history. Economic development is conceived
of as the process of transition from one type
of economic system to another, implying
both economic growth (increased production and increased per capita income) and
sociocultural change. Implicit in the idea of
development as it has been traditionally
formulated is the notion that societies or
nations may be placed on an EVOLUTIONARY
scale, with the Western or 'developed'
nations as the most advanced and the Third
World or 'underdeveloped' (or 'developing')
nations as those who have not yet undergone
the necessary transformations towards prosperity and economic growth. Conventional
development studies have focused on the
manner in which Third World nations may

effect the transition towards, for example,
more efficient agricultural methods, INDUS-
TRIALIZATION, URBANIZATION, and so
forth. Development studies resolve themselves therefore into the analysis of the
economic, political, social and cultural
characteristics of underdeveloped nations
which are impeding their progress, and the
manner in which developed nations may
diffuse or transfer technological, cultural or
other elements in favour of developing ones.
Analyses of the influence of social and
cultural factors in processes of technological
and economic change have often assumed
that hypotheses developed to account for the
process of industrialization in Western
nations may also apply to the development
process in Third World nations.

Much importance has been placed in
anthropological studies of development on
the relationship between attitudes, values
and economic change. Following WEBER's
emphasis on the primacy of ideological
factors in stimulating economic development
(1958), or following McLelland's concept of
ACHIEVEMENT MOTIVATION (1961), some
anthropologists have attempted to locate the
ideological factors (values, attitudes or cultural patterns) which may act as obstacles to
economic development. APPLIED ANTHRO-
POLOGY and ACCULTURATION studies have
attempted to resolve the contradictions between traditional sociocultural patterns and
the needs of economic and technological
development, often suggesting strategies for
the mutual accommodation and adaptation
of old and new.

Modern anthropology has presented an
increasingly critical attitude towards the
concept of development, and there are many
different strands of opposition to both conventional development studies and applied
anthropology. It has been repeatedly
pointed out by a range of critics that the
development concept is one which puts a
convenient label on a highly complex series
of variables, the analysis of which raises
problems of a theoretical, political and
ethical nature. Implicit in the development
concept is the evolutionary notion of societies which 'progress' and 'improve' and
which are more or less advanced along the
path of development. Both DEPENDENCY
theory and WORLD SYSTEMS theory have
pointed out that it is totally illusory to

attempt to study a Third World nation as an independently evolving unit: instead, we must consider the Third World and its 'underdevelopment' as a byproduct of the expansion of a CAPITALIST world system of COLONIAL and NEO-COLONIAL dominance. Marxist theorists have also criticized the development notion for distracting attention from the analysis of international power structures within capitalism and disguising the essentially predatory relationship of developed to underdeveloped nations. Marxist theory does however differ from world systems theory in that while the latter postulates a single world capitalist MODE OF PRODUCTION, Marxist analysts assess in any given situation all of the diverse modes of production which can be seen to co-exist there. The crucial difference between the two types of analysis is the degree of autonomy accorded to each sociopolitical formation within the world economy.

Similarly, the loose agglomeration of ideas of progress or increasing RATIONALITY which are associated with development theory do not provide a sound basis for the analysis of processes of social and economic CHANGE. Urbanization or industrialization, for example, are by no means always indices of increasing well-being or progress in Third World nations, and must be carefully examined in each context for their social, political and economic consequences. It is customary nowadays for the anthropologist to examine critically who benefits from the development process, and whether technological or economic 'advances' signify any overall improvement for the whole population, or merely increased profit for a national and/or foreign elite (*see*, for example, AGRIBUSINESS). Proponents of APPROPRIATE or INTERMEDIATE TECHNOLOGY have argued that the most appropriate technology at community level is often that which can be built and maintained locally at low cost and which is directed towards resolving basic community problems and needs, rather than imported high technology which is only available to wealthy elites and which will ultimately serve to increase the gap between rich and poor.

developmental cycle of the domestic group. This concept was developed by FORTES, who recognized the need to incorporate DIA-CHRONIC DATA into the essentially static or synchronic model of the DOMESTIC GROUP which was employed within the STRUCTURAL FUNCTIONALIST school. Faced with the variation in type of domestic group structure which may pertain within a given community at any one moment in time, Fortes suggested that they might be viewed as different phases in the developmental cycle of a single general form for each society. Due to demographic factors and to the different stages in the process of FAMILY reproduction, only a certain, perhaps small, percentage of domestic groups will conform to the ideal type at any one moment. This model links the individual life cycle to the structure of the family and domestic group, and the concept of the developmental cycle has become part of the standard anthropological procedure for the analysis of domestic group structure and KINSHIP systems. However, it provides an incomplete explanation of every type of variation in domestic group forms. Some variations may be due not to stages in the reproductive cycle of the family but to historical processes of change affecting family and domestic group organization. Similarly, there may be not one but several ideal types or patterns of domestic group organization within a given community, as different social groups or strata may have differing ideals and practices with regard to family and kinship, or may be affected differently by processes of sociocultural change.

deviance. Deviance is often defined as divergence from social NORMS, and is thus a broader category than CRIME which refers only to those acts which will attract a formal sanction. Deviance is, as social scientists since DURKHEIM have pointed out, a normal phenomenon in human society, and has been linked by some to the capacity for CREATIVITY and INNOVATION which is part of our human behavioural heritage. While Durkheim and the FUNCTIONALIST school pursued the analysis of deviance and the reactions to deviance as necessary and functional elements in the definition of social boundaries and the expression of social solidarity, conflict theorists on the other hand have investigated the manner in which the labelling and handling of 'deviance' in society is also a mechanism of SOCIAL

CONTROL and repression which lends itself to strategic manipulation by the dominant class in order to further their interests and maintain their position. Anthropologists have also explored the SYMBOLIC dimensions of deviance and its relationship to systems of cognition and CLASSIFICATION. APPLIED ANTHROPOLOGISTS have used anthropological methods and insights in the study of deviance within modern industrial society.

diachronic. Diachronic studies take into account the dimension of time. Diachronic studies may be HISTORICAL, EVOLUTIONARY or processual. Studies which do not take into account the time dimension are termed SYNCHRONIC.

dialect. A variant or version of a language, specific to a given local or social group, or category of persons. Often the term is reserved for variations from the 'standard' or written language, though in principle the standard language should itself be regarded as simply another dialect specific to a literate middle class. The boundary between what may be regarded as a separate language and what should be classified as a dialect of the same language is not always clear, since the distinction is an arbitrary one, for example, in the case of dialects (or languages) which are partly but not fully mutually intelligible.

dialectic. In philosophy, a method of reasoning which proceeds by the successive resolution of contradictions. The Ancient Greeks used the term to refer to the process of question and answer which permits us to arrive at the truth. In modern philosophy and other disciplines the concept owes much to the contributions of Hegel, who applied the dialectical principle not only to thought or reasoning but also to history. According to Hegel, the process of contradiction and development in thought determines the process of history. In thought, and therefore in reality, each concept or phenomenon generates its negation or contradiction, and the synthesis, which is the resolution of this contradiction, generates in turn a new contradiction. In Hegel's idealist philosophy of history it is the development of thought which determines the development of human society. Marx adopted Hegel's dia-

lectical method but rejected the idealist theory of history in favour of MATERIALISM.

dialectical materialism. This term is generally used to refer to the version of Marxist theory developed by Engels and others, which contends that dialectical laws determine all material phenomena and processes. Dialectical explanations must therefore account for natural as well as social and historical phenomena. The application of dialectical materialism to the specific field of human history and society is termed HISTORICAL MATERIALISM.

dichotomy. A division into two classes. (*See* BINARY OPPOSITION; DUALISM.)

dictatorship. This term is sometimes used as a synonym for DESPOTIC government, but it is more generally applied to any government not elected by DEMOCRATIC process. Anthropologists have mainly studied local level politics, and have not yet analysed the features of political power structures at the level of central government. We therefore lack studies of Third World central governments, many of which are termed dictatorships, and cannot establish the extent to which their governmental principles can be regarded as extensions of local level sociopolitical organization, or whether they exist in contradiction or opposition to such local structures. Studies of national ELITES and their relationship to local level social systems are also inadequate at present.

dictatorship of the proletariat. A transitional stage, according to Marxist theory, between capitalism and communism. This stage is characterized by state control of the means of production and centralized political power.

diffusion. A term introduced to anthropology by TYLOR, to refer to the transmission across space of cultural elements or TRAITS. This transmission of elements of material and non-material culture may take place due to migrations of their bearers into new territories, or by a process of transfer in CULTURE CONTACT. In 19th- and early 20th-century anthropology there was an important debate between the diffusionist theorists and theorists of EVOLUTION or independent invention. Evolutionary theo-rists held that universal psychological features had generated similar inventions in different parts of the world, while diffusio-nists believed that important cultural ele-ments had been invented in very few parts – or even in only one part – of the world and had spread outwards from there by dif-fusion. The British anthropologists G. Elliot Smith and W. Perry, for example, were proponents of the HELIOCENTRIC theory that culture was invented only once, in Egypt, and was diffused from there to the other continents. A less extreme version of diffu-sionist theory was developed by the KULTURKREIS school in Germany and by the CULTURE HISTORICAL school in the United States. These theorists preferred careful historical-geographical analysis of the rela-tionships between cultures and CULTURE AREAS to the 'speculative history' of the evolutionists. In modern anthropology the concern for historical reconstruction and the debate between diffusionism and evolutio-nism has largely given way to different kinds of study of social structure and historical process, though ACCULTURATION studies maintain an interest in the processes where-by cultural elements may be transferred from one group to another, and the manner in which such elements are transformed and adapted to their new context.

direct exchange. *See* ASYMMETRIC/SYM-METRIC ALLIANCE.

disasters. The anthropological study of such disasters as FAMINES and other situations of extreme physical and social disruption has repeatedly shown that these 'natural' events are in fact often in large part also social and political in their nature and origin. Many 'natural disasters' are to some degree caused by the intervention of humans in the natural environment and the ecosystem, and most if not all are predictable long before they reach crisis stage. Similarly lack of planning and provision for foreseeable crises makes their effects more severe, and we may perceive considerable differences in terms of econo-mic and social status in the differential effects which disasters have, for example, on middle class urban elites and on the urban or rural poor.

discrimination. The differential treatment of persons according to their classification as members of particular categories such as RACE, sex, age, social class etc. Discrimi-nation is thus distinguished from PREJUDICE, which is made up of unfavourable or discri-minatory attitudes (not actions) towards persons of different categories. Racial, sexual and other types of discrimination may exist at the level of personal relations and individual behaviour, and they may also be institutionalized as legal or administrative policy (*see* RACISM, GENDER). The concept of discrimination is used to refer to modern industrial societies which are characterized by a generalized ideology of equality of opportunities and rights, but which exclude from them certain categories of persons, sometimes small minorities, but often large and important ones or even majorities such as women.

disharmonic. *See* HARMONIC/DISHARMONIC.

disorganization. The failure of INSTITUTIONS or organizational arrangements in society to fulfil their stated goals, or to meet the minimum necessary requirements for the maintenance and reproduction of the group and its social system. We may also speak of disorganization where there are internal and external conflicts and contradictions in the different organizational arrangements within a society. The term is of course a relative one, and some degree of disorganization is a feature of any social system.

dispute settlement. The settlement of dis-putes is an important focus not only of the ANTHROPOLOGY OF LAW but also in POLI-TICAL ANTHROPOLOGY and in the study of POWER, since disputes and their resolution provide a guide to the points of strain and contradiction in a social system as well as to the structures of power and authority which are brought to bear on them. Disputes or episodes of CONFLICT may be resolved by means of a number of different procedural forms ranging from the informal to the formal legal mode. Self-help, often violent in nature, is one kind of dispute manage-ment in which the parties handle the conflict by fighting or feuding or by other actions of offence or retribution. This often leads to escalation of the original conflict, and for this reason many societies possess other kinds of mechanism which can be used to lead conflicts towards a peaceful resolution. In some groups disputes are settled by the process of ORDEALS or DIVINATION, and it is interesting in these cases to observe who is able to manipulate or define the outcome of these procedures.

Where a third party intervenes in the resolution of disputes or conflicts, we may distinguish several different modes of procedure, including MEDIATION, ADJUDICATION and ARBITRATION. Arbitration is a more formalized mode of mediation, in which the parties to the dispute agree to submit themselves to the decision of a qualified or appointed third party. Where there is no third party, we may distinguish the modes of NEGOTIATION and self-help or coercion as described above.

Anthropological analyses of disputes often focus on the manner in which situations of conflict reveal the structural alignments and divisions within the group. Differences and contradictions which are masked in everyday interaction are generally laid bare in conflicts, where persons are subject to pressure to define their loyalties. Disputes thus reveal important features of social organization, and the mechanisms which exist for their settlement likewise indicate points of authority and cohesive power within social and political systems.

distinctive features. In linguistic analysis, distinctive features are the minimal contrastive features which permit us to distinguish speech sounds from one another. (*See* PHONOLOGY.)

distribution. This term is used in two rather different senses: generally, it refers to the physical movement of goods to people, and in its strictly economic sense it refers to a system of product sharing which allocates goods to consumers according to certain principles. In NEO-CLASSICAL economics the study of distribution is reduced to the study of individual choices and decisions, while Marxist economists on the other hand stress that distribution must be analysed in terms of the EMBEDDEDNESS of the economy in society. They thus examine the manner in which distribution patterns reveal the forms of exploitation inherent in a given MODE OF PRODUCTION. In ECONOMIC ANTHROPOLOGY distribution patterns have typically been analysed as part of each group's total sociocultural configuration, revealing social relationships as well as cultural values, attitudes towards sharing and the rights and obligations of different persons with regard to the products of labour. POLANYI in an important study of distribution distinguishes three forms: RECIPROCITY, REDISTRIBUTION and MARKET exchange.

divination. The acquisition of information through the use of magic. There are a variety of means, from the interpretation of naturally occurring phenomena to a range of manipulative practices which are performed in order to arrive at a verdict or decision. Divination is typically employed to discover the identity of a criminal, to resolve a dispute regarding some offence, or to predict the outcome of a future event. When ancestors, spirits or divinities are believed to communicate with humans through the divinatory process we may speak of oracles which are consulted in order to obtain from a supernatural source information which is not empirically deducible. Divination is an important element in magical systems, and has been analysed anthropologically both for its revelations about social structure and for the way it constructs COSMOLOGICAL and SYMBOL SYSTEMS. EVANS-PRITCHARD's classic study of Azande WITCHCRAFT and divination (1937) established a tradition of STRUCTURAL FUNCTIONALIST interpretations of RELIGION and divinatory practices. These studies focused on how oracles, divination, and the manner of interpreting their results, reflect mechanisms of fission, fusion, social control and authority within the group. From the point of view of cosmological and symbolic systems, divinatory practices provide important insights into notions of the nature and origin of truth, as well as the intervention or influence of supernatural forces in the everyday life of human society. In some cases, divinatory and magical practices may form part of elaborate cosmological systems which are also scientific in nature: astronomical systems developed in many traditional cultures were both religious and divinatory astrological systems as well as products of scientific observation.

divinity. A property of SACREDNESS which derives from a god or gods who may also be termed divinities. (*See* RELIGION.)

division of labour. A universal feature of human societies, whereby different categories of work are assigned traditionally or typically to different categories of persons. In small-scale technologically simple societies the division of labour is generally restricted to the division of tasks according to sex (*see* SEXUAL DIVISION OF LABOUR) and AGE. In HUNTING AND GATHERING societies for example there is generally little specialization apart from that according to sex and age, and there are no full-time specialists nor formal occupational categories. The emergence of specialists in agricultural societies is linked to the existence of an agricultural surplus which permits the support of specialized craftsmen and in some cases priests, armies and nobilities (*see* CHIEFDOM; STATE; CLASS).

Economists in the 19th century had discussed the process of increasing occupational specialization in modern society, pointing out that it created greater efficiency and wealth in the economy. Marx, while accepting that specialization increased overall production, pointed to its negative or ALIENATING effects and to the fact that rather than increasing general prosperity the improvements in productive capacity contributed to increasing polarization of capital and labour. A major contribution to the anthropological study of the division of labour is DURKHEIM's *The Division of Labour in Society* (1893) which makes the distinction between two types of social system: that based on MECHANICAL and that based on organic solidarity. Organic solidarity is found in complex modern societies where the unity of the whole is produced by a series of complex interdependent relations between different specialists. Mechanical solidarity is found in small-scale societies where there is comparatively little division of labour and which are thus composed of a series of similar units performing similar functions. Durkheim believed that each of these types of solidarity implied a different kind of overall moral order in society, and to each corresponded a distinct form of CONSCIENCE COLLECTIVE.

divorce. The formal dissolution of the MARRIAGE tie, varying widely in nature and extent in different ethnographic contexts. One of the factors frequently mentioned as of importance in this respect is the nature of involvement of property transactions in the marriage relationship: it has been suggested that where MARRIAGE PAYMENTS are high divorce will tend to be uncommon, whereas when they are low or non-existent it will be more easily available. Goody (1958) however has refined this argument (*see* DOMESTIC GROUP) and has pointed out that the factors to be taken into account are not only marriage payments themselves but the total economic and kin context of the marriage relationship. Apart from the consideration of economic factors, some anthropologists have explained the frequency or infrequency of divorce in terms of regularities in affective systems or ATTITUDES, which are in turn linked to principles of social organization which may either place emphasis on the marriage relationship or alternatively favour other ties (brother–sister, parent–child, ties between groups of men and groups of women, and so on). In this latter case, it is argued, the marriage relationship and the nuclear FAMILY are marginal to social organization and therefore tend to be unstable. STRUCTURALIST theorists following LEVI-STRAUSS' analysis of the ATOMS OF KINSHIP have pointed out that such regularities and oppositions in attitudinal and relational systems should not be studied as agglomerations of individual relationships but rather in terms of an overall structure of 'relations between relations'.

Finally we should mention that the procedures and attitudes surrounding divorce are also an expression of GENDER relations and of the structural dominance of males. Discrimination against women in divorce is one of the ways in which men exert control over female sexuality and reproductive activity.

domestic group. This term has been widely employed in anthropology, partly due to the numerous difficulties encountered in attempting to define the alternative terms FAMILY and household which may be used to refer to the basic units of society. Many writers have preferred the more general or neutral term 'domestic', though any attempt to define this concept, or to delimit the structural or functional features which would distinguish a domestic unit, is likely to meet with the same difficulties. Generally speaking the core functions considered to define the domestic domain are two: those relating to the acquisition, preparation and consumption of FOOD and those relating to the procreation, rearing and socialization of children. Anthropologists who have examined this concept critically have however pointed out that many 'non-domestic' institutions in fact intervene in these core functions, and that the domestic group itself has important politico-economic functions within the wider society. In practice the term is usually used as a synonym for 'household', though the household as conventionally conceived of is not found in all societies, and the domestic functions mentioned above are distributed differently among the social institutions found within any given ethnographic context. It is perhaps more productive to focus on domestic relations or functions than on domestic groups as such. Following FORTES, many anthropologists have made use of a conceptual opposition between the domestic and the political or JURAL domains, often linking this to the opposition of male and female roles. This opposition may however be an artificial one, corresponding to a given ideology of sexual roles rather than the reality of social organization, and this conceptual scheme should in general be used with caution, as it may lead us to neglect the analysis of important relations and functions which cross-cut the conventional assignment of women to the domestic and men to the public domain.

Variations in domestic group organization within a single society have been analysed as products of the DEVELOPMENTAL CYCLE, but this model does not account for the possibility of demographic and historico-social processes which may produce changes in domestic group structures over time. These latter have frequently been analysed as the products of changes in economic relations and systems. Many writers therefore consider the means by which property is transmitted and controlled as determining factors in the structure of domestic groups. One of the most challenging theories of this type is that of J. Goody (1976), who has linked a cluster of factors including MARRIAGE PAY-MENTS, descent groups, KINSHIP TERMINOLOGIES and domestic group organization to the changing forms of the transmission of property. He contrasts bridewealth and dowry as forms of marriage transaction and of redistributing property, and traces a number of the consequences for kinship relations and domestic organization of such forms. For example, he suggests a link between dowry systems, bilateral kinship, and MONOGAMY and between bridewealth, unilinearity and POLYGYNY. Goody's thesis has stimulated considerable debate, and encouraged the presentation of ethnographic examples which would contradict the theory or demand its greater refinement.

Other than property transmission, the requirements of labour are also often cited as factors determining domestic organization. Thus in cultural ecology several writers have attempted to show regularities in domestic group organization according to the requirements imposed by given techno-environmental constraints. However we must recognize that production is socially organized and that labour relations exist on a community wide basis, not merely within the household (see DOMESTIC MODE OF PRODUCTION).

Finally, the importance of marriage alliance is also a central factor in the creation and nature of domestic groups. The marriage alliance is a political relationship, which allows us to link the study of domestic groups to the analysis of political power relationships within the community as a whole.

domestic mode of production. A theory of the economics of technologically simple societies developed by M. Sahlins (1972). Sahlins sought to account for the tendency to under-production or to less than full utilization of productive potential in these societies. In doing so he borrowed from the work of the Russian economist Chayanov, who had observed the tendency in peasant households to limit production to the requirements of the household or DOMESTIC GROUP. Once these requirements are met, there is no stimulus to further production. Sahlins' model of the domestic MODE OF PRODUCTION incorporates not only the idea that domestic groups produce in order to meet their needs, but also the notion of the domestic group's independence as the unit which controls the MEANS OF PRODUCTION and the labour process. Sahlins' description of the domestic mode of production details an ideal type of productive system in which domestic groups are autonomous politico-economic units. It implies an evolutionary model in which the most primitive societies and economies are those where there are few significant relationships between households. Inter-household ties, be these of kinship, political relationship, and so on, are seen as factors which will tend to militate against domestic group autonomy and stimulate surplus production over and above the requirements of the household, eventually culminating in the overthrow of the domestic mode of production as control of the means of production passes into the hands of extra-domestic groups. Sahlins' model has been criticized by those ECONOMIC ANTHROPO-LOGISTS who contend that production even in the most simple society is already controlled at a community level, and that there are always important political, economic and social relationships linking domestic groups with one another.

dominance. Dominance in human behaviour and relationships has been interpreted in two different ways. On the one hand anthropologists influenced by ETHOLOGY and SOCIOBIOLOGY – or other biologically-oriented models – have seen dominance as the expression and regulation of aggression. On the other, more socially- and culturally-oriented analysts regard dominance as the behavioural expression of social inequality and socioculturally structured POWER relations.

dominant mode of production. In Marxist theory, where there are situations of contact between different socioeconomic formations we may observe the phenomenon of ARTI-CULATION OF MODES OF PRODUCTION. In these situations the dominant MODE OF PRODUCTION is that which integrates the economic system as a whole, while the modes of production which are incorporated or articulated with this at a local level are regarded as subordinate or secondary.

ge. *See* DOWRY.

double unilineal descent. Also sometimes called bilineal DESCENT, describes the existence within one society of both PATRILINEAGES and MATRILINEAGES, which are employed for different purposes. An individual is thus a member of two descent groups or corporations, one through the maternal and the other through the paternal line.

dowry. A form of MARRIAGE PAYMENT made by the parents or kin group of the woman to the couple on marriage. It functions as a kind of anticipated inheritance: the woman receives on marriage the portion or share of her parents' wealth or property which corresponds to her.

drama. The study of drama in anthropology has links to the analysis of RITUAL and also to the anthropology of ART. Drama is itself a broad category, referring to many different ways of acting out roles or situations in a ceremonial or theatrical context. Many non-Western cultures have complex theatrical traditions, sometimes involving full-time specialists or professional actors; India and Japan are two notable examples. Such dramatic traditions may employ DANCE and musical elements as well as drawing on religious and cultural traditions within the wider society. Other dramatic performances may be staged by part-time specialists. There is also the type of drama which is not set apart as entertainment but contained within a ritual or ceremonial context. The acting out of roles and situations in ceremony and ritual may be analysed both for its dramatic properties and the manner in which it expresses and acts upon the dynamics of group and social relationships. Perhaps the principal exponent of this approach has been TURNER (1974), who employed the concept of 'social drama' in order to explore the symbolic and dynamic aspects of social relationships.

Dravidian kinship system. A mode of kinship classification which may be associated with symmetrical marriage alliances. Dravidian kinship systems are found in many parts of the world, including North and South America and the South Pacific, but the name is derived from their occurrence in South India and Sri Lanka. In the Dravidian system of kin classification, near as well as more distant relatives are defined as 'cross' and 'parallel'. This system of kin classification is commonly associated with a requirement that a male Ego marry a woman who falls into the category of CROSS-COUSIN. It is also often associated with an EQUIVALENCE in the terminology of affines with those consanguineal relatives who would be affines if cross-cousins consistently married one another. A man's wife is often classed with 'female cross-cousin', father-in-law with 'mother's brother' and mother-in-law with 'father's sister'. Because of these associations Dravidian terminologies have been interpreted as reflecting the existence of systems of symmetrical alliance. In these systems, which have also been referred to as 'two-section' systems, there is a rule or practice that two classes of people exchange wives. The two classes may be exogamous MOIETIES or they may be conceptualized as two kinds of relative such as kin and affines. Inspired by the ideas of LEVI-STRAUSS, the anthropologists L. Dumont (1953) and R. Needham (1966–7) pioneered the interpretation of Dravidian kin classification as the terminological expression of a two-section system. According to this approach, which is conventionally called ALLIANCE THEORY, the terminology embodies a theory of marriage linking two classes of people – kin and affines – through generations, and cross-cousin marriage is the means by which this alliance is maintained.

The close association of Dravidian terminologies with descent and marriage rules is questionable. Dravidian terminologies occur in association with varying kinship rules and practices, and can exist with or without exogamous moieties, lineages and descent groups, with or without a rule of cross-cousin marriage and even with asymmetrical marriage alliances. Symmetrical marriage alliance alone cannot therefore explain Dravidian kinship terminologies, for it does not necessarily occur with these terminologies.

Few, if any, Dravidian terminologies resemble the ideal type. They may occur alongside other modes of terminological classification or they may incorporate non-Dravidian characteristics. Early analyses of Dravidian terminologies have presented a relatively simple system, but as H.W. Scheffler (1973) has pointed out, the meaning of terms within such a system has not been adequately considered. Alliance theorists have tended to interpret terms in the light of a male Ego and have neglected the possibility that for a female Ego a term may have different meaning. In view of these problems it is unlikely that any one social institution or mode of behaviour can explain the occurrence of these systems of kinship classification.

dreams. Dreams and their interpretation play an important part in many cultures, and are often linked to supernatural or religious phenomena. In every culture there is some standardized way of interpreting dreams, though the importance accorded to them varies greatly from one culture to another. In some cultures they are regarded as sources of important information about the future, the supernatural or spirit world, or kinds of truth not available to ordinary consciousness. They thus may have a DIVINATORY or revelatory function, or may be regarded as a means of communicating with supernatural or spirit beings. In SHAMANISTIC religions dreams are often accorded especial importance as sources of information and spiritual influence. In modern Western culture the interpretation of dreams is generally in terms of psychological or psychoanalytic schemes, in which the dream is believed to reveal aspects of our subjective or inner world and its dynamics. Indigenous theories of dreams in non-Western cultures sometimes arrive at similar conclusions, but by means of relating dreams to a spiritual or supernatural world believed to exist outside the individual.

drinking. Most human groups possess an indigenous alcoholic beverage and employ it in certain social and ritual contexts. The use of alcohol in any particular group should be considered as part of its total range of consumption of DRUGS which may produce ALTERED STATES OF CONSCIOUSNESS and which are permitted or prescribed under certain culturally defined circumstances. There is often an elaborate symbolism involved in the choice of different intoxicatory or hallucinatory substances for different social and ceremonial occasions. For example, in many Amazonian native groups traditional *manioc* beer is the appropriate beverage for a communal work party and is associated with sociability, family and communal life; while *aguardiente* or the liquor obtained from the non-native patron is reserved for a less social, or even anti-social, drinking pattern, which is generally conducted among groups of men and is sometimes associated with such aggressive behaviour as fighting or arguing. Hallucinogenic drugs, on the other hand, are reserved for shamanistic and religious occasions and are a means of communicating with a non-ordinary reality governed by shamanistic spirits. The use of alcohol itself varies considerably from culture to culture. In some cultures its use may be religious, and drinking may accompany and mark sacred and ritual occasions. In others its use may be social or recreational, and in still others the social use of drinking may spill over into its anti-social use, especially when it is believed that it is permissible or understandable for a drunken person to have less control over certain impulses or reactions. Such elements as stereotypes of drunken behaviour, the degree of control a drunken person is expected to display, and the amount consumed in order to achieve the drunken state are likewise subject to cross-cultural variation.

drugs. Chemicals which are used to produce changes in the physical and/or mental state of the individual. These changes may be desired for medical (therapeutic) purposes (*see* MEDICAL ANTHROPOLOGY), or may be a part of the social and/or recreational use of drugs. A further category of drug consumption is that of drug abuse, where it is supposed that drugs are being employed in a manner which is harmful to the individual (also known as 'drug addiction' or 'drug dependence') or which leads to anti-social or criminal behaviour. Criticism of this type is however problematic, since in many modern societies certain drugs are picked out for social disapproval and criminal prosecution while others equally harmful like alcohol, are socially acceptable. All human groups possess a range of drugs which are employed both medicinally and to obtain desired mental states or sensations (*see* ALTERED STATES OF CONSCIOUSNESS). One of the most widespread drugs in the modern world is tobacco, which is used by many groups as a stimulant, and which taken by mouth in large doses, also has hallucinogenic effects.

Alcohol is also a virtually universal drug (*see* DRINKING). Apart from these two most common stimulants, a wide range of substances are in use to manipulate the psychophysical state of the individual, and which may be a part of RITUAL and ceremonial settings in some groups, while in others their use is an everyday routine. In the high altitudes of the Andes mountains in South America, indigenous peoples have since pre-Hispanic times made use of the coca leaf to avoid cold and fatigue in the extreme conditions under which they work. In recent decades the international demand for refined cocaine has created a whole new system of coca production, refinement and transportation, which operates illegally but constitutes a major political and economic force in the Andean nations. This juxtaposition of traditional and modern systems using stimulants with the same base substance brings home forcefully the need for careful examination of drugs in their social and cultural context.

In Western industrial society drug users' subcultures have been studied anthropologically, and attention has been given to the manner in which users define, interpret and attempt to manipulate the effects of drugs or of combinations of drugs, as well as classifying of different types of drug user according to participation in, and attitudes to, the 'drug scene' and in the wider society. A particularly notable phenomenon in the changing patterns of drug use associated with modern industrial society compared to its traditional counterpart is the consistent tendency for the DESACRALIZATION of drugs, as those substances whose original use and purpose was religious or ritual are adopted for recreational purposes. Anthropological popularization has played a part in this process in recent years.

dualism. Dualism as a general principle may take several different forms: that of an overall conceptual division into two great classes (such as the Chinese Yin and Yang), that of BINARY OPPOSITIONS or CODES, or in social systems that of MOIETIES or so-called DUAL ORGANIZATION. Despite dualism's universality as a feature of human CLASSIFICATORY systems, it is arguable that it cannot be directly translated into a principle of social organization.

dual organization. A type of social organization which has been observed mainly in Indonesia and in the Amazonian region, where the community is divided into two all-encompassing units termed MOIETIES. In the conventional model of dual organization these moieties are exogamous wife-exchanging units (see ASYMMETRIC/SYMMETRIC ALLIANCE) which have in addition certain clearly defined rights and obligations of a ceremonial nature with regard to one another. These rights and obligations may involve the performance by one moiety of certain rituals (such as MORTUARY rites or INITIATION rites) on behalf of the other. LEVI-STRAUSS, in an analysis of dual organizations (1963), has pointed out that they are not as simple in reality as the classic model suggests. He examines ethnographic data regarding dual organizations from different parts of the world, and shows that in fact they are a mixture of three types of model: diametric dualism, which divides the community along a diametric axis into two complementary halves; concentric dualism, which divides it into centre and periphery; and triadic structures, which underlie dualistic manifestations. He argues therefore that the basic structure of these systems is triadic, and this structure in its turn generates concentric and diametric dualisms. He sees diametric dualism as a static form which cannot represent the basic underlying structure, and suggests that this conclusion may be extended further to the theory of generalized and restricted EXCHANGE. In doing so he suggests a modification to the original theory of ELEMENTARY STRUCTURES, for if a triadic structure always underlies and generates a dualistic manifestation, so restricted exchange should be considered simply as a special case of generalized exchange.

DuBois, Cora (1903–). An anthropologist who worked within the CULTURE AND PERSONALITY school, and who published an influential study of *The People of Alor* (1960) in which she employed the concept of MODAL PERSONALITY.

duolocal. A residence rule in which each spouse continues to reside with his or her kin after the marriage.

Durkheim, Emile (1858–1917). French sociologist and social philosopher whose works have been profoundly influential in all areas of the social sciences and who is regarded as a founding father by both sociology and anthropology. Different aspects of his work have influenced different areas of social scientific thinking. In sociology, the works of T. Parsons have provided an influential interpretation of Durkheim's FUNCTIONALIST theory of society, and in anthropology too the STRUCTURAL FUNCTIONALIST tradition was heavily influenced by Durkheim, originally through the medium of RADCLIFFE-BROWN and later through a series of social anthropologists who have drawn upon Durkheim's ideas. Durkheim's work has also pioneered other areas, including the sociology and anthropology of KNOWLEDGE, the study of DEVIANCE and the sociology of education. Another strand of Durkheim's work is formed by his studies of CLASSIFICATION (see MAUSS) which have been influential, along with other areas of his work, in the development of STRUCTURALISM and SYMBOLIC ANTHROPOLOGY. It is evident that there are very many different, sometimes contradictory, strands in Durkheim's work. Stephen Lukes, in an important study of Durkheim's work as a whole (1973), isolates a number of basic concepts which are central to his thought. The idea of CONSCIENCE COLLECTIVE, which refers to the totality of cognitive, moral and religious elements which comprise the consciousness and/or conscience of the social group is an example. Later he modified this concept to incorporate the notion of COLLECTIVE REPRESENTATIONS which are specific states of the *conscience collective*. Like Durkheim's other important formulation, SOCIAL FACTS, collective representations have an independent existence: that is to say, they cannot be analysed in terms of the psychological characteristics of the individual persons or states of mind which constitute them. In this manner Durkheim attempted to establish a clear division between the field of psychology and that of sociology, and argued for the development of a distinct set of sociological theories for the explanation and analysis of social facts. Among important conceptual dichotomies elaborated by Durkheim Lukes mentions the opposition between SACRED and PROFANE and that between the NORMAL and the pathological.

Major works by Durkheim include *The Division of Labour in Society* (1902; trans. 1933) (*see* DIVISION OF LABOUR); *The Rules of Sociological Method* (1895; trans. 1938); *Suicide* (1897; trans. 1951); *Primitive Classification* (1903; trans. 1963); and *The Elementary Forms of the Religious Life* (1912; trans. 1925).

dyad. A personal relationship which links two ACTORS. The analysis of dyads and the manner in which these combine and ramify within a social system is central to the study of social NETWORKS.

dyadic contract. The anthropologist FOSTER has employed this concept in his study (1961) of the Mexican villagers of Tzintzuntzan. Dyadic contracts are exchange relationships, voluntarily entered into and cultivated by villagers both with status equals and with persons of higher status, in order to maximize security in an uncertain environment. In common with other forms of relationship involving RECIPROCITY, it is necessary in

these dyadic contracts that the interchange of goods and services never be balanced. There must always be a debt, since to balance the 'account' would be to terminate the relationship (*see* GIFT). Foster notes that since the formal possibilities of the kinship system give the individual more potential allies or associates than he can in fact employ it is through the choice of particular individuals with whom to enter into exchange relationships that an individual organizes actual allies or associates. As Foster puts it, 'by means of the dyadic contract, implemented through reciprocity, he patterns his real behaviour'.

dynasty. A family of hereditary rulers. The dynasty is part of an ARISTOCRATIC class.

dysfunction. In FUNCTIONALIST theory, a distinction is made between eufunctions, which are positive elements contributing to overall EQUILIBRIUM, and dysfunctions, which are those elements which are maladaptive or contribute to disequilibrium.

E

early anthropology. While anthropology as a specialized discipline is a fairly recent development in intellectual history, it has its roots in much earlier traditions of philosophical, historical, and other scientific enquiry. ETHNOGRAPHY as a distinct genre has similarly been developed largely since 1940, but owes a great deal to earlier ETHNOLOGICAL and geographical accounts. The tracing and examination of the historical and philosophical roots of modern anthropology is an important element in our assessment of our own ETHNOCENTRISM and of the degree to which our own cultural and intellectual heritage may be shaping our perception of other cultures. Some anthropological theories and concerns can be traced back to the classical philosopher-historians with their concern for the relationships between geographical factors (especially climate), national character, the rise and fall of nations and the ideal moral order which ought to obtain in society. Elements of FUNCTIONALIST social theory, for example, can be linked to the Graeco-Roman organic model of social harmony.

In the European Renaissance, scholars were influenced not only by the rediscovery of Graeco-Roman thought but also by the fresh evidence of peoples in the New World with different customs and cultures, as well as by a growing spirit of scientific enquiry. Renaissance scholars attempted to account for the existence and characteristics of primitive peoples in terms of Christian theological notions and biblical history. At the same time, political philosophers made use of notions of the primitive or 'savage' society as contrasted with European society. MONTAIGNE formulated the concept of the noble and natural savage, while HOBBES and LOCKE contrasted the poverty and brutality of the state of nature with the virtues and benefits of civil society.

The origin of anthropology as a general science of human society and culture is to be found in 18th- and 19th-century developments of EVOLUTIONARY theory, and the subsequent emergence of schools of thought which may properly be called anthropological.

ecodevelopment. A concept which has emerged from ecological and sociocultural studies and which is put forward as an alternative model of DEVELOPMENT strategy opposed to conventional development programmes which are often ecologically and ethnically destructive. The notion of ecodevelopment embraces that of APPROPRIATE TECHNOLOGY as well as that of environmental sensitivity and conservation, and advocates the assessment of technological strategies in terms of their long-term environmental consequences and their socio-cultural implications rather than simply in terms of short-term maximization of profits or exploitation of limited resource bases. Ecodevelopment strategies give priority to the satisfaction of the needs of the local population and the adaptation of the technology to be employed to the characteristics of the ecosystem, rather than the adaptation of the ecosystem to the technology.

ecological anthropology. *See* CULTURAL ECOLOGY.

economic anthropology. A field which currently has a number of diverse foci of interest, including the study of production, DISTRIBUTION and EXCHANGE in a comparative perspective, the ethnographic description of specific economic systems, the analysis of pre-capitalist or 'mixed' economic formations, and the analysis of national, multinational and world economic systems and their impact on small-scale or peasant communities. One of the factors which has impeded the development of economic anthropology is the wide empirical and conceptual gulf which exists between capitalist and pre-capitalist economic formations. This has led both to a lack of exchanges of knowledge between the disciplines of economics and anthropology, and to considerable theoretical debate within economic anthropology about the applicability or relevance of concepts developed to assess capitalism when employed within the context of the pre-capitalist or mixed systems that anthropologists study.

Economic anthropology consequently confined itself traditionally to the study of small-scale tribal or peasant economies, though many would now argue that it can and should contribute to an overall comparative theory of economic formations. Economics and economic history on the other hand generally take as their conceptual starting point the capitalist economic formation, paying little or no attention to 'primitive' or tribal economies and analysing peasant and feudal ones as transitions towards capitalism. Even Marx, with his theoretical concern for pre-capitalist formations, in fact gives few guidelines for their analysis. Within MARXIST ANTHROPOLOGY, therefore, there has been considerable debate as to how pre-capitalist formations are to be assessed and interpreted.

The emergence of economic anthropology as a subdiscipline coincided with the appearance of modern fieldwork techniques which obliged anthropologists to confront both anthropological and economic theories with the realities of production, distribution and exchange in the small-scale tribal or peasant economies which they studied. In this phase of economic anthropology, little attention was paid to HUNTING AND GATHERING societies, which indeed appear to defy most of the conventional notions developed with reference to other social types. Through the works of MALINOWSKI, FIRTH and RICHARDS in Britain and those of HERSKOVITS and TAX in the United States, tribal and peasant economies provided the context for the analysis of economics as part of holistic social or cultural systems. These studies were focused on systems of distribution and exchange, or RECIPROCITY, with less attention being paid to the study and classification of systems of production. In Marxist economic anthropology, on the other hand, more

attention has usually been paid to describing and classifying MODES OF PRODUCTION and less to systems of distribution and exchange.

The early studies by anthropologists within the STRUCTURAL FUNCTIONALIST perspective had already demonstrated that in order to understand RATIONALITY in economic decision making in a tribal society it was necessary to place the economic in the context of the social. Decisions which within a capitalist or a socialist system we would conventionally define as purely economic must be regarded in pre-capitalist systems as EMBEDDED within the contexts of kinship, religion, ceremonial, politics and so forth. In non-monetary economies (see MONEY) the exchange of labour and goods is often bound up with rights and obligations between kinsmen, or between leaders and followers, rulers and subjects, and so on. Similarly ceremonial occasions or transactions such as MARRIAGE PAYMENTS involve exchanges or consumption of large amounts of goods. The notion of monetary or material profit cannot be applied here, since we must consider the social and ritual obligations and needs which also carry weight in individual decisions about the deployment of resources.

In later economic anthropology, however, considerable debate was generated about how precisely the concept of economics was to be broadened out in the study of pre-capitalist societies. The economic historian POLANYI initiated this debate when he charged earlier economic anthropologists with uncritical adoption of the notions of neo-classical economics in the study of pre-capitalist formations. Polanyi argued that there were radical differences not only of degree but of kind between capitalist economies dominated by MARKET exchange and pre-capitalist ones where GIFT or ceremonial exchange predominated. He divided systems of distribution into three types: reciprocity, redistribution and market exchange, and argued that for each of these types a separate set of analytical concepts should be employed. Polanyi and his followers, who became known as the substantivist school, waged a continuing battle with the formalist economic anthropologists who continued to claim the applicability of neo-classical economic concepts, with due modification, to pre-capitalist economies. Marxist theory remains at the margin of this debate, rejecting together with the substantivists the universal applicability of so-called economic 'laws' which are in fact specific to capitalism; it insists instead, however, on the integrated analysis of capitalist and pre-capitalist economic formations according to historical materialist principles (*see* FORMALISM/SUBSTANTIVISM).

One factor which has led to the decline of the formalist-substantivist debate is the realization that neo-classical economic laws are not sufficient for the analysis and interpretation of either capitalist or post-capitalist economies. The focus thus shifts from establishing a separate set of analytical principles for the different types of economy, towards developing a conceptual scheme for the interpretation of the relationships between economy and social system in different contexts, and at different levels of technological and productive development. The supposed discreteness of a capitalist economy is shown to be largely artificial and illusory: capitalist economies, too, are in fact embedded in sociopolitical systems and are subject to a whole range of non-market influences. The difference between a modern and a traditional society would therefore be that while traditional societies give priority to domains such as kinship or religion through which they express social (and economic) relations, modern societies privilege the economic domain for the expression of relatiohships which are partly economic but primarily social.

Marxist and neo-Marxist theories of anthropological economics have generally rejected the neo-classical division of production, distribution and consumption in favour of the overall integrating concept of mode of production which in theory encompasses all of these domains, though as we have already noted Marxists have in practice paid too little attention to systems of distribution. In Marxist theory, all the elements which enter into the process of production – land, materials and tools, capital, knowledge and expertise, and so on – are grouped together under the generic term MEANS OF PRODUCTION. Access to, ownership of and control of the means of production are differentially distributed among the population as a result of the SOCIAL RELATIONS OF PRODUCTION. The means of production together with the social relations of production

constitute the mode of production, and in its turn determines the nature of the total SOCIOECONOMIC FORMATION. There have been different suggestions of means in which the concept of the mode of production may be applied to pre-capitalist society. Thus we have some authors who retain the term PRIMITIVE COMMUNISM, while others refer to the LINEAGE mode of production and still others to the DOMESTIC MODE OF PRODUCTION, each stressing different aspects of community, kin group or household control over the means of production and the labour process.

Marxist economic anthropologists have also focused on questions regarding the process of social REPRODUCTION: that is to say, the manner in which societies and productive systems are maintained and perpetuated across time. Thus as B. O'Laughlin points out (1975), we must look beyond the 'level of immediate production' in examining an economic system, in order to take into account the demands of social reproduction. In any productive system there is always some surplus over and above the needs of SUBSISTENCE, a surplus which is necessary for the purposes of reproducing social, ideological and productive resources.

According to classic Marxist theory, there is always a contradiction in any socioeconomic formation between the forces of production, which tend to develop, and the relations of production, which tend to ossify or stagnate around traditional forms. This contradiction eventually culminates in the overthrow of the old relations of production in favour of new ones more appropriate to the developing productive forces. Apart from SAHLINS' (1972) pioneering attempts to apply this notion to the evolution of small-scale societies, there has been little systematic application of this idea to the anthropological domain.

Another area of debate in economic anthropology has been the relationships between small-scale societies and capitalist penetration. (*See* CAPITALISM; COLONIALISM; DEVELOPMENT.)

economic man. A theoretical construct employed in neo-classical economics, the economic man is an idealized individual decision maker who acts in his own interest within the economic system as far as his information and his potential for operation in the market permit. The concept of economic man, which is closely linked to that of RATIONALITY, has been criticized as an inadequate model of human behaviour, since it fails to take into account both social groups and relations and the extra-economic or extra-financial constraints and considerations which enter into the determination of individual decisions and strategies. (*See* ECONOMIC ANTHROPOLOGY.)

ecosystem. See CULTURAL ECOLOGY.

education. A term with a broad range of meaning, embracing both the notion of SOCIALIZATION or ENCULTURATION in general and the specific process of formal education which may also be called 'schooling'. The growth of formal educational institutions is generally linked to increasing division of labour and role specialization in society and to the development of LITE-RACY. Formal educational institutions are usually only found in a developed stage in state societies, where the type and amount of education considered suitable for each social class or sector of society are important indicators of class relations. Formal education has both intended or conscious purposes and unintended ones: what is taught or learned in the formal curriculum may be in fact less important than the values and attitudes which are being inculcated, and which arise from the structure of educational institutions and the patterns of social interaction they create.

Formal education in state societies is generally designed predominantly with technical and occupational needs in mind, and its stated purpose is to prepare students to fill available occupational roles, as well as to encourage certain values and attitudes (patriotism, good citizenship, leadership, co-operativeness or competitiveness, and so on) the definition of which varies greatly according to cultural context and social class factors. However the unstated function of schools or educational institutions is also to exclude certain persons from access to specific occupational or social positions. Critical analysts of educational theory and practice have pointed out that educational institutions generally function to reproduce structures of class dominance and their ideological justification, excluding subordinate classes and minorities from access to occupational and intellectual preparation, or providing them with a restricted education which reinforces their marginal position in society. This critique of traditional formal education has led to the attempt to develop radical alternatives which break free from dominant class structures by allowing the oppressed sectors of society to search actively for appropriate educational practice rather than be passive objects of an educational system designed for them by the dominant class. Education is consequently linked to political liberation, to class consciousness and the overthrow of oppressive political structures. Such radical educational theory may be more or less revolutionary, depending upon whether primacy is placed on intellectual preparation and consciousness raising or on sociopolitical action.

Unlike informal education, which arises spontaneously from social interaction and from the learning situations generated by everyday economic and social activities, formal education may embody values and knowledge not possessed by the community as a whole, and may therefore be used to inculcate new attitudes or values as well as to impart new skills to the younger generation. There is accordingly often latent or manifest conflict between the formal educational system and some parts of the community it serves. In ethnographic contexts widely distributed around the world we may observe many such conflicts, from the obvious cases of imposed MISSIONARY education in tribal communities to the more subtle processes of ideological, social and cultural conflicts or discrepancies between community values and the values of formal education.

An analysis of education and educational institutions must take into account the political and ideological functions of education, and also the existence of opposing and contradictory currents in educational theory and practice, many of which are linked to political positions or programmes.

egalitarianism. *See* STRATIFICATION.

Eggan, Fred R. (1906–) This US anthropologist was considerably influenced by RADCLIFFE-BROWN's theory of STRUCTU-RAL FUNCTIONALIST anthropology. He was the author of several influential studies of

North American Indian social organization and culture (1937), and advocated the method of 'controlled comparison' (*see* CROSS-CULTURAL COMPARISON) as a means of integrating structural and historical data in the study of culture (1975).

Ego. In the study of KINSHIP, the term Ego is used to refer to the person who is taken to be the centre or focal point for the reckoning of relationships: thus KINSHIP TERMINOLOGIES are conventionally presented as systems of terms of address and reference employed by 'male Ego' and 'female Ego' respectively. In Freudian psychology, the term is used to refer to the reasoning self which acts to maintain the individual in the face of the conflicting demands of reality and internal drives or impulses.

Ego focus. In KINSHIP studies, we may distinguish Ego-focused kinship reckoning from ANCESTOR-focused kinship reckoning. Ego-focused kinship networks or groups are those which are traced outwards from a living person, rather than downwards from a common ancestor.

elementary structures. In LEVI-STRAUSS' original formulation of this concept (1949), he defined elementary structures of KINSHIP as 'those systems in which the nomenclature permits the immediate determination of the circle of kin and that of affines, that is, those systems which prescribe marriage with a certain type of relative'. COMPLEX STRUCTURES, on the other hand, were defined as 'systems which limit themselves to the defining of the circle of relatives and leave the determination of the spouse to other mechanisms, economic or psychological'. This was interpreted by many anthropologists as a dichotomous and mutually exclusive classification of kinship systems, with the CROW and OMAHA systems as a kind of middle term or intermediate type, since in these systems the universe of spouses is relatively definitely bound because there are extensive INCEST taboos within a limited social space, even though there are no marriage PRESCRIPTIONS as such. However, later Levi-Strauss (1965) modified his formulation of the contrast between elementary and complex structures, stating that 'the notions of "elementary structures" and "complex structures" are purely heuristic – they provide a tool for investigation – and they cannot be used alone to define a system...Similarly all systems have a "complex" aspect, deriving from the fact that more than one individual can usually meet the requirements of even the most prescriptive systems, thus allowing for some freedom of choice'. (*See* ALLIANCE THEORY.)

elites. A group of privileged persons or power holders. Elites exist within many different social contexts and at different levels of analysis: we may refer to a ruling group as a whole as an elite, while at another level we may discern an elite of more powerful persons within this group. In political philosophy and in sociology, there have been a number of attempts to formulate theories of political and social organization using the concept of elites as a central one. These theories are controversial in their political implications, and have often been implicitly or explicitly opposed to Marxist theory and class analysis and also to democratic political philosophy. Some of these theories see elites as desirable because of their supposed functional advantages for society as a whole, since they accord special power and privilege to a specially prepared or trained group, while others view the concentration of power in the hands of a few individuals as inevitable due to their superior personal qualities or their ability to organize themselves into a ruling group, while still others denounce this process of elite formation. In order to understand the functioning of elite groups within society it is necessary to combine NETWORK analysis with analysis of class structures and overall systems of social and political STRATIFICATION. Elites form and operate within the social and political space accorded to them by a given society, and while we may acknowledge the universal tendency for power groups to crystallize out of any given situation, this tendency must be interpreted within the context of a given class structure or type of political system. (*See* POLITICAL ANTHROPOLOGY.)

Elliott-Smith, Grafton (1831–1937). An Australian surgeon and anatomist, who was impressed by the complexity of ancient

Egyptian culture and formulated the theory that all civilization had diffused from one point of origin in Egypt. A popular exponent of this so-called HELIOCENTRIC theory was PERRY. (*See* DIFFUSION.)

embeddedness. A term from ECONOMIC ANTHROPOLOGY. It is used of economic institutions which in modern society are regarded as analytically independent or autonomous; in pre-capitalist economies such institutions are seen as 'embedded' in kinship, religious systems, or other aspects of social relations. (*See* FORMALISM/SUB-STANTIVISM.)

emic/etic. Originally coined by the linguist Kenneth Pike (1967) and derived from the words 'phonetic' and 'phonemic'. Phonetic accounts of language are based on the observer's measurement of physical sound differences, while phonemic accounts are those based on speakers' conscious or unconscious models of sound differences. The distinction between emics and etics in anthropology became popular for a time, used for the contrast between the explication and presentation of indigenous models of reality on the one hand and the description and comparison of sociocultural systems according to the observer's criteria on the other. Emic analyses are therefore those which stress the subjective meanings shared by a social group and their culturally specific model of experience, while etic analysis refers to the development and application of models derived from the analyst's theoretical and formal categories. This contrast was linked to the debate about CULTURAL RELATIVISM and opposing positions in anthropology. However, it is generally recognized that the emic/etic distinction is not one that can be too straightforwardly employed in anthropology, since what distinguishes the discipline is precisely its combination of different kinds of 'native model' (including the observer's own native models derived from his culture and society) with different kinds of attempt at theoretical synthesis or generalization. The emic/etic distinction, while it cannot be used to classify or divide anthropological aproaches into neat categories, nevertheless points to a crucial area of controversy and of great theoretical importance within the discipline.

emotion. Most anthropologists would agree that there is a universal biopsychological basis or potential repertoire of emotional reactions in human beings, but opinions differ as to the extent to which the learning and expression of emotion is cross-culturally variable. Weston LaBarre has argued (1970), for example, that there is no universal cross-culturally valid interpretative scheme or language of the emotions, and that each culture attaches specific and variable meanings to expressions or gestures conveying emotion. Other researchers have argued that facial expressions of emotion are universal in their meanings, though culturally variable in the contexts in which they are employed and in the intensity of their expression. Studies of emotions in cross-cultural perspective form part of PSYCHOLOGICAL ANTHROPOLOGY and have also been of importance in SOCIALIZATION studies and in the CULTURE AND PERSONALITY school.

empiricism. In philosophy, the accordance of priority to experience and observable reality, as opposed to logical reasoning or *a priori* categories. In the social sciences, the meaning is rather of models and theories which seek the explanation of regularities in behaviour, social organization, and so on at the level of the phenomena themselves. This approach has been criticized among others by STRUCTURALISTS who argue that regularities occur not 'on the ground' but as underlying structural principles which are to be inferred from observable reality. British SOCIAL ANTHROPOLOGY has often been characterized as 'empiricist' in its orientation.

enculturation. Introduced in US cultural anthropology as a substitute or alternative for SOCIALIZATION. In practice the two terms are not systematically distinguished from one another, and the introduction of 'enculturation' is probably due above all to the prevalence of the culture concept in US anthropology over that of social structure or social system, implied by the term 'socialization'. It is probably not fruitful to attempt to distinguish rigidly between the two concepts, since in the process of role-learning and development of the individual it is evidently true to say that he is becoming both a cultural and a social being. The concept of enculturation implies that the process of becoming incorporated into a specific culture and learning its norms and patterns is one which continues beyond childhood into adult life, and may include the incorporation of migrants or persons in situations of contact and change into new cultural configurations at any moment in their lives. Similarly the learning of one's own culture is not a process limited to childhood, but continues throughout adult life as one is incorporated into new roles and statuses in family and kinship networks, in community or political structures and in new work roles. Like socialization, enculturation is generally considered to be informal learning or learning which arises out of social interaction, and is thus distinguished in practice from formal EDUCATION or schooling. However in its broadest sense enculturation or socialization would include both formal and informal mechanisms.

endocannibalism. *See* CANNABALISM.

endogamy. The converse of EXOGAMY, that is to say, the norm or rule of MARRIAGE within a given group. As LEVI-STRAUSS has pointed out, all marriage alliance systems are both endogamous and exogamous since all define a circle of persons within which marriage is permitted as well as one within which it is prohibited (*see* INCEST). Modern studies of marriage alliance and KINDRED organization have shown however that it is important to distinguish different types of endogamy, and that in certain systems endogamy is not simply the opposite of exogamy but is a positive organizing principle. We should therefore distinguish kin group endogamy (marriage with a certain category of relative) from alliance endogamy (marriage with a person defined in terms of an alliance category) and local group endogamy. These principles may or nor coincide, and it is important to define the operation and limits of each.

energy. The concept of energy is of great importance in biological and ecological theories and has been applied to anthropological interpretation in the field of ecological anthropology and in the theories of WHITE and other anthropologists concerned with the relationship between energy, culture and EVOLUTION. White viewed culture as a mechanism by which humans capture energy, and he based his theory of cultural evolution on the criterion of increasing per capita use of energy. As cultures develop, the total amount of energy they capture from the environment increases, as does the amount of inequality in the social distribution of energy flow (*see* POWER). Ecological anthropologists such as Odum (1971) have developed methods for analysing and diagramming the flow of energy in ecosystems, taking into account humans and their culture. Critics of the energy-based theory of cultural development have pointed out that biological and ecological models of energy flow and energy use cannot be unthinkingly extended to human sociocultural systems, since between humans and natural resources there intervenes a complex area of social and cultural structures and systems which cannot be reduced to a crude materialist explanation.

Engels, Friedrich (1820–95). Engels was born in Germany but lived for many years in England, where he was a close friend and collaborator of MARX. Engels' contributions to Marxist thought and his interpretation and development of Marxism have been extremely influential, especially in the formation of Soviet orthodox Marxism, though within Marxist thought Engels has also been heavily criticized for producing an over-deterministic and crude 'scientistic' version of Marx's theories. Thus many modern Marxists would reject the form of Engels' systematization of the theories of DIALECTICAL MATERIALISM and HISTORICAL MATERIALISM as over-simplistic. Engels' *The Origins of the Family, Private Property and the State* (1884) draws on MORGAN's evolutionary scheme, combining it with Marxist theory, but this work has been perhaps less influential within anthropology itself than within socialist political thought, where it is often accepted and cited as a programmatic statement regarding the evolution of society.

Enlightenment. A period in European intellectual history from the late 17th to the 18th century, during which there was a revival and development both of humanistic and scientific ideas. Enlightenment social philosophers influenced the development of the social sciences in general and of anthropology in particular (*see* EARLY ANTHROPOLOGY). ROUSSEAU was one of the important Enlightenment thinkers to speculate regarding the nature of primitive humans, formulating the celebrated notion of the 'noble savage'. HOBBES on the other hand is well known for his opposing formulation of natural or primitive life as 'solitary, poor, nasty, brutish and short'. Another influential thinker, LOCKE, formulated the idea of the *tabula rasa* or blank slate upon which learning and experience would write the nature of human personality and behaviour. All the Enlightenment thinkers held in common however a humanistic tendency and an orientation towards the importance of education as well as towards scientific investigation of the human species as a part of the natural world. Other important figures in the French Enlightenment include MONTESQUIEU and CONDORCET. Montesquieu, in his *L'Esprit des lois* (1748), emphasized the influence of environment on the development of different systems of law. He also stated a position of cultural relativism, arguing that moral criteria were relative to the characteristics and norms of each society. He introduced the classification of social types into savagery, barbarism and civilization, a classification later adopted within EVOLUTIONARY theory.

Condorcet emphasized the role of the human intellect and its development in the determination of the course of human history and progress. In the Scottish Enlightenment, HUME argued for the primacy of empirical observation as the basis for what he called the 'moral sciences'. FERGUSON developed the notion of social progress as consisting of a series of stages, and analysed the process of rise and decline of nations as well as such factors as the impact of environment and patterns of socialization.

From this brief sampling, it is clear that the Enlightenment social philosophers laid important foundations for the study of the diversity of social forms, prefiguring many vital issues in anthropological theory regarding the origins and development as well as the nature and characteristics of social institutions.

entrepreneur. In economic analysis, the entrepreneur is an agent who takes risks and decisions and anticipates market factors in order to organize productive activities. The entrepreneurial role is typical of CAPITALISM, though in certain pre-capitalist contexts we may point to similar forms of behaviour within different institutional settings.

environment. *See* CULTURAL ECOLOGY.

environmental determinism. *See* CULTURAL ECOLOGY.

epistemology. In philosophy, the theory of knowledge. Epistemology is contrasted with ontology which is the study of the nature of things. (*See* ETHNOPHILOSOPHY.)

equality. *See* STRATIFICATION.

equilibrium. Equilibrium, or 'balance', is a concept widely employed in SYSTEMS THEORY, ecological anthropology (*see* CULTURAL ECOLOGY), CYBERNETICS and also in FUNCTIONALIST social theory to refer to a property of systems, which are assumed to seek to establish a stable or steady state. This steady state implies a functional equilibrium between the internal dynamics of the system and a given environment. As critics of functionalist theory have pointed out, the concept of equilibrium or disequilibrium cannot be employed as an explanatory principle in sociological analysis, since to point to the adaptive or non-adaptive consequences of a behaviour or institution does not constitute an explanation of its existence or maintenance within a given historical context where actors may or may not be aware of such functional implications.

equivalence. *See* EXCHANGE; GIFT; MONEY.

Eskimo. In KINSHIP studies, the Eskimo or Eskimo type system of KINSHIP TERMINOLOGY is that in which all cousins are equated but distinguished from siblings.

estate. In the study of social STRATIFICATION, a distinction is often made between three major types of social stratum: CASTE; CLASS and estate. The estate type corresponds to FEUDAL and post-feudal societies. Like social class, estate is based on economic criteria, since it relates to land and property rights. Unlike social class, however, estate is a status intrinsic to one's structural position and defined by law. Thus the statuses of vassal, serf, or lord are fixed and ascribed by birth into a given socioeconomic category.

ethics. The question of ethics in anthropological research is one which has generated considerable debate, and there are three main areas of concern. The first is concerned with controversial uses of APPLIED ANTHROPOLOGY for political, military or other strategic purposes (in Vietnam or in Chile, for example). The second relates to the position the anthropologist should adopt on tribal peoples threatened with extinction (*see* ETHNOCIDE). The third area is perhaps the most general and could be held to include the first two, concerning as it does the political commitment or neutrality of the professional anthropologist and the relationship of his research to the needs and demands of specific communities or interest groups (*see* CRITICAL ANTHROPOLOGY; MARXIST ANTHROPOLOGY). Perhaps the most common, or at least the traditional, position among the majority of anthropologists is to separate the area of academic research from the area of personal commitment and to consider that questions of ethics are to be decided by the anthropologist according to personal criteria and apart from academic considerations. However within critical anthropology and Marxist anthropology this position has been criticized since, it is argued, there is no such thing as a politically or ideologically neutral study in the social sciences. According to this position, an anthropologist who makes a study of 'traditional social structure' among a tribal people threatened with extinction is actually making a political statement by choosing not to analyse the power structures and historical processes which are leading to the destruction or modification of this particular social system. Whether he intends it or not, this anthropologist aids in the creation of a stereotype of unchanging and unchangeable tribal cultures which are to be regarded as museum pieces inevitably swept aside in the march of progress. Thus, as pointed out by the critical anthropologist Stefano Varese, the anthropologist reproduces in his work the marginalization of native peoples from

participation in national history and political life which is created by centralized structures of political dominance.

In general the training of anthropologists includes relatively little instruction, guidance or debate over ethical issues arising in the fieldwork situation itself or the broader relationship between anthropological research and political commitment. This is unfortunate, since many anthropologists carry out their research in Third World countries characterized by political instability and among poor or oppressed sectors of the community. The lack of preparation to face the ethical and political dilemmas of the FIELDWORK situation may lead anthropologists to isolate themselves from many aspects of the social system which they should be taking into account as part of the total reality they study.

ethnic group. Any group of people who set themselves apart and are set apart from other groups with whom they interact or coexist in terms of some distinctive criterion or criteria which may be linguistic, racial or cultural. The term is thus a very broad one, which has been used to include social CLASSES as well as racial or national minority groups in urban and industrial societies, and also to distinguish different cultural and social groupings among indigenous populations. The concept of the ethnic group thus combines both social and cultural criteria, and the study of ETHNICITY focuses precisely on the interrelation of cultural and social process in the identification of and interaction between such groups.

ethnicity. The key features of this concept are the identification and labelling of any grouping or any category of people, and the explicit or implicit contrasts made between the identified group and another group or category. There must always be a we/they dichotomy to apply a concept of ethnicity. The features of labelling and contrast are dynamic, subject to contextual reinterpretation, and exist variously at different levels. Boundaries established by both labelling and contrast do not prohibit individuals from moving back and forth between respective groupings or categories, nor do they prohibit peoples from identifying or being identified differently as they move back and forth.

Frequently the 'we/they' contrast is stipulated or ascribed in a given social system or nation state in terms of negative categories (for example 'non-whites'). Ethnic identities are often part of an explicit or implicit paradigm of multiple contrast groupings, with a central dynamic established ideologically to merge the contrast groups or categories. 'Melting pot' ideology in the United States is one example. Another example is *mestizaje* in many Latin American nations. Here the concepts of *indio* (Indian) and *negro* (black) contrast fundamentally with *blanco* (white) within an ideology of racial mingling that asserts, as part of the structure of elite domination, that all peoples are becoming increasingly similar, increasingly civilized, and increasingly national, due to the 'lightening' (and enlightening) emergence of the *mestizo* or mixed person. Nonetheless, when the criteria of labelling and contrast are applied to situations in nations such as Colombia, Venezuela or Peru, we find that the concepts of 'Indian' and 'black' contrast quite strongly with *mestizo*.

Ethnicity may be objective or subjective, implicit or explicit, manifest or latent, acceptable or unacceptable to a given grouping or category of people. Paradox and ambiguity often characterize ethnic designations, tying such designations to ideas about culture, society, class, RACE, or nation. For example, in Guyana the concepts of 'black' and 'Amerind' contrast, and the latter term is used because those classed as 'Indian' have come from India. But there are 'black Amerinds' in Guyana, many of whom speak Arawak, a native American language. Ethnically, for non-Arawaks, who regard themselves as 'human', identification by language places them in an 'Amerind' category while identification by physical features could place members of the same Arawak family in contrasting categories (Amerind and black).

A label accepted by a given people in circumstances of resource competition or bargaining over political power may be completely rejected by them in another context. For example, indigenous leaders in Bolivia or Ecuador may speak for 'all Indians', using the Spanish word *indio* to embrace not only those whom national developers label 'Indian' but all poor, lower-class, mixed categories of people as well. In other contexts, however, while such leaders are speaking native languages, they may use terms that signal a natioñship of confederacy involving dozens of distinct categories of native peoples, speaking multiple languages, and condemning as racist the persistence of such terms as *indio*.

The study of ethnicity in modern anthropology involves understanding the development and bases of labelling and contrast applied to groups and categories of peoples. Ethnicity study cannot be separated from the study of self-identity systems, stereotyping, class systems, systems of resource competition, and systems of political and economic domination and change. The study of ethnicity relates to cultural persistence and CHANGE, the maintenance and crossing of all established boundaries, and the construction of boundaries that both separate and bind people in a myriad of ways. Self-identification and stereotyping are viewed through the lens of ethnicity as complementary, dynamic and mutually supportive phenomena.

ethno-. The prefix ethno- is extensively used in modern anthropology to indicate either that the topic so prefixed is being considered within cross-cultural or anthropological perspective, or that it is being analysed from the point of view of folk, popular or indigenous classifications, or both. It would be impossible to list in the present work all the terms which have been created using this prefix, but the reader will find here a representative sample.

ethnobotany. A part of ETHNOSCIENCE or ETHNOTAXONOMY which studies the way in which a given human group classifies the botanical resources within its environment. Ethnobotanical studies such as those carried out by Brent Berlin in Mexico and Peru have shown the complexity and scientific nature of indigenous botanical classifications. In the Amazon Basin rainforests, native peoples possess botanical classifications more detailed than those of modern Western science, often distinguishing several different species where existing Western taxonomy recognizes only one. Ethnobotany in its widest sense also embraces the study of the uses of plants and the importance of plant classifications in cosmological and mythic systems.

ethnocentrism. This term was introduced into anthropology by SUMNER to refer to the habit or tendency to judge or interpret other cultures according to the criteria of one's own culture. It is a universal tendency, though in different ethnographic and historical contexts we may observe greater and lesser degrees of tolerance or relativistic attitudes towards other ethnic groups. One of the main concerns of anthropology is to examine and set aside conscious and unconscious ethnocentrisms in the study of human cultures, and anthropology has an important potential influence on public opinion in the sense that it can relativize assumptions and values implicit in our culture by contrasting them with the different assumptions and values of other cultures. Perhaps a more complex issue is that of whether anthropologists should also combat ethnocentrism in the peoples they study: should 'native ethnocentrism' be respected as part of the indigenous world view, or should the anthropologist combat prejudice and misinterpretation in the community by providing more information about the values and customs of other peoples?

ethnocide. The sociocultural analogue of GENOCIDE, a term first applied to the systematic attempt by the Nazis of Germany to annihilate all of the Jewish people within their sphere of control. The concept of ethnocide, implying cultural extermination, is a powerful and evocative one that is often used by anthropologists to protest the denigration of cultural and social pluralism in contemporary nation states. Ethnocide is the systematic attempt to destroy completely the culture of a people. Ethnocidal programmes carried out as a facet of 'modernization' or DEVELOPMENT in contemporary nations often have the unintended consequence of strengthening ethnic boundaries and may even lead to processes of cultural revitalization, social reproduction of and heightened consciousness of varied customs, and ETHNOGENESIS.

ethnodevelopment. This concept, which has been advanced within Latin American CRITICAL ANTHROPOLOGY, refers to the partici-

pation of ethnic groups in the formation and implementation of DEVELOPMENT projects in accordance with their own needs and aspirations. Ethnodevelopment (*etnodesarrollo*) takes the form of 'ethnic projects' which are designed by rather than for the people concerned, and which imply the revaluation of their own culture as the basis upon which future development is to be constructed. Ethnodevelopment is thus opposed to ETHNOCIDAL development projects imposed upon local communities by dominant national elites. (*See* ETHNOGENESIS.)

ethnoecology. The study of indigenous knowledge of ecological resources and their exploitation. Such knowledge may provide a more rational basis for DEVELOPMENT projects (*see* ETHNODEVELOPMENT) than imposed techniques derived from Western science which may not be appropriate to the ecological, cultural and social conditions of a given region or locality. Ethnoecological studies have shown that indigenous ecological knowledge is often complex and advanced, as for example in the case of the Amazon Basin rainforest environment where traditional systems of SWIDDEN AGRICULTURE have maintained intact the rainforest ecosystem for thousands of years, in sharp contrast to the devastating effects of non-native incursions into the same environment.

ethnogenesis. The construction of group identity and resuscitation or persistence of cultural features of a people undergoing rapid and radical change. It may also be used to refer to a new ethnic system emerging out of an amalgamation of other groups. The criteria of labelling and contrast (*see* ETHNICITY) are crucial in understanding this phenomenon. The concept itself comes from the Soviet Union where scholars and ideologues constantly confront the underpinnings of cultural persistence and social consciousness of 'being' Lithuanian, Latvian, Ukranian, Armenian, Tazik, Uzbek, Yakut, Chukchi or Tartar, in spite of, or as a consequence of, large scale application of ETHNOCIDAL policies.

The concept of ethnogenesis may also be applied to the overcoming of certain ethnic boundaries (for example, those constructed on political, dialect or ecosystem bases) and affirming the oneness of a people according to a given criterion. Examples would include the emergence of a pan-Quechua-speaking solidarity in the Andes and Upper Amazonia, Pan-Africanism in the Old and New World, of the Ghost Dance religion among the Sioux and other native Americans in the United States in the first part of the 1800s.

The term is not a common one in North America or England, but it is employed by critical anthropologists in Latin America. Recently, it has become linked with arguments about ETHNODEVELOPMENT (*etnodesarrollo*) which stress cultural transformation of a given people, on their own terms, by supporting various ethnic categories and groups in various and novel ways so as to avoid the ethnocide/ethnogenesis paradox that permeates so many of the world's developmental plans and practices.

ethnographic film. The use of film in ethnographic fieldwork and in the promotion of anthropology to the public or as an educational tool is a field which dates back to the early classic ethnographic films such as *Nanook of the North* (1922) by Robert Flaherty. The recent availability of videotape technology has given a new impetus to this field by reducing the costs dramatically, but only recently within VISUAL ANTHROPOLOGY have anthropologists begun to examine systematically the possibilities and the limitations of film as a research and educational medium. One of the most interesting developments in modern ethnographic filmmaking is the training of informants to handle filming equipment, thus permitting them to structure the material according to their own conceptual schemes.

ethnographic present. A convention which was common in ETHNOGRAPHIC WRITING until fairly recently, and which involved the suspension of historical consciousness for the purposes of reconstructing an image of a 'traditional' or 'primitive' society as a functioning whole at a given point in time. Thus the ethnographer referred to the social or cultural system of the people studied in a generalized present tense, without specifying the historical moment to which his observation applied. This convention has been largely rejected in modern anthropology in favour of a more careful historical

relativization of the data presented. (*See* FUNCTIONALISM; CRITICAL ANTHROPOLOGY; HISTORY AND ANTHROPOLOGY).

ethnographic semantics. *See* COGNITIVE ANTHROPOLOGY; FORMAL ANALYSIS.

ethnographic writing. Anthropologists have generally paid little explicit attention to ethnographies as texts, often treating ETHNOGRAPHY as synonymous with FIELDWORK or as a method rather than a product of research. Marcus and Cushman in a review of this topic (1982) describe the 'ethnographic realism' which has been the accepted genre of ethnographic writing over the past 60 years, both in British and US circles. This ethnographic realism, influenced in part by the tradition of the travel account and in part by that of the scientific monograph, embodied a tacit agreement not to overtly question or analyse the rhetorical or narrative dimensions of ethnography. Marcus and Cushman distinguish this from the 'experimental ethnography' which in recent years has begun to experiment with narrative forms and give more explicit consideration to the conventions of ethnographic writing. This experimental ethnography is stimulated in part by philosophical and literary theory and in part by a questioning of the traditional mystification of the 'art of ethnography' which has discouraged closer examination of this central anthropological activity. The work of Clifford Geertz has been especially influential in the development of an experimental ethnography which, while it continues to perform the traditional task of the interpretation of culture, also becomes a forum for discourse regarding theoretical, philosophical and epistemological issues. Ethnographers such as BATESON had also offered novel methods of textual presentation, innovations which are continued and developed in the works of anthropologists sensitive to philosophical and literary trends as well as within CRITICAL ANTHROPOLOGY.

ethnography. This term is used with two distinct senses: that of ethnographic research (*see also* FIELDWORK) and that of an ethnographic monograph (*see* ETHNOGRAPHIC WRITING). As a category of anthropological research, ethnography is characterized by the first-hand study of a small community or ethnic group. Such studies combine to a varying degree descriptive and analytical elements, but the central characteristic of conventional ethnographies is that they focus on one specific CULTURE or SOCIETY and consider theoretical or comparative generalizations from the standpoint of the ethnographic example. The origin of the modern ethnographic research tradition is generally traced to MALINOWSKI, who as part of his FUNCTIONALIST theory of society stressed the primacy of field research and PARTICIPANT OBSERVATION, and to BOAS who like Malinowski reacted against the 'speculative history' of EVOLUTIONARY theory and advocated the careful description of specific cultures.

Ethnography in both US cultural and British social anthropology from the postwar period until recently had acquired a generally anti-historical or at least ahistorical perspective, concentrating on the reconstruction of a specific cultural or social system without regard to its historical development, and relegating historical considerations to a separate area labelled as the study of social or cultural CHANGE, as if this were somehow an aberrant rather than a normal feature of human groups. A related tendency in this type of ethnography is the tendency to artificially isolate the unit of study (the TRIBE, the HUNTING AND GATHERING band, the PEASANT community), considering it as a self-contained culture or society and failing to consider regional, national and international politico-economic and social structures with which the local community interacts. These tendencies in conventional ethnography have been amply criticized from many directions and by many divergent theoretical perspectives which reject both STRUCTURAL FUNCTIONALIST and CULTURAL RELATIVIST positions, and seek to establish a new type of ethnography which is conscious both of historical process and of regional, national and international power structures as these impinge on the local community (see CRITICAL ANTHROPOLOGY; MARXIST ANTHROPOLOGY; DEPENDENCY; WORLD SYSTEMS). Within COGNITIVE ANTHROPOLOGY a different kind of critique of traditional ethnography has been developed. This so-called New Ethnography, influenced in large part by linguistic

method, has developed more sophisticated and rigorously controlled methods for the study of indigenous TAXONOMIES and systems of CLASSIFICATION. However, as critics of FORMAL ANALYSIS point out, the refinement of these techniques does not in itself constitute an adequate theoretical basis for anthropological enquiry or generalization.

Finally, it should be noted that the distinction between ethnography and anthropology is questioned within the tradition of ETHNOLOGY, where it is regarded as a spurious one since it is argued that there can be no general 'science of man' apart from the comparative and historical study of peoples.

ethnohistory. Anthropology and history are combined in ethnohistory, which joins the theoretical framework of anthropology to the methods of historiographic research for the study of cultural and social process. Where historians have concentrated by and large on the 'great tradition', anthropologists and ethnohistorians have devoted attention to the 'little tradition' and to the history of non-Western peoples. Ethnohistory has strong connections with new developments in popular and local history, which stress the study of history 'from below' rather than the history that is shaped by interpretations based on ideological impositions emanating from the dominant classes. The term 'ethnohistory' also has a rather different though overlapping sense, that of the study of a people's own representations of their history, linked to the study of ORAL TRADITION. These two senses of the term, the search for historical data on ethnic groups and the ethnic group's own representation of their history, may be separated by referring to the former as 'historical ethnology' or 'historical anthropology'. (See HISTORY AND ANTHROPOLOGY.)

ethnology. The comparative and historical study of cultures or peoples. Its basic unit of study, as defined in Soviet or European ethnology, is the ETHNOS. KROEBER defined the field of study of ethnology as embracing culture, history and geography. RADCLIFFE-BROWN distinguished ethnology, meaning the historical-geographical study of peoples, from the functional study of social systems which he termed SOCIAL ANTHROPOLOGY. In many European – and especially East

European – countries the term 'ethnology' is used rather than anthropology, since it is considered that there can be no general 'science of man' without or apart from the comparative and historical study of peoples. Ethnology thus combines historical and field study of popular, FOLK and tribal cultures with CROSS-CULTURAL COMPARISON and generalization.

ethnomathematics. The study of systems of NUMBERS and of mathematical operations within a given sociocultural context. There are two mains strands to this type of enquiry: one which explores the ritual and symbolic significance of numbers, and the other which explores the relationship between the complexity of mathematical operations and the level and type of technological development of the group.

ethnomedicine. The study of indigenous or popular healing practices and of beliefs, attitudes and strategies regarding health and disease. The term is also sometimes used as an alternative to MEDICAL ANTHROPOLOGY. Some authors prefer to use 'ethnomedicine' since it suggests the primacy of folk categories and interpretations in the study of health and disease.

ethnomethodology. An approach associated with the sociologist H. Garfinkel, who was influenced by phenomenological philosophy into directing sociological analysis to the structure of everyday reality and social interaction. Ethnomethodology sees the goals of social actors as central, and studies the manner in which speech and social organization emerge from social interaction, which is seen as a process by means of which actors define, seek and achieve their goals. The discipline thus studies the methods by which actors come to understand and produce structures of social interaction. Social norms, as expressed in utterances, are seen not so much as reflections of a fixed moral-social order, but as continuing achievements in a process of actor's formulations of desired definitions of social order. Weider's study of prison language shows that the convicts' 'code' is more a method of persuasion and justification than it is a reflection of an organized way of life. Ethnomethodology has drawn from both anthropology and sociology as well as linguistic analysis, and its most notable achievements have been in the field of conversational analysis.

ethnomusicology. The study and cross-cultural comparison of musical systems in non-Western contexts and of the relationship between music and cultural or social factors. Early studies of non-Western music include Baker's study of Seneca music (1882), which employed Western techniques of comparative musicology and supplied some cultural data in addition to the recording of native music, and Sachs' attempts to place musical data in an evolutionary sequence (1962). DIFFUSIONIST and KULTURKREIS theorists employed musical data to support their hypotheses. BOAS was influential in encouraging his students to record musical and other artistic data as a source of information about culture, and to explore the relationship between musical and cultural phenomena. Following Boas, HERSKOVITS examined the relationship between music and culture in African and New World contexts. Subsequent studies of African and Afro-American music have demonstrated the extraordinary conservatism of certain musical forms even when transposed to entirely new contexts.

Alan LOMAX, who has also studied DANCE in cross-cultural perspective, has attempted to delineate worldwide 'music areas' (*see* CULTURE AREAS) and also to develop a cross-culturally valid system of musical notation called CANTOMETRICS (1977). He relates musical expression to cultural pattern in general and also to the degree of social stratification, which he argues is correlated with the complexity of musical systems. Modern trends in ethnomusicology have been strongly influenced by linguistic models and methods, employing models from structural linguistics in order to understand musical forms or attempting to correlate musical and linguistic features within given cultural contexts.

McLeod in a review of this topic (1974) points out that music in general is a highly structured and highly redundant sound system which is always related to RITUAL and is always 'context-sensitive'. McLeod argues for the careful study of this context sensitivity and of the phenomenon of borrowing and conservatism in music. Music is responsive to cultural change and may at times express conflict, discontent or instability, but is at the same time borrowed from culture to culture and conserves its form. Uses and functions of music range from ritual to recreational, and include the expression of group solidarity or personal creativity as well as that of anxiety, protest or conflict.

ethnopharmacology. The classification and use of medicinal plants in indigenous or popular culture, involving elements of ETHNOBOTANICAL and ETHNOMEDICAL methods.

ethnophilosophy. Dupré, in his study in this field (1975), mentions three principal aspects of ethnophilosophy, which is generally defined as the study of indigenous philosophical notions and also of the philosophical implications of the anthropological endeavour (philosophical anthropology, as some prefer to call it). Firstly, there are issues in anthropology which require the clarification and consideration of their philosophical implications if they are to be resolved, as we may easily observe if we examine the philosophical confusions implicit in many theoretical debates in modern anthropology. Secondly, cultural anthropology provides important data for philosophy, since cultural data like historical data permits philosophers to clarify concepts and better comprehend reality. Thirdly, the philosophical or critical examination of the ideological roots of anthropology itself is a vital area.

ethnopsychiatry. The study of mental illness in cross-cultural perspective, including the study of the definition, classification and treatment of mentally ill persons in different cultural contexts. There is considerable debate among anthropologists about the extent to which certain mental illnesses are universal and the extent to which cultural factors intervene in the definition of mental illness and the determination of its symptoms. Anthropologists who have made special studies of this field include M.K. OPLER, who examined the manner in which mental disorders are patterned and influenced by the 'normal' behaviours within given ethnic groups; and A.F.C. Wallace, who has put forward the theory that many

culturally specific mental disorders may have a bionutritional basis. (*See* PSYCHOLOGICAL ANTHROPOLOGY; MEDICAL ANTHROPOLOGY; CULTURE AND PERSONALITY.)

ethnos. From the Greek, meaning a tribe, people or nation other than the Greeks; adopted in Soviet and European ETHNOLOGY to refer to distinctive cultural units characterized by a common tradition, the units of study of ethnology.

ethnoscience. The study generally of the systems of CLASSIFICATION and TAXONOMIES employed by different societies. (*See* COGNITIVE ANTHROPOLOGY.)

ethnosemantics. Ethnosemantics or ethnographic semantics refers to the field of study of folk or indigenous systems of meaning and CLASSIFICATION within the perspective of COGNITIVE ANTHROPOLOGY or the 'New Ethnography'. Ethnosemantics was influenced in its development by both structural linguistics and cognitive psychology, and aims to analyse and interpret the thought patterns of peoples in different cultures. A basic concern of ethnosemantics is the accurate description and recording both of systems of communication and of TAXONOMIES and systems of classification. Ethnosemantics is concerned with the representation of knowledge in taxonomic form, the semantics of folk classifications, and also with models of indigenous decision making or the study of cognitive schemata in use.

ethnotaxonomy. The study of indigenous or folk TAXONOMIES within COGNITIVE ANTHROPOLOGY or ETHNOSEMANTICS.

ethology. The essence of this field of study which was pioneered by Konrad Lorenz (1966) and Nikolaas Tinbergen (1972) is the idea that the theory of evolution may serve as a paradigm for the analysis of all life, including human life and human behaviour. Early ethological research focused on identifying instinctive and adaptive behaviours, including instinctively programmed learning patterns, in animals. Ethological studies were important in stimulating a range of popular works speculating upon the importance of instinctive and adaptive behaviours in shaping human personality and culture, as well as more serious and cautious studies in the fields of SOCIOBIOLOGY and PHYSICAL ANTHROPOLOGY.

etic. *See* EMIC/ETIC.

etiquette. A formal code of manners and behaviours appropriate to a series of different situations of social interaction. It may be analysed as a mechanism by which a dominant social class marks itself off from subordinate classes who do not have access to or opportunity to practise such a code, and historical changes in codes of etiquette are due in part to the process whereby aspiring or upwardly mobile groups imitate the etiquette of a traditional ruling class, thereby obliging the latter to invent new refinements, or alternatively to the overthrow of a traditional code of etiquette in favour of a new one associated with the newly dominant group. The cognitive and symbolic dimensions of codes of etiquette are also subject to anthropological interpretation, and they may be seen as systems for the classification, interpretation and management of different social situations and persons.

Evans-Pritchard, Sir **Edward Evan** (1902–73). This British social anthropologist is often associated with the STRUCTURAL FUNCTIONALIST school of anthropology, though in fact upon analysing his works it is clear that there are very many differences between his position and that of either RADCLIFFE-BROWN or MALINOWSKI, and in this as in many other cases the grouping together of anthropologists under a theoretical banner often leads to the failure to consider the distinctive theoretical contribution of each and the real diversity of opinions between them. However, there is no doubt that Evans-Pritchard's pioneering ethnographies did indeed have an extremely important influence on the development of what is loosely termed the structural functionalist tradition or phase in social anthropology, particularly in the areas of kinship studies (*see* LINEAGE THEORY) and the study of RELIGION. Evans-Pritchard insisted on the links between HISTORY AND ANTHROPOLOGY and identified anthropology as essentially a humanistic and descriptive study whose task was to interpret and translate other cultures. He thus remained unreceptive to attempts within functionalist or structural functionalist theory to formulate laws or general theories of society. His main works include *Witchcraft, Magic and Oracles among the Azande* (1937), *The Nuer* (1940), and *Essays in Social Anthropology* (1964).

evil eye. A widespread folk concept of a harmful influence which emanates involuntarily from certain persons. In Latin America, for example, the evil eye (*mal de ojo*) is believed to be the result principally of unexpressed sentiments of envy or jealousy and especially affects young children, causing them to become sick. Under certain circumstances to admire a baby or child (especially if the admirer is childless) may be interpreted as a potentially aggressive or harmful act, since it suggests underlying envy and the possibility of the evil eye.

evolution. The process by which a species or a population of individual organisms undergoes structural modifications over time as a result of the process of interaction with its environment. Different theories of evolution put forward different views of the relative contribution and interaction of environmental and hereditary factors in the process of evolution. It is generally assumed that the overall trend in the evolution of organisms is towards increasing adaptation to their environment, and also towards the increasing complexity and differentiation or diversification of species as each adapts to specific environmental conditions. This line of reasoning accounts for the overall trend towards the diversification of species and the development of more complex from simpler forms. Biologists and physical anthropologists distinguish between macroevolution, the long-term structural change in species, and microevolution, the continuing modification that may be observed in modern populations. Within the reduced timescale of microevolution, we may observe reversals of or variations from long term evolutionary trends, and it is important to bear in mind when we study theories of social or cultural evolution too that macroevolutionary trends do not always account for any given historical or geographical variation which we may observe.

By extension, the concept of evolution has also been applied in the analysis of the development of human society and culture (*see* EVOLUTION, SOCIOCULTURAL). The concept of evolution has bridged the natural and social sciences, and has been central both to biological and anthropological enquiry since it was first advanced in the writings of Charles Darwin and Herbert SPENCER. These two writers are widely regarded as the founders of evolutionary theory, Darwin in the natural and Spencer in the social sciences, though it has often been pointed out that their ideas were naturally enough anticipated in the works of previous investigators. Darwin's own theory of biological evolution was closely paralleled by that of Alfred Russell Wallace, who however never shared the public recognition accorded to Darwin as the founder of evolutionary theory. In the field of natural history, important elements of evolutionary theory were contributed by Lamarck. Lamarck's theory of evolution relied on the notion of environmental influences affecting the organism, which was then able to pass on these modifications to its offspring (the inheritance of acquired characteristics). Darwin however disputed this point, and argued that evolution was proceeded by a mechanism of natural selection, which caused certain random mutations to survive because they were more fitted to the environment while others died out because they were less adaptive. He therefore argued that the hereditary individual variation between members of a particular species was random, and unrelated to environmental pressure. Since individuals vary slightly from one another, and some of these random variations confer adaptive advantages given specific environmental conditions and pressures, more of the individuals possessing the adaptive characteristic will survive to breed and pass on this characteristic to their offspring, thus bringing about a gradual modification in the species as a whole. Darwin's theory also relied in great measure on the prior task of classification of plants and animals which had been carried out by the naturalist Linnaeus, and which permitted him to conceptualize the relationship between different species as one of gradual development of related forms.

It has been pointed out that while Darwin's theory was regarded when he first advanced it as being revolutionary and potentially anti-Christian, since it provided scientific evidence of the inaccuracy of the Biblical theory of creation, it in fact owes much to philosophical and religious notions of his time. The notions of progress and perfection implied in natural selection of species are for example surely not unrelated to the historical moment and to broader intellectual and philosophical trends which represented change and human history as a progression towards technological and moral perfection. The conservative reaction against Darwinism and its eventual adoption as a paradigm in the natural and social sciences must be understood in terms of philosophical and intellectual responses to the social change accompanying the industrial revolution. Similarly the recent upsurge, especially in the United States, of 'creationist' theories which regard the Bible as literal truth and oppose Darwinian theory, reviving a debate which ten or twenty years ago was regarded as a non-issue, must also be analysed in terms of current political and intellectual trends and conflicts.

It would not be appropriate here to enter into the debate within the biological sciences about theories of evolution and the contributions which have been made to genetic and biological theory since Darwin. However it is important to mention that Darwinian and neo-Darwinian evolutionary theory, while it has been accepted widely as orthodoxy in scientific circles, is nevertheless not without its opponents, nor is it a complete account of the process of development and modification of species. One of the major problems for conventional evolutionary theory is how to account for structural changes which are not gradual and quantitative but drastic and qualitative. For example, it is hard to conceive of a process by which organisms could gradually modify their physiology over the generations and become warm-blooded rather than cold-blooded. Certain developments are revolutionary rather than evolutionary: that is to say, they are either/or alternatives which imply radical changes in structure and functioning of the organism and which are difficult to account for in terms of orthodox notions of natural selection or random genetic mutation.

evolution, human. The study of human evolution is part of the province of PHYSICAL ANTHROPOLOGY and is a field in which recent and current discoveries of fossil remains of early human or HOMINID forms are still contributing towards the reconstruction of an as yet incomplete evolutionary record. S.L. Washburn and R. Moore provide an introductory overview of this field in their *Ape into Human: A Study of Human Evolution* (1980) but one must consult the specialist journals such as the *Yearbook of Physical Anthropology* in order to obtain an up-to-date view of present research. Many of the crucial questions about the emergence of distinctively human characteristics such as speech and culture or social organization remain unanswered within the study of human evolution. While comparative studies of primate behaviour may provide some of the answers or at least indicators of them, there is nothing in the primate world which approaches the complexity and diversity of human communicative and cultural systems.

The earliest identifiable hominid form in the fossil record is generally agreed to be *Ramapithecus*, a tropical forest dwelling form found in Africa and South Asia and dating from the period between 15 and 10 million BP. There is some disagreement as to whether *Ramapithecus* is to be regarded as the first distinctively hominid ancestor or whether certain apes (chimps and gorillas specifically) also descended from this form, with the divergence of the hominid line proper coming later on in the period 10 to 5 million BP. Unequivocal findings of a distinctive hominid line emerge with *Australopithecus*, found mainly in Africa, and with a time span of 5.5 to 2.5 million (possibly 1.5 million) BP. The studies of the Leakeys at Olduvai Gorge have made the australopithecines well-known. The range and variation of findings have led to a number of different classificatory schemes and theories of the evolution of australopithecine forms. Several different species or varieties have been identified, but all share a relatively humanlike bodily structure, combined with a skull retaining many apelike characteristics and a small cranial capacity (less than half that of modern *Homo sapiens*). The emergence of the first tools in hominid populations is traced to the period between 3 and 2 million BC, and is associated with the form classified as *Homo habilis* or *Australopithecus habilis*. These ancient humans or proto-humans lived in organized social groups and hunted large animals 'as well as employing and manufacturing stone tools (and presumably wooden and bone ones).

The next stage of human evolution is the species *Homo erectus*, which is found in a wide variety of geographical locations (Africa, Asia and Europe) and dates from the period 1 million to 300,000 BP. *Homo erectus* evolved over its time span a cranial capacity approaching that of modern humans, and developed more sophisticated hunting techniques as well as a wider range of tools. Later *Homo erectus* populations used fire, and there is some evidence of CANNIBALISM which would indicate the development of ceremonial systems. The next form to emerge is the celebrated Neanderthal, which is found in the period 100,000 to 40,000 BP. Neanderthals are nowadays classified as the first *Homo sapiens* form, *Homo sapiens neanderthalensis*. There is considerable debate, however, about the exact progression from *Homo erectus* to Neanderthals and modern humans, and the degree of regional variation in these widespread forms makes it difficult to discern macroevolutionary trends. There is consequently disagreement as to whether Neanderthals are ancestors of modern humans or parallel but separate developments from the *Homo erectus* line. The main feature of Neanderthal populations is the evident proliferation of regional technological traditions, as well as the increasing complexity of tool kits and the further development of ceremonial and religious systems. There is argument about whether Neanderthals possessed speech, and if so in what form.

Modern *Homo sapiens sapiens* emerges in the fossil record from about 40,000 to 25,000 BP in Europe, Africa and Asia, and there is considerable controversy over the possibility of independent and parallel evolutionary developments or conversely of migrations which could account for the early widespread distribution of modern human populations. Some theorists regard as diacritical in the emergence and differentiation of modern humans the phenomenon of speech and the cultural and social consequences of human communicative and symbolizing capacity as diacritical in the emergence and differentiation of modern humans. (*See* LINGUISTICS AND ANTHROPOLOGY.)

evolution, sociocultural. An important and often controversial concept in the social sciences, the notion of evolution has been applied by a large number of sociological and anthropological theorists in order to account for the historical progression from simpler to more complex social and cultural systems. One of the first such evolutionary theorists was SPENCER, who coined the phrase 'survival of the fittest'. At first anticipating and later drawing on the theories of Darwin, Spencer argued that there was a continuum which united inorganic, organic and superorganic evolution, and that the same laws could be applied to society and its progress as were applied to the natural world. This approach came to be called 'SOCIAL DARWINISM', and rested on two basic propositions. The first of these was that societies, like organisms, were composite wholes made up of functionally integrated parts, and underwent growth, decline, differentiation and integration. Spencer argued that social forms, like biological organisms, gradually evolved from simple homogenous undifferentiated structures into more complex and internally differentiated forms. The second basic premise was linked to Victorian *laissez-faire* INDIVIDUALISM, and consisted in the application of the principle of natural selection to humans in society. The poor, sick or less able were regarded as 'unfit', and it was thought that they should be allowed to die out in order to permit society's natural progress. This argument became in some circles an ideological support for *laissez-faire* policies.

Of course the notion of evolutionary progression of society was not original to Spencer: he simply brought it into new prominence by attempting to unify notions of social evolution with the biological theory of organic evolution. However the idea of a progressive advance of social forms was already widespread in the ENLIGHTENMENT, and both French and Scottish social and moral philosophers were employing evolutionary schemata in the 18th century. MONTESQUIEU had proposed an evolutionary scheme consisting of three stages: hunting or savagery, herding or barbarism, and civilization, which became very popular among 19th-century social theorists. MORGAN and TYLOR were two among many who adopted it. COMTE employed a different scheme, focusing on psychological rather than technological criteria: his three stages were the theological, the metaphysical and the scientific. To each of these three stages a type of mental state corresponded, together with a kind of knowledge, and a specific form of social structure. Among the Scottish Enlightenment thinkers, FERGUSON had also developed a theory of sociocultural evolution, distinguishing the stage of barbarism from that of savagery by the emergence of private property, and the stage of civilization or 'civil society' by the emergence of moral refinement and non-despotic political systems. Adam Smith on the other hand located the key distinction between evolutionary stages in the mode of subsistence characterizing each: hunting and fishing, pastoralism, agriculture and commerce.

New impetus was given to these theories in the 19th century by the publication of Darwin's works, and a whole generation of evolutionary anthropologists emerged whose works were to have a profound and lasting influence on the discipline. Drawing on Enlightenment thought and on new cross-cultural, historical and archaeological evidence, such theorists developed rival schemes of overall social and cultural progress as well as of the origins of different specific institutions such as RELIGION, MARRIAGE, the FAMILY, and so on. Morgan was one of the most influential evolutionary theorists of the 19th century, adopting as he did Montesquieu's stages. His theory was to influence the works of MARX and ENGELS as well as a wide range of later anthropological evolutionary theory. Morgan (1877) divided savagery and barbarism each into three stages (Lower, Middle and Upper) and provided contemporary ethnographic examples of each of these stages. Each separate stage was distinguished in the scheme by a technological development such as the use of fire, the bow and arrow or pottery, and was correlated with developments in patterns of subsistence activity, family and marriage and political organization. Tylor and FRAZER on the other hand focused especially on the evolution of religion and viewed the progress of society or culture from the viewpoint of the evolution of psychological or mental systems. Other evolutionary theorists who put forward different schemes of development of society and of religious, kinship or legal institutions include MAINE, MCLENNAN, and BACHOFEN.

These early evolutionary schemes are referred to as 'unilineal', since they argue more or less categorically for a single series of stages along which it is assumed that all human groups will progress although at uneven rates. Thus a contemporary 'primitive' group may be taken as representative of an earlier stage of development of more advanced types (*see* SURVIVAL). These unilinear evolutionary schemes fell into disfavour in the 20th century, partly as a result of the constant controversy between evolutionist and DIFFUSIONIST theories and partly because of the newly accumulating evidence about the diversity of specific sociocultural systems which made it impossible to sustain the largely 'armchair' speculations of these early theorists. Under the influence of BOAS in the USA and that of MALINOWSKI and RADCLIFFE-BROWN in Britain, new schools of anthropology were founded which were largely hostile to unilinear evolutionary schemes (*see* CULTURE HISTORY; STRUCTURAL FUNCTIONALISM) and concentrated on the elucidation and description of each social or cultural system as a functioning whole with its own internal logic and system. Thus many cultural and social anthropologists believed – and continue to believe – that to impose an overall evolutionary scheme is to do violence to the particular history of each sociocultural system and the system of unique meanings and events which this creates (*see* CULTURAL RELATIVISM).

Evolutionism was not entirely abandoned however, and within both MARXIST ANTHROPOLOGY and US cultural evolutionism and cultural ecology there are continuing research and theoretical traditions focusing on sociocultural evolution. In contemporary US evolutionism there are two main currents of thought: the unilinear evolutionism associated with WHITE and his students such as SERVICE and SAHLINS, and the multilinear evolutionism proposed by STEWARD. White (1959) posited that the overall development of human culture was to be understood in terms of the increase in levels of ENERGY use. Steward (1955) pro-

posed his theory of multilinear evolution in order to reconcile evolutionary theory with the growing evidence of cultural and social diversity available as a result of the advances of modern ethnography and CROSS-CULTURAL COMPARATIVE studies. Steward still employed an overall scheme of evolutionary progress through the stages of BAND, TRIBE, CHIEFDOM and STATE, but he combined this general scheme with the study of specific ecological adaptations and their variability (*see* LEVELS OF SOCIOCULTURAL INTEGRATION). Service (1975) and Sahlins (1972) similarly attempt to reconcile the contradiction between a broad evolutionary scheme accounting for the sweep of human history and the real diversity of contemporary sociocultural forms by distinguishing between general evolution and specific evolution. 'General evolution' is defined as the overall or dominant trend in human sociocultural development, while 'specific evolution' is characterized by variations from and reversals of this overall trend due to specific historical, geographical or ecological conditions.

In contemporary ecological anthropology or cultural ecology, the prevailing view of cultural evolution tends to be non-unilineal. Ecological anthropologists such as Marvin Harris (1979), Roy Rappaport (1968) and Andrew Vayda (1969) have produced new theories emphasizing the importance of environmental factors in influencing sociocultural adaptation and change. Employing CYBERNETIC and ecological theory, the new cultural ecologists are examining more closely the interrelations between humans, culture and ecosystems and the possible short term or long term consequences of different adaptive responses. Inasmuch as these theories may be classed as environmental determinism, they are fundamentally opposed to evolutionary schemes employed within Marxist or neo-Marxist anthropology, which stress the role of social organization and social transformation or REVOLUTION in the determination of sociocultural change and progress (*see* CHILDE).

exchange. This concept, which is closely linked to that of RECIPROCITY and also to that of COMMUNICATION, refers to the establishment and maintenance of relationships between persons. In order for social relationships to exist we must exchange something – whether it is the communicative exchange of language, the economic and/or ceremonial exchange of goods or the exchange of spouses. Exchanges may be equal or unequal, equivalent or nonequivalent, and the study of exchange mechanisms, patterns of exchange and circulation, and exchange relationships leads us straight to the heart of social and cultural organization. In this broad sense the study of exchange is the study of anthropology itself, and exchange theory is fundamental to areas as diverse as ECONOMIC ANTHROPOLOGY, KINSHIP and ALLIANCE THEORY, STRUCTURALISM, POLITICAL ANTHROPOLOGY, ACTION THEORY, NETWORK analysis and so on. In the works of LEVI-STRAUSS and other anthropologists influenced by structuralist theory there is a tendency to unify different domains such as marriage exchange, economic exchange and linguistic communication, accounting for all these different domains in terms of similar structural models. Thus the exchange of words, goods and women may all be equated as expressions of similar underlying exchange models. However this approach has been criticized for failing to take into account the political and strategic dimensions of exchange relationships, dimensions which are analysed for example in network analysis and action theory. Recently anthropologists like Victor TURNER, Norman Whitten, Fredrik Barth and Abner Cohen among others have attempted to unite these two perspectives by studying ADAPTIVE STRATEGIES and the manipulation of cognitive-symbolic domains within political contexts.

exchange value. The exchange theory of value is associated with neo-classical economics and is that which defines the value of a commodity as the value for which it can be exchanged. Marx's critique of exchange value and his alternative LABOUR THEORY OF VALUE are important elements in Marxist economic theory. (*See* VALUE; COMMODITY FETISHISM; ECONOMIC ANTHROPOLOGY.)

exegesis. The explication or elucidation of sacred texts. In anthropology the term 'native exegesis' is sometimes used to refer to the explanations or interpretations of MYTH, RITUAL or SYMBOLISM which is pro-

vided by informants themselves to the ethnographer. Some cultures are characterized by developed indigenous exegesis within a native philosophical tradition: a celebrated example is the Dogon philosopher Ogotommeli, or the complex COSMOLOGICAL schemes of certain Australian aboriginal peoples. In other cultures, however, there is a more pragmatic orientation and there may be little interest in the explication or discussion of cosmology. Apart from the differences between cultures, it is interesting to analyse the differences within cultures and the factors which may lead to the development of individuals with specialized KNOWLEDGE of cosmological or symbolic domains.

existentialism. A philosophical movement tracing its roots to the philosophers Kierkegaard and Heidegger and associated principally with Sartre and Merlau-Ponty in France. Existentialism with its emphasis on individual existence, consciousness, decisions and freedom has had few direct links to anthropology but as an important philosophical and critical trend has indirect influences and echoes in areas as diverse as CRITICAL THEORY, ETHNOMETHODOLOGY and ACTION THEORY.

exocannibalism. *See* CANNIBALISM.

exogamy. The practice of marrying out of a given social group or category. The converse of exogamy is ENDOGAMY or the obligation to marry within specified social limits. All systems of MARRIAGE alliance are both exogamous and endogamous, and the terms cannot be employed as general descriptions of marriage patterns without specifying the level of local group, kin group, class, caste, ethnic or other category to which the marriage prescriptions or proscriptions relate. (*See* INCEST; ALLIANCE THEORY.)

experience. The subjective perception of events by the individual, who interprets these events according to his or her cognitive and psychological characteristics. Experience thus becomes part of the personal life history of the individual. There is evidently a dialectical and mutually reciprocal relationship between cultural pattern and individual experience, since cultural forms mould and shape our interpretation of events while at the same time the sum of individual experiences is part of the content of our culture. Distinctive or special personal experiences of certain culturally standardized types (*see* ALTERED STATES OF CONSCIOUSNESS) are taken up within cultural traditions and form the basis for the collective creation of MYTH, LEGEND and ORAL TRADITION. Similarly the sociological and psychological effects of RITUAL and ART rely on a merging of cultural form and individual experience.

experiment. A mode of scientific investigation which attempts to verify or falsify hypotheses by means of maximal control over the variables under investigation. Such control is generally impossible to exercise in the social sciences, and the laboratory experiment is thus limited to the fields of natural science and psychology. Under certain circumstances it may be possible to construct quasi-experiments under partially controlled conditions in the social sciences, but more commonly the sociologist or anthropologist must rely on processes of interpretation and analysis of uncontrolled data available from the historical record or obtained by social scientific research techniques. (*See* RESEARCH DESIGN.)

exploitation. Used in an ecological sense to refer to the utilization of a given resource or resources in the environment. In its economic sense, it is the extraction of SURPLUS value from producers. According to Marx, exploitation arises in class-based societies as a result of the ability of the dominant class, who control the MEANS OF PRODUCTION, to extract from the producer more than is needed for the latter's basic subsistence needs or payment. In the sense defined by Marx exploitation is in itself a morally neutral term, since it is the degree, nature and utilization of surplus product rather than its existence *per se* which determines the progressive or retrograde nature of the overall system of class relations. In common usage, however, the term has acquired pejorative connotations and refers rather to the existence of unjust or abusive labour policies.

expression. A concept which links the notion of COMMUNICATION to that of CREATIVITY.

The expressive dimension of culture includes such fields as ART, DANCE, RITUAL, MYTH and in general the areas which have been studied from the viewpoint of SYMBOLISM as domains which link individual EXPERIENCE and cultural form.

expropriation. The taking of private property without compensation to its owner. Expropriation may be carried out by the state as part of programmes of LAND REFORM or as part of nationalization schemes affecting foreign or national private capital enterprises. In many cases however such schemes are accompanied by some form of compensation to the owner, though this may not represent the real value of the property. (*See* REVOLUTION.)

extended family. The extension of FAMILY membership beyond the confines of the nuclear family. This extension may be inter- or intra-generational. Extended family forms may be classified according to the links between the nuclear families which compose them: for example, sororal or fraternal, MATRILINEAL or PATRILINEAL extended family forms may be distinguished. The classification of family types as extended and nuclear has been commonly employed in sociology, but in anthropology is not generally regarded as of analytical value, since anthropological studies of KINSHIP groups and networks employ a series of more sophisticated classifications and categories rather than the crude distinction between nuclear and extended.

extension of kinship terms. The hypothesis that KINSHIP TERMS have a single central or core referent which is then extended to include other kinsmen. This has been the focus of controversy between different approaches to the study of KINSHIP. Buchler and Selby, reviewing this topic (1968), distinguish two main approaches to the extension of kinship terms: that based on social learning theory and that based on semantic or linguistic theory. The former approach, adopted by such theorists as EVANS-PRITCHARD, MALINOWSKI, RADCLIFFE-BROWN and FORTES, assumes that the basic meaning of a CLASSIFICATORY kin term is its closest biological referent, and addresses itself to the mechanisms by which this term is extended to other kinsmen by virtue of

social or psychological factors, role similarities, and so on. Thus it is assumed that a
child first learns the kinship terms which
relate to members of the nuclear family, and
comes to associate these terms with specific
attitudes and kinds of emotional and social
relationship. Subsequently he extends these
terms to other persons perceived as in some
way similar to the 'core' referents of each
term. This approach has been widely criticized for assuming that the learning of kin
terms by children during the SOCIALIZATION
process and the extension of sentiments and
attitudes acquired in the nuclear family
context to the wider society may be held to
explain the structure of kinship terminology.
As critics point out, the child does not create
anew the system of kinship terms: he or she
learns a system already in existence.

Opponents of social learning theory fall
into two classes. On one hand structural
theorists have rejected the notion of the
extension of kin terms, claiming that these
are category terms with no single primary
referent, and denouncing as ethnocentric the
assumption of the universal psychological
primacy of nuclear family relations. Leach
(1959) claims for example that 'kinship
terms are category words by means of which
the individual is taught to recognize the
significant groupings in the social structure'.
On the other hand, the semantic or linguistic
approach, instead of focusing on how kinship terms are learned, attempts to isolate by
FORMAL ANALYSIS the principles of kin
classification. In the work of Scheffler and
Lounsbury (1971) the technique of componential analyis is linked to the attempt to
confirm the theory of the extension of
sentiments, but in fact the componential or
formal method does not require or prove the
extensionist hypothesis. As Schneider has
pointed out (1965), much of the debate rests
on logical confusions and failure to define
the questions which may be resolved with
reference to specific kinds of data.

F

factions. Political action groups which are characterized as non-corporate and leadership-oriented (or leader-centred). In the study of POLITICAL ANTHROPOLOGY, approaches within ACTION THEORY have stressed the importance of such informal groups as factions, as against the emphasis on CORPORATE GROUPS characteristic of STRUCTURAL FUNCTIONALIST theory. Factions exist mainly within small-scale political ARENAS, since they are essentially personal groupings based on the abilities or CHARISMA of their leader, and are fluid or unstable in their composition. In general, factions are considered to be pragmatic and opportunistic groupings which exist to pursue the interest of members and leaders and/or to oppose those of other factions. However, there may also be differences of ideology between factional groupings, and it would be erroneous to consider them as solely interest groups defined in opposition to one another, though this may in fact be their main function.

In the study of political anthropology we may distinguish certain types of political system characterized by the overwhelming importance of factional allegiances: for example the BIG MAN systems of Melanesia and similar factional political systems in Amazonian and other indigenous groups. SEGMENTARY lineage systems can also be studied in terms of the formation of factional allegiances and its influence on processes of fission and fusion. Within state societies, the emergence of political factions is regarded by some as a pathological phenomenon indicative of the breakdown of normal structures of political AUTHORITY, while others regard it as normal for factions to co-exist at local level with centralized political structures.

family. A controversial term in anthropology with a definition beset by difficulty and disagreement, though like the related term household it is often employed loosely and without precise definition. Yanagisako, reviewing this topic (1979), provides an excellent summary of many of the main issues involved in the debate about these concepts. There is general agreement that the essence of the family is KINSHIP relations while the essence of the household is DOMESTIC activities. Thus families and households are analytically distinguishable and often empirically different. In studies of PEASANT communities, the term 'family' is often used to refer to jurally defined corporate kin groups whose central function is control over property (especially land) but such a functional definition of the family cannot be employed in a wide range of societies (either tribal or industrial) where property and land holding or other economic functions are performed by groups other than the family. Other functional definitions have been attempted, including those which define the family with reference to sexual, reproductive, socializing or other domestic functions. However as Yanigasako points out there is no single function or set of functions which is universally performed by one set of consanguineal kinsmen which could thus be defined as 'the family'. Thus many anthropologists have rejected functional definitions in favour of structural ones. Goodenough (1970) defines the universal nuclear family group as that composed of a woman and her dependent children. When the family also contains the woman's husband, he calls this the 'elementary conjugal family'. When the woman's consanguineal relatives (other than children) are included this is the 'consanguine family'. Goodenough does not however specify the functional components of these relationships.

FORTES (1969) formulated a definition which would meet with the agreement of many anthropologists, when he considered the family to be the 'reproductive nucleus' of the DOMESTIC GROUP. This reproductive nucleus may or may not contain at any given time the woman's husband. Wider consanguineal and affinal ties are thus analysed under the more general rubric of KINSHIP, which does not presuppose the primacy of any one group or unit. LEVI-STRAUSS has argued that the concept of the nuclear family as conventionally employed is analytically innappropriate and incomplete, since the ELEMENTARY STRUCTURE of kin relations always contains the wife-giving or alliance relationship as an integral part.

The nuclear family as MURDOCK originally defined it (1949), composed of mother, mother's husband and children, is not universally present in all societies, as we know from such ethnographic examples as the Nayars of South India, where marriage is a minimal institution and the mother-children unit has no significant bonds to father or mother's husband (see MATRIFOCAL). The tendency, inherited from MALINOWSKI and other genealogically-oriented anthropologists, to focus always on the reproductive function as the essence of the family unit can make us fail to examine the cross-cultural variability in the significance and sociocultural interpretation of this function. Yanigasako argues that treatments of family in anthropology have often been both ethnocentric and androcentric, ignoring both the political component of female relationships and the female viewpoint on family structure and process (see GENDER; FEMINISM; WOMEN AND ANTHROPOLOGY).

Considerable research has been devoted to the examination of cross-cultural variability in family functions and forms, despite the lack of an agreed cross-culturally valid definition of the family. Thus various competing typologies exist, some of them concerned with the testing of hypotheses relating to psychosocial universals, others with evolutionary hypotheses. Underlying many anthropological studies of family and domestic structure is an evolutionary and/or psychological postulate: that the (nuclear) family is the basic and universal productive, reproductive and social unit upon which other kinship, locality or political groupings are historically superimposed. In the work of Fortes, this is linked to psychoanalytical theory regarding the primacy of the mother-

child bond, from which all other emotional and social relations are held to stem. Opposing this position are the STRUCTURALIST and alliance theorists (notably LEACH and Needham) who argue that the basis of kinship systems is category relationship and not psychological universals (see EXTENSION OF KINSHIP TERMS).

The distinction common in sociology between nuclear and extended family forms has been little applied in anthropology, where it gives way to a more sophisticated examination and classification of the numerous types of family and domestic group which may be observed cross-culturally. However much debate regarding the family has centred on the nuclear–extended dichotomy and the supposed breakdown of extended family ties with INDUSTRIALIZATION. As Yanigasako points out, much of this debate is spurious since it rests on an over crude dichotomization of nuclear and extended forms and the failure to define what is meant by extended family ties. It is necessary, therefore, to reformulate this debate in terms of a more careful study of continuity and transformation in family forms and functions in the contexts of industrialization and social change.

Debate about the future of the family in industrial society has been stimulated in part by anthropological evidence of the cultural relativity of family forms and supposed 'natural' family relations, and has centred also on the relationship which exists between family, socialization and political or ideological systems. This is a complex issue, since family historical research has shown there are both contradictions and consistencies between family forms and values and wider political, economic and religious institutions. Families in some respects perpetuate through the socialization process the ideological and value systems of the wider society, but in some respects and in some contexts they may also oppose or contradict these: especially in periods of social change or in the formation of SUBCULTURES.

family cycle. See DEVELOPMENTAL CYCLE OF THE DOMESTIC GROUP.

family, joint. A term generally used to refer to a type of composite or extended family composed of nuclear families linked together by sibling ties.

family of marriage. Also called 'family of procreation'. The nuclear family formed by Ego upon marriage and the birth of Ego's children.

family of orientation. Also called 'family of origin', this refers to the nuclear family group within which Ego was born and/or raised.

famine. The scarcity of food and resulting malnutrition and starvation among the poorer sectors of the community are often attributed to climatic factors or natural DISASTERS such as drought, flood, and earthquake. Famines should be studied as the result not only of such natural occurrences but also as consequences of the breakdown of socioeconomic systems: as in the case of famines resulting from situations of warfare, political instability or violence. The differential effects of famine among a given population are particularly relevant to anthropological analysis, revealing the variations in access to power and scarcity of resources among its number. It should also be noted that victims of famine are not the passive objects journalistic treatments of this subject often represent them as being. They are active human beings who have reached the limit of personal, social and politico-economic resources, and the famine they endure is itself an extreme example of the types of food scarcity often encountered in anthropological research, and which severely test the networks of reciprocity and social relationship of many communities. Famine, like POVERTY and hunger in general, should be regarded not as a natural but a social phenomenon, and it is part of anthropology's responsibility and legitimate field of study to document and analyse critically the structures of politico-economic and social class dominance which deny certain sectors of the population access to basic subsistence resources. (*See* DEVELOPMENT; CRITICAL ANTHROPOLOGY.)

farming. *See* AGRICULTURE.

farming systems research. A field in which APPLIED ANTHROPOLOGISTS have increa-

singly intervened in recent years, and which involves a systematic approach to agricultural DEVELOPMENT. In farming systems research the farmer, the agricultural extension worker, the agricultural engineer and the development worker or social scientist work together in a team in order to resolve local level problems. Farming systems research involves the use or development of APPROPRIATE TECHNOLOGY and computers are being employed more and more to assist the farmer with specific problems.

fascism. This term is often used in a rather general sense to refer to extreme right-wing political movements or tendencies. In a more limited sense it refers to specific political movements in the histories of Italy and Germany, and their ideological or political descendants. The term derives from the Latin *fasces*, a bundle of rods which was a symbol of the authority of magistrates in Ancient Rome, and the first Fascist Party was founded by Mussolini in Italy. The term was subsequently extended to Nazi Germany, and to Spain under Franco, though it is important to recognize that historical analysis has amply demonstrated that there are considerable differences between each of these examples of fascism in government. In general, the main characteristics common to all types of fascism are considered to be its opposition to working class organizations and to socialist or communist parties, combined with a nationalist and/or racist ideology, a cult of leadership focused on a central figure, and a tendency towards the use of violence of both the legal-military and illegal, or mass, kind. Psychological and social-psychological analyses of fascism have concentrated on its appeal to alienated or marginal sectors of society and to the authoritarian personality, while historical analyses have put forward a number of different hypotheses about the relationship between fascist movements and particular historico-social conditions and forces. Fascist-type political movements are present in most modern nations, with more or less prominence, and may at times emerge as parties of government. The conditions of their rise to power may be influenced both by internal factors such as the disorganization of other political parties, the breakdown of social CONSENSUS, economic crises, the growth of a marginal or disaffected sector of society due to migrations, and lack of economic opportunity. They may also be decisively influenced by external support for extreme right-wing parties or governments. The United States, for example, has tended in the past to support right-wing and neo-Fascist governments in Third World nations, a policy which it justifies by claiming that it is opposing the spread of communism, and these governments have in turn established economic and military agreements favourable to the United States and to a small ruling group but unfavourable to the interests of the majority of the population. (*See* IMPERIALISM; DEVELOPMENT; DEPENDENCY; CAPITALISM.)

fashion. The essence of fashion is its voluntary and historically changeable nature. It is thus diametrically opposed to TRADITION and to the forms of dress and bodily adornment which are obligatory and fixed signs of social identity or status in certain traditional societies. Because fashion changes periodically and because the individual may follow it more or less assiduously, it is essentially competitive and lends itself to the display of affluence or personal prestige, or indications of leisure. It is consequently less developed in pre-class and more developed in class societies, functioning in the latter both to mark off the different classes according to the fashions appropriate to each, and as a part of intra-class rivalry or competition for prestige.

fatalism. It is sometimes claimed that PEASANT or traditional societies are characterized by fatalistic attitudes towards life: in other words, that their members regard their own actions as powerless to influence the course of events. This is in turn claimed to be related to peasant CONSERVATISM and other aspects of the peasant WORLD VIEW (*see* LIMITED GOOD). However it has been shown within community studies of groups such as the Mesoamerican peasants, that such attitudes or values as fatalism are not universal characteristics of peasant communities. Different geographical regions and different historical moments may be characterized by a variety of prevailing attitudes, and we should perhaps regard fatalism not as an absolute value of peasant society but

rather as one of a set or repertoire of traditional attitudes which may come to the fore under varying circumstances. These include active participation and decision-making which will affect the environment and alter the course of events. It is therefore necessary to contextualize generalizations about peasant attitudes and values, and to consider the specific circumstances which elicit responses of fatalism or active strategy.

feast. Feasts are characteristic social events of central importance in certain ethnographic areas (Amazonia, Northwest Coast, and New Guinea, for example). Ecological anthropologists have examined feasts as mechanisms of REDISTRIBUTION with adaptive advantages since they serve to even out differences in food production. Rappaport (1968) has provided us with a sophisticated account of the Tsembaga Maring pig feast as part of a complex flow of information and activity which operates as a means of maintaining the population in equilibrium with its environment and the natural resources exploited by humans. Rappaport also indicates in his analysis the multiple functions of feasting and its links to other social institutions. The feast is important in terms of ceremonial systems and is connected with the establishment of marriage alliances, the development of political relationships, and so on. Each of these aspects may be analysed in its own right, since the feast in these societies is a complete social institution, and a context in which many important social relationships and transactions are revealed. The prevailing tendency has been to regard feasting as characteristic of egalitarian societies and as a mechanism which militates against the accumulation of wealth by particular persons or families. This view has however been challenged by those who argue that it may be an element in the creation of political prestige and power, and its redistributory aspect may be more apparent than real. The leader who holds a feast invests a certain amount of production (often production resulting from the labour of wives and kinsmen or allies) in a ceremonial activity, but at the same time he gains both prestige and position, further securing his status as the centre of a redistributive network which may allow him to receive more than he gives out. Feasting within the context of BIG MAN-type political systems does contain within itself the possibility of increasing differentiation of the leader in terms of wealth and power, a potential which may or may not be realized within a given ethnographic context.

feedback. In CYBERNETIC theory, feedback mechanisms are those where information outputs from a given system are 'fed back' into that system as information inputs. Feedback mechanisms may be positive or negative: positive feedback amplifies or intensifies the activity of the system and may throw it into disequilibrium or malfunction, while negative feedback acts to limit the activity of the system or maintain it in equilibrium. The concept of feedback has been employed especially in CULTURAL ECOLOGY as a means of conceptualizing the adaptive or maladaptive consequences of given processes or actions.

feminism, feminist anthropology. The term 'feminism' embraces a variety of movements and ideologies concerned with the emancipation or liberation of women, the establishment of equal rights for women, and opposition to forms of male dominance. Within this field there are a great diversity of feminist movements and positions. From its origins in the late 18th and 19th centuries feminism has never been a united or homogeneous movement, and over the past 20 years an increasing diversification of feminist viewpoints and strategies has been apparent. One aspect of the feminist movement has always been the struggle for equal rights for women under the law, another the struggle for equal opportunities and access to education and occupational roles: both of these continue to be of importance, since the laws of modern nations continue to discriminate against women in a variety of contexts and a number of different ways. Another aspect of feminism concerns the question of female sexuality: here there have been a number of very different positions all classifiable as 'feminist' but sometimes radically contradictory. The birth control or family planning movement has been associated with feminism since its origin, and feminists today continue to insist on a woman's right to control over her own body and reproductive functions as a key element in female libe-

ration. However there are differing views within feminism as to the extent to which institutions such as marriage, the family, and patterns of heterosexual behaviour should be challenged. Some radical feminists argue for the overthrow of all these PATRIARCHAL forms, while others argue for a redistribution of the rights and obligations of males, females and the state within a basically traditional family structure. While feminists may all be in agreement in their rejection of male-imposed attitudes and roles in the domains of sexuality, reproduction and childrearing, there are a number of different views as to how women themselves should redefine these roles and values.

The relationship between feminism and Marxism or socialism is also one which is subject to debate and a variety of differing opinions. Conventional Marxist theory deriving from Engels' *Origins of the Family, Private Property and the State* (1884) relates male dominance or patriarchy to CAPITALISM, and assumes that the liberation of women will be achieved automatically with the establishment of socialism. However, both Marxist and non-Marxist feminist critiques have led to the emergence of contradictory positions. Marxist feminists have pointed to the necessity for a more careful analysis of the relationships between capitalism and female subordination, as well as to the differential effects of exploitation and subordination of women according to social class. It is pointed out, for instance, that working-class women within capitalism suffer more from the effects of male dominance than middle-class women do. Working-class women are society's least favoured sector as far as the distribution of opportunities and benefits is concerned, and due to the double oppression of sexism and their position in the class structure do not have the opportunity to express their situation or feelings which is provided to middle-class women. This has led to Marxist feminist critiques of those bourgeois feminist movements which focus on problems essentially felt by the middle-class woman and on the subjective or personal aspect of liberation rather than its social and political roots.

Marxism is thus opposed to certain elements of feminism in so far as they perpetuate existing structures of class dominance, restricting 'liberation' to educated middle-class women and adopting modes of action and debate which effectively exclude the participation of those working-class women who are in fact the prime victims of sexist attitudes and male dominance. Marxist feminists have also examined the ways in which capitalism both depends upon and reinforces sexism and male supremacy. Subordinate women perform a series of functions essential to the capitalist system: by means of their control over the socialization of children they reproduce the ideological structures of capitalism and the political passivity or false consciousness upon which it rests. They also perform free of charge essential domestic services, as well as constituting a reserve army of docile labour which can be utilized when required and sent back to the domestic domain when not needed. In response to prevailing sexist attitudes within Marxist and socialist political and intellectual movements, and to the persistence of sexism within socialist countries, feminists have pointed to the need for a critique within Marxism and socialism of assumptions regarding female roles, and the institutions of family and marriage. According to Marxist feminism the critical analysis and rejection of male dominance, patriarchal attitudes and their institutions become integral parts of any revolutionary or socialist programme, without which the overthrow of capitalism would be impossible, since patriarchy and male dominance are essential elements in capitalist ideology. Some radical feminists have opposed the Marxist view of male dominance as a product of capitalism. They have argued that male dominance is prior to capitalism, and is in fact the original form of subordination of one human being or class of human beings to another, and possibly the origin of all other forms of social inequality. They accordingly oppose Marxist and other theorists who state that female subordination is absent in pre-class societies. Some of these proponents of the universality of female subordination locate its roots in the biological nature of woman and the reproductive function and the corresponding biologically determined aggressiveness of males. Others however stress that it is an essentially social and cultural phenomenon. In this debate the anthropological evidence regarding pre-class societies has been important, though there is no general agreement

among feminist or other anthropologists about the existence or explanation of universal female subordination (*see* GENDER; SEXUAL DIVISION OF LABOUR).

In the Third World, feminist movements have also taken a variety of forms, though a similar division into Marxist or socialist feminist ideologies and bourgeois feminism can be made. Marxist or socialist ideologies focus on feminism as a part of overall political programmes opposing the capitalist system; bourgeois feminism concentrates more deeply on ideologies of male dominance and on the subjective liberation of the middle-class woman. A cross-cultural and anthropologically sensitive re-examination of feminist goals and attitudes towards family, marriage, children, and so on is urgently needed in the light of the experiences and values of women in the Third World. Anthropological studies of women's status (*see* WOMEN AND ANTHROPOLOGY) have so far neglected this area of study. Many have examined the situation of women in other cultures and societies, but few have considered the potential there for new feminist movements or women's organizations, or their emergence. Nor have they considered the relationship between their goals and those defined by Western middle-class feminism. Feminist anthropology is beginning to tackle these questions in its treatment of such topics as DEVLOPEMENT, INDUSTRIALIZATION, and so on, where it is necessary to consider the effects of processes of CHANGE on women and the extent and nature of their participation in the determination of strategies and responses to change.

Ferguson, Adam (1723–1816). One of the leading figures in the Scottish ENLIGHTENMENT, whose works focused on the history and development of ethical, political and social systems. In *An Essay on Civil Society* (1767) Ferguson described the progress of human history from savagery through barbarism to modern civil society (*see* EVOLUTION, SOCIOCULTURAL). Ferguson defined the difference between savagery and barbarism as the emergence of private property, which gave rise to commercial society characterized by the pursuit of individual self-interest and wealth. Civil society, on the other hand, represented the overcoming of barbaric individualism and the establishment of the social bond based on refined moral and ethical sentiments.

feud. Feuding is akin to WARFARE, but is generally distinguished from it inasmuch as the feud is a continuing state of hostilities marked by sporadic outbursts of violence. The feud is thus less generalized or less intensive than a state of war, and may be a constant state of relations between communities or between kin groups, marked, as in a blood-feud, by periodic attacks or revenge killings.

feudalism. In its main sense this term refers to the system of social and politico-economic relations prevalent in medieval Europe, though it has been extended by some authors to other historical and geographical contexts such as Japan, Eastern Europe, and post-conquest Latin America. Debate about the concept of feudalism has centred on whether it is best regarded primarily as a MODE OF PRODUCTION, as a political system, or as a legal system. Emphasis on the legal and normative aspects of feudalism has led to the study of the characteristic sets of rights and obligations relating to service, obedience and loyalty which existed between different social categories such as monarchs, lords, vassals and serfs (*see* ESTATE). In European feudalism, the granting of land as a reward for military service and political loyalty (the 'fief') formed the basis of a network of lords and vassals, of such complexity that the vassals of great lords became lords in their own right to lesser vassals. WEBER, emphasizing the political aspect of feudalism, stressed the possibility of local autonomy created by this system, and argued that the fundamental characteristic of feudalism was the decentralization of power and authority. He contrasted feudalism with patrimonialism which he defined as a system based on a centralized ruling class or ARISTOCRACY. The historian Marc Bloch (1949) however argued that centralization or decentralization is not the key issue in defining feudalism, since within feudal societies sharing basically the same characteristics strong and weak monarchies with more or less central power vied for that power against a degree of local autonomy. Authors who stress feudalism as a mode of production have also placed less emphasis on the internal relations of the ruling class and the distribution of power between monarchy and lords, and more on feudalism as a system of CLASS relations based on the extraction of surplus from PEASANT producers by the landholding class in general. The essential characteristic of feudalism for these analysts is thus the fact that political power was based on the ownership of land, enabling the landholder to extract surplus from the producer. From this point of view the legal-normative aspect of feudalism is regarded as a secondary or ideological development serving to justify the system of class relations.

The debate regarding the concept of feudalism in anthropology has centred on whether it is a historically specific mode characteristic of Europe during a certain phase of development, or whether it can be applied as a more general analytical category. Wallerstein points out that 'there is a fundamental difference between the feudalism of medieval Europe and the "feudalisms" of 16th century eastern Europe and Hispanic America'. He calls the latter 'coerced cash crop labour', a form of labour control in capitalist, not feudal, economies. In European feudalism there was no strong centralized authority as in systems of ORIENTAL DESPOTISM (*see* ASIATIC MODE OF PRODUCTION) since local powerholders controlled strategic elements of production and were able to intercept tribute to the centre and organize their own local regional alliances both against central power and against each other. Eric Wolf has suggested that neither the Asiatic nor the feudal systems should be reified as types, but rather that both should be regarded as examples of a 'tributary mode of production', the Asiatic more centralized and the feudal with more local and regional power. The essential common characteristic of these modes of production would thus be the extraction of tribute from producers by political and military means.

fictive kinship. This term has been applied to forms of social relationship such as blood brotherhood or the relations of godparents and godchildren which are modelled on natural kinship relations. Some anthropologists have argued that the term is misleading since such relations do not pretend to be natural ones, but rather are contrasted with and set aside from natural or biological kinship. Such authors have preferred the terms RITUAL KINSHIP or spiritual kinship. (*See* COMPADRAZGO.)

fieldwork. Research undertaken by the anthropologist or ETHNOLOGIST in a given ethnographic area or COMMUNITY. Such an ethnographic area in modern anthropology is not necessarily limited to the traditional tribal or peasant community, and may embrace studies of URBAN, industrial or other settings which the anthropologist selects for the purposes of intensive research. The anthropological perspective has similarly been employed in the study of SUB-CULTURES and in institutional research within modern industrial society. So, while it was once true to say that anthropology was the study of peoples considered to be PRIMITIVE, of exotic and little-known tribal cultures, and of peasant communities, modern anthropological research can no longer be defined by this criterion and must be defined instead by the application of its distinctive methods of fieldwork and analysis. In many cases, however, disciplinary boundaries become blurred in the study of modern industrial and urban society, due to the emergence of novel theoretical and methodological syntheses resulting from interdisciplinary collaboration and interchange. Such interdisciplinary influences are also to be seen in the anthropological study of traditional tribal and peasant communities, where modern anthropologists increasingly draw on historical, economic, political and sociological theories, amongst others, in order to provide an adequate account of local sociocultural systems and their interrelations both with one another and with national and international power structures (*see* CRITICAL ANTHROPOLOGY; DEVELOPMENT).

Apart from problems of RESEARCH DESIGN, methods and theoretical approach, fieldwork involves in itself some characteristic difficulties for which many researchers are initially unprepared wherever they choose to carry it out. The ethnographer may experience CULTURE SHOCK or a sense of disorientation when first arriving in the fieldwork setting, caused by the difference in codes of values and behaviour of the people

he or she is studying. This state of disorientation is perhaps necessary, and is in the long term a productive one, since like a RITE OF PASSAGE it prepares the ethnographer for the imaginative leap involved in coming to terms with an alien culture or way of life. The anthropologist's prior preparation, both formal and informal, may have given him or her unrealistic expectations of the community . A conscious or unconscious romanticism regarding 'the primitive', which may form an important or essential element in his or her motivation towards the profession, is met with the rude shock of the reality of a Third World nation of which the chosen community or people is a part. Many anthropologists react by rejecting the national or dominant society and taking refuge 'in the bush', regarding as tedious and unproductive any time they must spend, for example, negotiating fieldwork permits or waiting in capital or provincial cities. As a result, the ethnographer may fail to study the national and regional system of which a local community forms a part, and to neglect to document the way in which national and international power structures impinge upon the field of study.

There are other problems involved in fieldwork for the ethnographer, including the difficulties involved in establishing a role within the community and rapport with informants. Sometimes anthropologists find that it is difficult to explain their presence or the nature of their investigations to the people concerned, and some have found it easier to invent a false identity which the local community will more easily accept. Many would question the ETHICS of this practice, and the researcher faced with this difficulty should perhaps attempt instead to negotiate his or her status in the community pragmatically, openly declaring research interests but at the same time offering to perform some useful or valued service in return for the collaboration he or she requires. Increasingly in both tribal and peasant communities the role of the anthropologist is subject to questioning by the community itself, as well as to critical appraisal within national intellectual and political circles. The researcher should not assume that he or she has an automatic right to carry out investigations, and should be prepared to offer something in return to the community, as well as to share the results of research with local anthropologists, social scientists or administrators who may be able as a result to enrich and add to their knowledge of national sociocultural and ethnic diversity.

Fieldwork itself, including the negotiation and manipulation of the ethnographer's own status and role in the community, is increasingly regarded within critical anthropology as a legitimate and essential object of analysis, and many modern ethnographers argue that the ethnographer must state and fully examine his or her participation (or non-participation) in the community in order to evaluate the results of such research (*see* ETHNOGRAPHIC WRITING). These writers therefore assess critically the concept of PARTICIPANT OBSERVATION upon which ethnographic research is conventionally said to be based, pointing out that this is an inherently problematic notion.

Another area of difficulty which most ethnographers encounter concerns the attitude that they should take towards internal cleavages and divisions within the community or population they study. It is not always possible to resolve this dilemma, and it is generally true to say that the anthropologist must sacrifice either breadth of coverage and contacts to intensity of relations with one or two informants or families, or vice versa. It is impossible to be all things to all people in the field, and it is especially true of small-scale societies marked by FACTIONAL alliances that the population will force the anthropologist to 'take sides' even if he or she had no intention of doing so, the only alternative being to remain at the margins of the community, unable to perform adequate research. To be assigned an identity or a role is to be separated from other identities or roles, and though the anthropologist may exploit an ambiguous or marginal status to some extent in order to explore multiple social fields, he or she may not always be able to conserve neutrality or may under certain circumstances feel that neutrality is not an ethically acceptable position.

Many difficulties arise from a failure to define adequately the anthropologist's position as far as the community studied, and the aims of his or her research are concerned. Anthropologists are sometimes unsure about the relationship between supposedly academic or 'pure' research and their ethical or political commitment to defend and further the interests of the oppressed and impoverished sectors of society they study. In many Third World nations, intellectuals and representatives of indigenous peoples and other oppressed or subordinate groups share the general view of Western anthropology either as a form of espionage or an account of 'folklore' and exotic customs perpetuating a totally false image of their national reality and the real problems of their minority groups. Anthropologists also enjoy a poor reputation for ethical behaviour, and have been criticized principally for their lack of commitment to the welfare of the people they study, and the failure to share the results of their research and to communicate with local universities and intellectuals. It is natural enough for people who observe the anthropologist, comparatively wealthy by local standards and apparently free to pursue the line of research he or she chooses, to resent what they regard as the exploitation of the local community for the purposes of advancing his or her own career at home, placing the goals of his or her individual research project over and above any commitment to the aspirations and basic needs of the local population. And it is only to be expected that communities and peoples of the Third World will come more and more to reject this type of investigation and demand that the anthropologist contribute something in return for his or her presence. The profession itself will have to respond to these critiques, and intensify its internal and external debate about the coherence of its position as far as the conventional contexts of its investigations – poverty, oppression and social marginality – are concerned, if it is not to become increasingly removed from the reality it pretends to investigate.

fieldwork methods. *See* RESEARCH DESIGN; RESEARCH METHODS.

fighting. *See* FEUD; WARFARE; DISPUTE SETTLEMENT.

filiation. This term refers to the social recognition of relationships between parents and children. FORTES and other DESCENT theorists have contrasted descent, which refers to LINEAGE or CORPORATE GROUP membership, with filiation which refers simply to the link or relationship from parents to their children (*see* COMPLEMENTARY FILIATION). Other writers however do not distinguish the terms descent and filiation.

Firth, Sir **Raymond** (1902–   ). British social anthropologist who has made major contributions both in ethnographic research in Oceania and in several important areas of anthropological theory. Like LEACH, Firth made a notable divergence from the prevailing orthodoxy of STRUCTURAL FUNCTIONALIST theory in British anthropology during the postwar years, exploring many areas which were later to be taken up by younger scholars in search of fresh approaches. He employed the concept of SOCIAL ORGANIZATION as distinct from SOCIAL STRUCTURE, and his studies in this field were influential in the development of ACTION THEORY approaches in anthropology. In the field of ECONOMIC ANTHROPOLOGY, he was associated with the FORMALIST school of theorists who argued for the applicability, with due modifications, of neo-classical economic models to pre-capitalist and peasant economies. Firth has made also important contributions in the field of KINSHIP to the study of NON-UNILINEAL DESCENT. He is currently engaged in the preparation of a dictionary of the Tikopia language. Major works include *We, The Tikopia* (1936), *Malay Fishermen: Their Peasant Economy* (1946), *Elements of Social Organization* (1956), *Economics of the New Zealand Maori* (1959), *Social Change Among the Tikopia* (1959), *Essays on Social Organization and Values* (1964), *Themes in Economic Anthropology* (1967).

fishing. There has been some debate as to whether cultures based on fishing can be considered as a 'type' in a similar sense as pastoralists, HORTICULTURALISTS, and so on. However the variety of fishing techniques and technologies ranging from simple traps, spears, arrows and so on among indigenous peoples, to the different kinds and sizes of boats and nets employed in small-scale or in industrial fishing, render the attempt to formulate a type of general fishing or maritime culture extremely problematic. Within sociological studies of the so-called 'extreme occupations' fishing communities have been analysed in terms of their distinctive values and social organization, linked to the special demands of the occupational role. In small-scale or traditional societies, fishing activities sometimes share many of the characteristics of hunting: danger, uncertainty, the use of physical strength, and so on. In other cases they resemble more closely the gathering of a reliable and easily captured resource. The Northwest Coast area is perhaps the best-known example of a region where the comparative abundance and reliability of aquatic resources permitted a level of social development normally only associated with agricultural societies.

fission. The splitting of a social group or community into two or more opposing or separate groups, or FACTIONS. The term usually refers to the physical separation of such opposing groups, and is characteristic of small-scale societies where residence patterns are variable in accordance with political and kinship ties and with economic and ecological factors. Processes of fission (and also of fusion or aggregation) have been studied from the point of view of ecological adaptation as well as from that of cycles of political relationships. Some cultural ecologists view fission as the product of a complex series of 'messages' and interactions between humans, their culture and their environment, in such a way that ceremonial, political and social mechanisms act to regulate the relationship and distribution of population and resources in a given environment. Others criticize such arguments as a type of environmental determinism, contending rather that sociological and/or cultural factors are of primary importance in determining residence patterns and processes of growth or decline in community size. (*See* SCHISM; WARFARE; BIG MAN; SEGMENTARY.)

fitness. *See* EVOLUTION; ADAPTATION.

flexibility. One of the major criticisms which has been raised against both the British school of STRUCTURAL FUNCTIONALIST anthropology and US CULTURAL RELATI-

120   **folk**

VISM or CULTURAL DETERMINISM is their failure to account for the flexibility and individual variability of attitudes and values as well as norms of social behaviour. Both the British concept of social structure and the US concept of culture tended to become reified as systems considered to be above and beyond the individual and in some way to determine his or her behaviour and attitudes or values. Both approaches consequently tended to assume a high degree of uniformity and CONSENSUS as characteristic of 'primitive' or traditional societies. Critics have pointed out that these assumptions lead us to neglect both the actual degree of variation and disagreement found in any real population, and the possibility of flexibility, creativity and change in sociocultural systems. Approaches within ACTION THEORY, on the other hand, have tended instead to emphasize rather the flexibility or relativity of norms and values, and the creation of ongoing social systems as a result of the sum of individual decisions and actions. Within STRUCTURALISM there is an attempt to relate the variability of 'surface' manifestations of culture and social structure to underlying generative and/or analytical models or structures.

folk. A term used in ETHNOLOGY and anthropology to refer loosely to traditional rural peasant societies in which an ORAL TRADITION predominates. In his concept of the FOLK-URBAN CONTINUUM, REDFIELD attempted to endow this term with more precise analytical value. In the 19th century, the folk stratum was considered to be an inferior and backward residue existing within a modern nation, and folk culture was therefore treated as a collection of survivals from earlier evolutionary stages of society. Because of the pejorative connotations of the term, many modern anthropologists have avoided its use and that of such terms as FOLKLORE and FOLKWAYS. Many writers have therefore preferred the terms 'oral tradition' and ORAL LITERATURE, and more recently the prefix ETHNO-, to indicate the study of popular or pre-literate traditions.

The notion of 'folk' played a part in European nationalistic ideologies, where the 'folk' represented the repository of customs and values which expressed the spirit of a nation. In order to rid the concept of nationalistic or ethnocentric overtones, many modern folklorists have widened the definition of the term 'folk' to include any speech community or social group, and the study of folklore when widely defined in this way does not differ fundamentally from the study of oral tradition, CULTURE or SUBCULTURE in anthropology in general. In European ethnology, however, the terms 'folk' and 'folklife' are retained to refer to the study of rural peasant peoples.

folklife. Within the tradition of European ETHNOLOGY, this term refers to the study of the traditional everyday culture of the FOLK. This is generally considered to be the culture of pre-literate rural peasant peoples, dominated by the ORAL TRADITION, and is distinguished from the literate urban cultural tradition with which it coexists.

folklore. Originally applied to the study of aspects of rural peasant culture, this term has been extended to refer to other cultures and subcultures. The study of folklore embraces the examination of traditional knowledge, customs, oral and artistic traditions among any community (or sector of the community) united by some common factor, such as a common occupation, co-residence, or a common language or ethnic identity. We may thus speak of the folklore of an occupational group, a religious group, an institution, and so on. The essence of folklore is its spontaneous or organic nature: that is to say, it is a result of the experiences and interpretations of experience of persons engaged in social interaction. It may often be in conflict, therefore, with the information, values or knowledge imparted by formal educational institutions or which derive from the dominant literate culture of an elite. Recent developments in the analysis of MYTH and in areas such as LINGUISTICS and anthropology and ETHNOMETHODOLOGY, have made important contributions to the study of folklore as an examination of the creation of 'alternative' or folk systems of interpretation and expression of reality. Elements of folklore are often taken up within the dominant literate tradition, where they can be a source of both artistic and social innovation. (*See* ETHNICITY; ORAL LITERATURE; ORAL TRADITION.)

folkloristics. The study of FOLKLORE.

folk-urban continuum. One of the major theoretical constructs of the anthropologist REDFIELD, who developed it in order to account for the differences which he observed among various Mexican communities. According to Redfield the 'folk society' is characterized by its small size, physical isolation, a high degree of social homogeneity and group solidarity, and the absence of literacy. Urban society on the other hand is characterized by its greater size and its contact and communication between population centres, more role diversification and individualism, and literacy. Kinship ties prevail in folk society and behaviour is personal and traditional. The sacred, rather than the secular, is the dominant mode of experience and action. In urban society kinship ties are disorganized and the secular mode predominates. A community could be placed at a given position along the folk-urban continuum according to the extent to which it possessed the features regarded as characteristic of the fok or urban ideal types. As well as being a descriptive scheme, the continuum was also conceptualized as an account of the evolution of social forms, from the simpler to the more complex.

The notion of the folk-urban continuum has been criticized from various perspectives. It has been pointed out that the folk and urban types are abstractions which do not correspond to any real community. Critics have also argued that the creation of these two opposing poles, conceived of as evolutionary extremes, distracts attention from the need to study the interrelationships of folk and urban society, since they are in reality part of a single social and politico-economic system. Other critiques have focused on the priority that Redfield gives to VALUES and WORLD VIEW as the defining and determining characteristics of social types, and his consequent neglect of politico-economic and power structures. (*See* PEASANT.)

folkways. A term used to describe the CUSTOMS and habits, or typical behaviour patterns, characteristic of a given community or FOLK. It was employed by SUMNER in his *Folkways* (1909), but has not passed into general usage in British or US anthropology.

food. Given the importance of activities concerned with the obtaining, preparation, sharing and consumption of food and the time devoted to them, this topic has received little explicit attention from anthropologists, although practices, beliefs and customs relating to food are mentioned constantly as examples or illustrations in fields as diverse as KINSHIP, ECONOMIC ANTHROPOLOGY and SYMBOLIC ANTHROPOLOGY. G. Levitas (1983) provides in a review of this topic a survey of anthropological contributions both to the study of food and to specific aspects of the relationship between diet, nutrition and culture. FRAZER and TYLOR, among other 19th-century anthropologists, focused attention on food TABOOS as survivals of earlier evolutionary stages and stressed them in their theories of the origins of RELIGION (*see* TOTEMISM). Later British social anthropology under the influence of DURKHEIM and RADCLIFFE-BROWN developed the study of the moral value of food, and its use as a symbolic element in social relationships, where it helped to maintain the social structure. At the same time, American anthropologists under the influence of MALINOWSKI's functional theory of culture began to study how practices relating to food functioned, and the effects of these practices on the psychology and culture of the group. Cultural ecology has developed this approach further, and has also attempted to show that seemingly irrational food taboos and ritual practices are in fact adaptive mechanisms, which help to maintain the equilibrium between humans and resources in a given environment (*see* CULTURAL MATERIALISM).

The anthropological study of food was given a new direction by LEVI-STRAUSS who used it as a metaphor for his model of structural oppositions. In accordance with his theory that all the products of the human mind display a common cognitive structure, he uses the example of food to demonstrate how this structure is worked out in a context which has often been regarded as governed solely by practical or biological necessities. Combining the STRUCTURALIST approach with elements of British STRUCTURAL FUNCTIONALISM, Mary Douglas (1970) has sought to delineate the rules which generate food behaviour, as well as linking food taboos to social organization and structural categories.

These developments in structural anthropology were parallelled by the study of nutrition in tribal and peasant societies inspired by an interest in MEDICAL ANTHROPOLOGY. This generated a series of works examining the relationship between diet, nutrition, deficiency diseases and sociocultural factors. The approach taken in these studies, like that of the ecological anthropologists, tends to oppose the structuralist and social structuralist view of food practices as symbolic and/or social structural elements.

The resolution of this opposition may perhaps be found, as Levitas suggests, in the development of a historical approach which recognizes that ADAPTIVE STRATEGIES concerning food also involve the manipulation of cognitive-symbolic domains. Jack Goody's study (1982) therefore breaks new ground by taking into account the historical perspective. Goody explores the relationship between food systems and socioeconomic structures, linking food habits to specific MODES OF PRODUCTION and systems of COMMUNICATION. He views the culture of food accordingly not solely as a symbolic or normative structure, but rather as a product of specific historical processes, such that changes in food habits are therefore seen as products of changing social and class relations.

foraging. A term equivalent to the term GATHERING which is applied to the food-seeking activities or strategies of animals and also of humans.

forces of production. See MATERIAL FORCES OF PRODUCTION.

Forde, Daryll (1902–73). A scholar known for the breadth of his interests and especially for his wide-ranging contributions to the anthropology of Africa. Forde explored in his works – among other areas – the fields of kinship and marriage, the relations between environment and society, and the manner in which anthropology as practised by members of dominant cultures should stimulate and interact with anthropology as practised by indigenous scholars. Major works include *Marriage and Family among the Yako* (1941), *The Context of Belief* (1958), *Habitat, Economy and Society* (1963), and *Yako Studies* (1964).

formal analysis. A series of techniques for the analysis of ETHNOTAXONOMIES. Formal analyses have been applied to the study of KINSHIP TERMINOLOGIES, COLOUR TERMS, and ETHNOBOTANY, to name a few well-known examples, and potentially, they may be applied to any cognitive-linguistic domain. Formal analyses, also called 'formal semantic analyses' because they focus on areas of particular SEMANTIC significance, have been developed as tools of ETHNOGRAPHIC research and interpretation within COGNITIVE ANTHROPOLOGY. When addressing themselves to the problems of cross-cultural TRANSLATION, cognitive anthropologists employ these techniques to avoid the pitfalls of ethnocentric or otherwise incomplete interpretations of the linguistic – and therefore cultural – systems of other peoples. Formal analyses aim to delineate the range of meanings or referents of each term in an indigenous taxonomy or terminology as exactly as possible, avoiding the tendency to translate terms to their nearest equivalent in the ethnographer's language wihout taking into account that their exact range of reference is considerably different. For example, in the study of kin terms, formal analyses aim to specify the exact range of persons referred to by each term, without prejudging the 'meaning' of the term on the basis of one of its referents. Formal techniques such as COMPONENTIAL ANALYSIS and transformational analysis have the advantage of allowing us to perceive relationships between the properties of kinship terminologies which are otherwise conceptualized as abstract structures. Buchler and Selby (1968), referring to the overall aims which characterize such analyses, remark that meaning has been restricted to attempts to map precisely the semantic components necessary to define kin-class assignment, attempts that owe much of their inspiration to modern linguistics, both structural and generative and add that the object has been, first, to discover the least number of criteria that would distinguish one kin term from another: 'Next, an analysis of the system is made, in which various formal orderings of the data are used to describe the relationships between classes of kin. The hope is that such structuring of the data will make it easier to understand and compare, and also that the anthropologist's arrangements correspond to and are predictive of natural ordering, that is, the ordering that "makes sense" to the native informant.'

As this statement makes quite clear, formal analysis is merely a technique or a tool which does not in itself supply the necessary theoretical or interpretative model upon which the anthropological hypothesis is built. However, much of the opposition to formal analyses in kinship studies has been in reality opposition not to the technique itself but to the theoretical positions with which it has been associated, as when Scheffler and Lounsbury employ it in support of their hypothesis on the EXTENSION OF KINSHIP TERMS.

Formal semantic analyses essentially aim to discover the dimensions of semantic contrast which are employed by the native speaker, and a formal analysis of a terminology should generate a model which replicates the original data, presenting it both as a set of basic elements and a set of rules for operating upon these elements, so that the entire system may be generated in as economical a manner as possible.

formalism/substantivism. A debate within ECONOMIC ANTHROPOLOGY which was prominent for a time, between the formalist position, which held that neo-classical economic models could with due modification be applied to pre-capitalist economies, and the substantivist position, which argued that radically different models of economic behaviour and structure needed to be developed for pre-capitalist economies. Formalists such as FIRTH and Robbins Burling therefore argued that any economic system can be viewed as the outcome of MARKET forces, reflecting the cumulative effects of MAXIMIZATION by individuals. Substantivists, on the other hand, following POLANYI, claimed that these principles of neo-classical economics applied only to market-dominated economies, not to those dominated by REDISTRIBUTION or RECIPROCITY. Marxist economic anthropology remained at the margin of this debate, regarding the issue of RATIONALITY or non-rationality as irrelevant, since individual maximization could for them determine the structure of economic systems in no instance, as that structure is in fact a product of institutional and class structures.

formal semantic analysis. See COMPONENTIAL ANALYSIS; FORMAL ANALYSIS; TRANSFORMATIONAL LINGUISTICS.

Fortes, Meyer (1906–83). British social anthropologist who was trained by SELIGMAN, MALINOWKSI and FIRTH and later worked closely with EVANS-PRITCHARD, RADCLIFFE-BROWN and GLUCKMAN. Fortes had previously been trained in psychology, and his psychological interests continued to manifest themselves in his studies of family and kinship. His classic studies of the Tallensi and later the Ashanti were seminal in the development of British STRUCTURAL FUNCTIONAL and DESCENT theory. These interpretations of Tallensi and Ashanti society strongly coloured his theoretical approach in such areas as LINEAGE THEORY, the study of RELIGION and ANCESTOR worship, and he has been charged by LEACH among others with elevating to the level of general anthropological theory the particular observations that he made in these ethnographic contexts. Major works include *The Dynamics of Clanship among the Tallensi* (1945), *The Web of Kinship among the Tallensi* (1959), *Oedipus and Job in West African Religion* (1959), *Kinship and the Social Order* (1969), and *Time and Social Structure* (1970).

Fortune, Reo Franklin (1903–79). British social anthropologist who made important contributions to Oceanian anthropology. His best-known work is *Sorcerers of Dobu* (1932).

Foster, George McClelland (1913–). This North American cultural anthropologist is well-known for his studies of Mesoamerican communities and his hypotheses regarding PEASANT culture in general (*see* LIMITED GOOD).

Fourth World. A further subdivision of the conventional categorization of nations according to their degree of DEVELOPMENT (*see* THIRD WORLD). The Fourth World is composed of those lesser-developed nations which have the lowest levels of per capita income, generally those which have no access to important natural resources and/or those with extremely low local levels of manufacturing industry development. Those countries generally considered as part of the Fourth World are the lesser-developed nations of Africa and Asia.

Foustel de Coulanges, Numa-Denys (1830–89). French scholar whose work on religion and society, *The Ancient City* (1864), was influential in the development of DURKHEIM's functionalist theory.

fraternal polyandry. *See* ADELPHIC POLYANDRY.

Frazer, Sir **James George** (1854–1941). Scottish classicist who extended his field of study to include ethnographic data from a vast range of sources in his attempt at the construction of a universal theory of the evolution of MAGIC, RELIGION and SOCIETY. Frazer had a great influence on the literary and intellectual culture of his day, but in anthropology itself he has been much criticized for the idealist and non-empirical nature of his work. Anthropologists like MALINOWSKI in Britain and BOAS in the USA strongly rejected the 'speculative history' and 'armchair anthropology' which he epitomized in favour of research strategies of detailed ethnographic enquiry and documentation. Major works by Frazer include *The Golden Bough* (1926–36), which is his most celebrated and wide ranging synthesis of worldwide examples of the development of religion, and *Totemism and Exogamy* (1910).

Freud, Sigmund (1856–1939). Austrian physician who specialized in nervous disorders, and whose theories of individual psychology and of mental illness have had profound and far-reaching effects in modern intellectual culture. Freud founded PSYCHOANALYSIS, and the ramifications and influences of many of the fundamental concepts he developed in this area may be traced in a number of intellectual fields far wider than the limited circle of 'orthodox Freudian' thinking within psychiatry. In the social sciences, most of Freud's writings directly about the origins and nature of society have not been widely influential, and have been dismissed by many as dubious extensions of his theories of individual psychology. However, his indirect influence here – as in all fields of intellectual enquiry – cannot be denied, and in the anthropological field his theories of individual psychology have been of great importance in the development of PSYCHOLOGICAL ANTHROPOLOGY, the anthropology of RELIGION and KINSHIP studies.

The study of hysteria among his patients prompted Freud early in his career to focus on the functions of fantasy and dreams, and on the existence of sexual drives in the pre-adult stages of development. This exploration of infantile sexuality was to prove the most controversial element in his work in many circles. He contended however that experiences in early childhood were decisive in forming the adult personality and its dynamics. Freud employed what has been termed a 'hydraulic model' of the basic drives or instincts underlying mental phenomena. These drives (the sexual and reproductive instinct or *eros* and the destructive and aggressive instinct or THANATOS) generate energy which, it is assumed, seeks an outlet or expression in the behaviour of the individual. The discharge of this psychic energy he termed *cathexis*, and in his theory of the psychosexual development of the individual he traced the stages through which the focusing of this energy normally progressed: from the oral stage, through the anal stage, to the genital stage of sexuality. Early in his work Freud introduced the distinction between conscious, pre-conscious and unconscious areas of mental activity, and initiated the development of therapeutic techniques for the study of the unconscious domain, an area not normally available to ordinary consciousness. Prominent among these techniques are those of dream analysis and free association. Later Freud refined his model, distinguishing the id, ego and superego. The id is the unconscious reservoir of basic instincts or drives, and operates according to the pleasure principle. The ego or conscious self represents the reality principle and develops as a result of interaction with the environment. The superego develops as a result of processes of identification with parental figures and internalization of their values or expectations.

In his study of the development of society, the family and religion, Freud posited that early evolutionary stages of society paralleled stages of individual psychological development. He extended, for example, his theory of the Oedipus complex to the development of the INCEST taboo in human society, arguing that this was instituted as a result of early man's guilt at the crime of parricide committed in order to secure sexual access to the mother. Freud's theories of the universality of the Oedipus conflict were called into question and subjected to cross-cultural testing by a variety of ethnographers from the 1930s on.

His major works of interest to anthropology include *The Interpretation of Dreams* (1900), *Totem and Taboo* (1913), *The Future of an Illusion* (1927), and *Civilisation and its Discontents* (1929).

friendship. Friendship has been little studied in cross-cultural perspective, and ethnographers have perhaps paid most attention to institutions such as 'formal friendship' where the obligations and rights of each partner are carefully specified, than to informal and diffuse relationships or NETWORKS of friends. Formal friendships may take the form of trading partnerships with specified obligations, of working partnerships, or of RITUAL KINSHIP. Friendship might be regarded by many as an illegitimate or useless anthropological category, since the definition of friendship and the uses to which it is put in different cultures are so variable, and since behaviour of a type which we in Western society would identify as friendship may be associated in other cultures with specific social institutions such as AGE SETS or other kinds of voluntary and involuntary association. The basic common characteristics of relations of friendship in Western society are first of all their optional nature in that they are not prescribed by the structure of kin or other social relations but are formed by individuals as a result of their inclinations and choices, and secondly the altruistic or mutually supportive behaviour which is expected between friends. The study of friendship is part of the study of social networks, of RECIPROCITY, and of the relationships created by individuals in the social space which is left undetermined by the system of kin or other obligatory relationships. We might thus assume friendship to be more highly developed in those societies where there is a wider range of persons not classified as kinsmen or not standing in another type of fixed or obligatory relationship to Ego. However there is little cross-cultural evidence of the extent and nature of friendships, nor of the different cultural definitions of friendship in comparison with other types of relationship in small-scale or pre-capitalist societies, upon which to base such a hypothesis.

frontier. The concept of frontier has been employed in the study of inter-ethnic relations to conceptualize the penetration and interpenetration of different ethnic groups or culture-bearers in processes of MIGRATION and DEVELOPMENT. The frontier may be a demographic one, when one population or ethnic group expands into the territory of another, for example; an economic one, where a territory is exploited by, or annexed to, another for the purposes of extractive or other economic activities; a military or political one if military or political institutions are extended to a new territory; an ideological one if missionizing, educational or propaganda activities are being carried out, and so on. Of course, all of these different kinds of frontier may be present in any one empirical context. The differentiation of kinds of frontier allows us to conceptualize separate aspects of the process of colonization, or of domination of one territory or population by another. Frontier social relationships are of special interest to anthropologists concerned with culture contact and with ETHNICITY and development.

function. This term has several different meanings, and the failure to define it with sufficient precision has led to considerable confusion and debate about functionalist theory in the social sciences. In mathematics, 'function' refers to the association between variables: one variable which depends upon another is said to be a function of it. In biology, it refers to the contribution made by one organ, or part of an organism, to the life of the organism as a whole. In the social sciences, early functionalist theory such as that of SPENCER in Britain and that of DURKHEIM in France employed the biological or organic analogy in their studies of human society, and this was taken up by RADCLIFFE-BROWN and MALINOWSKI, who suggested that the constituent parts of society or social institutions functioned together and in mutual dependence as an integrated whole. The notion of function thus embraces several different though overlapping areas of enquiry: the contribution which each part makes to the functioning of the whole, the functional interrelationships which exist between different parts within a total organism or system, and in addition the functional equilibrium or disequilibrium of a total system or organism. (*See* FUNCTIONALISM.)

functionalism. A term applied to theories or models in the social sciences which explain social and cultural institutions, relations and behaviour in terms of the functions which they perform in sociocultural systems. Functionalist theory in anthropology may be traced back at least to SPENCER, who was one of the first social theorists to employ the ORGANIC ANALOGY in his interpretation of sociocultural EVOLUTION. In France, DURKHEIM also laid the foundations for functionalist theory in the social sciences, contributing many key concepts which were later to influence the British STRUCTURAL FUNCTIONALIST school in particular. While 19th-century theorists like Spencer employed the organic analogy in conjunction with evolutionary theories of social development, modern functionalist theory in anthropology is associated especially with MALINOWSKI who rejected the evolutionary speculations of the early social theorists and put forward instead a functionalist theory which has often been criticized as ahistorical. Malinowski (1926) argued that the existence of any custom, social institution or social relation should be interpreted in terms of its function: that is to say, in terms of its contribution to the satisfaction of 'needs' (both primary physiological and emotional needs and also secondary or social needs). The method of PARTICIPANT OBSERVATION pioneered by Malinowski is also often associated with functionalist theory, though evidently there is no necessary link between participant observation as a method and the acceptance of all the implications of a functionalist approach. In the work of the structural functionalists influenced by Durkheim, the theory of SOCIAL FACTS and Durkheim's insistence on the independence of sociological explanation led to the interpretation of social systems as wholes without reference to psychological, environmental or other types of 'need'.

While in British social anthropology functionalism is generally linked to the ahistoricism of Malinowski and the structural functionalist school represented by RADCLIFFE-BROWN, FORTES and others, in US cultural anthropology functionalist and 'neo-functionalist' theories have been associated instead with evolutionary and ecological anthropology. However the theoretical problems of combining functionalist models with their assumptions of EQUILIBRIUM and evolutionary or processual models have not been satisfactorily resolved as yet in these fields, and functional theories continue to be criticized as either tautological, teleological or trivial. They are tautological or circular in the sense that since they emphasize the systematic interconnectedness of sociocultural elements, elements are invoked to explain each other. They are teleological (explaining a cause by its effect) where they explain a phenomenon in terms of its contribution to the stability or 'needs' of the total system, disregarding the immediate causes and motivations which are necessary in order to give rise to the phenomenon. And finally they are trivial where the analyst, aware of the pitfalls of tautology and teleology, creates so many subcategories and surrounds the analysis with so many cautionary observations that it explains nothing.

A common criticism of functionalist theory is that it fails to take into account the phenomena of CONFLICT and disintegrative forces in society, since it always tends to assume the harmonious functioning of the whole. Thus ACTION THEORY and MARXIST ANTHROPOLOGY among others have contested the functionalist perspective, arguing for the study of individual, group and class conflict and competition as factors leading to social and historical change.

fundamentalism. A term generally employed to refer to certain religious SECTS which share a belief in the literal truth of the Bible and its account of the creation of the universe and the human species. The controversy concerning EVOLUTIONARY versus biblical accounts of creation was widely regarded as a dead issue until 10 or 15 years ago, when there was in the USA an upsurge of fundamentalist or 'creationist' movements which declared their opposition to the teaching of evolutionary theory in schools and universities. This anti-scientific trend must be understood in terms of its historical and ideological contexts. In both the USA and the Third World fundamentalism is linked through the activities of MISSIONARY organizations such as the Summer Institute of Linguistics to authoritarian and reactionary political positions. Such institutions portray CAPITALISM and the American Way of Life as divinely ordained, and argue that it is necessary to intervene in both religious and political spheres in order to combat the works of the devil. These are assumed to manifest themselves principally as COMMU-NISM or other forms of anti-religious ideology. In social and political action fundamentalist sects define all that opposes them as demonic, and consider all that aids them to be evidence of the hand of God. The success and popularity of such sects, with their opposition to scientific enquiry and secular ideologies of all kinds, is symptomatic of deep-rooted contradictions in modern North American society, which has always appeared to place high value on scientific and technological achievements.

funeral. *See* MORTUARY RITES.

G

Galton's problem. A recurrent issue in the research of CROSS-CULTURAL COMPARISON. Sir Francis Galton raised an objection to TYLOR's notion of ADHESIONS, or correlations, in cross-cultural research. Basically, Galton's objection concerned the proposed method for ensuring that units selected for comparison were genuinely independent and equivalent. He pointed out that Tylor had not specified how traits which were diffused from one area to another should be distinguished from those which were independently invented, since there was no definition in the method of how population units were to be designated and differentiated for the purposes of comparison.

gambling. Games of chance or skill in which the participants must risk some form of stake, which they stand to lose or multiply dependent upon their success in the game. The gamblers may play the game themelves, or they may simply gamble upon the chances of others or upon the outcome of any given event or activity. James Woodburn has pointed out that gambling may be a major pastime among HUNTING AND GATHERING peoples such as the Hadza of Tanzania, who have plenty of free time left over from basic subsistence activities. Some forms of DIVINATION are akin to gambling in that they submit decisions, judgments, and so on to chance, supposing that divine or spiritual intervention will determine the outcome. Recreational forms of gambling are found in many different kinds of society, but within modern capitalist systems gambling has acquired a special and ambiguous status. On the one hand it is regarded as immoral, while on the other it is at least partly institutionalized. Countries vary, however, in the amount and types of gambling (such as lotteries, horse racing, casinos) which are permitted within the framework of

the state or of legitimate business enterprise. Gambling is one of the activities which is both approved and disapproved of by the dominant classes, since on the one hand it offers the possibility of financial gain without work because it militates against the 'work ethic' but on the other it is a useful palliative and a distraction from the root causes of the inequality of wealth. State and privately-run lotteries are with other gambling activities with a popular and important institution in many countries among the lower and lower-middle classes, using the image of ordinary people who suddenly become rich as a distraction from real social and economic problems. Gambling among the rich performs a different function as a form of conspicuous or prestige consumption only available to the wealthy, and takes different forms from those found among the poorer sectors. There are as yet few anthropological studies of gambling and of the links between the many forms it takes, its popularity, and other aspects of attitudes and WORLD VIEW. It would be interesting, for example, to examine cross-culturally the notions of chance and profit and the items or commodities which are or not liable to be wagered.

game. *See* PLAY.

game theory. A theory of individual decision-making or strategy in which the subject has only an imperfect knowledge of the outcome. The game model assumes that a number of persons are in competition for some desired reward or resource, and that there are a limited number of available strategies, but that each player is unaware of the strategy to be adopted by any of the others. Game theory thus extends conventional microeconomic theory of decision-making to situations where more than one 'player' or 'firm' is involved, and where there is a degree of uncertainty about the outcome of any given decision, since the unknown strategy of others may affect the result. Games are defined either as 'zero-sum', where one player's gain is the other's loss (*see* LIMITED GOOD), or 'non-zero-sum', where co-operative strategies or coalitions may produce benefits for both, some or all of the participants. One of the important concepts developed within game theory is that of MINIMAX strategies which bring about an intermediate result by minimizing possible losses and maximizing possible gains at the same time. Game theory is most useful in its expansion of the decision-making model to account for co-operative and conflictive behaviour, and the balance between the two in the determination of individual strategies.

gathering. Gathering or foraging is a subsistence strategy involving the collection of wild or naturally-occurring food resources such as plants, eggs, and small animals. Societies entirely dependent on HUNTING AND GATHERING are nowadays comparatively rare, since AGRICULTURAL techniques of one sort or another have been either diffused throughout, or imposed upon, most of the world's regions. However, in some areas such as the Amazon basin hunting and gathering persist among the majority of indigenous groups as important elements of subsistence alongside HORTICULTURE, while some of the more isolated groups continue to subsist by hunting and gathering alone. In the debate and discussion about hunting and gathering societies, it has been argued by some that excessive emphasis has been placed on the social, symbolic and nutritional importance of hunting, a predominantly masculine activity, and insufficient emphasis on the predominantly female activity of food gathering. Such critics point out that in the so-called 'hunting' societies a large proportion of the food consumed is in fact contributed by women's gathering activities, though often little prestige is accorded to these in comparison with male hunting. Those writers who emphasize the importance of protein resources in hunting and gathering societies as determining factors in population distribution and density have contended that the superior prestige accorded to hunting reflects the greater importance of animal protein in comparison with the carbohydrates provided mainly by gathered foodstuffs, and it has also been pointed out that hunting is often a more dangerous, less routine and more uncertain activity than gathering. It is argued, therefore, that it tends to attract more prestige and symbolic or magical importance. (*See* GENDER.)

Gemeinschaft/Gesellschaft. A conceptual dichotomy developed by the German sociologist Ferdinand Tonnies (1887; trans. 1955), and variously translated as community and society, community and organization, or community and association. *Gemeinschaft* or community is characterized by Tonnies as dominated by kinship and moral bonds, producing a relatively homogeneous, cohesive and traditional social order. *Gesellschaft* on the other hand refers to a social order where impersonal contractual relationships predominate, as in urban industrial society. These concepts influenced REDFIELD's formulation of the FOLK-URBAN CONTINUUM.

gender. In modern anthropology this term has increasingly replaced the term 'sex' in discussions of socially and culturally determined differences in the behaviour, role and status of men and women. The term 'gender' when used with reference to languages, is applied to the classification of nouns into categories conventionally called masculine, feminine or neutral. More recently it has been used to refer to the social, cultural and psychological patterning of differences between males and females. The distinction between sex, which is a biological phenomenon, and gender, which is a cultural classification, allows for the separation of the biological and cultural aspects of differences between males and females, thus avoiding a biological determinist position. Gender identity is conveyed and structured by both verbal and non-verbal means, and recent interest has focused on, among other things, the manner in which gender classifications are influenced by the semantic structure of language. Thus Lakoff (1975) has suggested that generic terms in language may influence cognitive structures and attitudes towards gender. Where the generic term for a class or entity which may be sexually differentiated is the male one, and the female term is the 'marked' one of the pair, it is argued that this language both reflects and helps to perpetuate attitudes of male dominance and superiority. The use of the term 'man' to mean human beings in general, while 'woman' refers only to females, is a good example. Studies of the changes in gender-marked terms in Indo-European languages have shown that female terms consistently tend to undergo changes in meaning, acquiring pejorative connotations, while male ones do not. This phenomenon may be observed in the terms 'bachelor' and 'spinster': 'bachelor' conserves its original meaning of single man, while 'spinster' has acquired the negative or pejorative connotation of 'old maid'.

Lakoff has studied sex differences in the use of American English, claiming to find differences in vocabulary (for example the greater use by women of 'empty' adjectives such as 'cute'), more use of question forms where men tend to use affirmations, more polite forms, more 'hedging' and also more 'correct' forms, and so on. Empirical testing of these claims is incomplete and the results somewhat contradictory, but Lakoff has pioneered an important area which requires further investigation and more sophisticated testing methods in order to ascertain the relationships between social position (including social class and other factors besides gender identity) and language use. (*See* WOMEN AND ANTHROPOLOGY; LINGUISTIC ANTHROPOLOGY; SEXUAL DIVISION OF LABOUR.)

genealogical amnesia. In societies where GENEALOGY is of importance, certain genealogical links or ancestors may be omitted from genealogical reckoning or 'forgotten'. It is often assumed that the suppression of certain persons from accounts of ancestry generally follows a regular pattern: those who do not have descendants or who are not important points of reference as far as the present-day social and kinship structure are concerned tend to be those who are most readily forgotten. This may not always be so, however, and the empirical evidence in any given case must always be investigated. (*See* DESCENT; LINEAGE THEORY.)

genealogical fiction. A phenomenon related to GENEALOGICAL AMNESIA, whereby genealogies may be adjusted to suit better the requirements of the present-day social and kinship structure or the interests of the person or group concerned. Actual genea-

logical ties may be forgotten or suppressed and new ones substituted. This process of readjustment or reconstruction of genealogies reveals aspects of the interplay between the 'ideal models' of kinship structure and the realities of relationships between persons and groups. (*See* DESCENT; LINEAGE THEORY.)

genealogy. A record or account of relationships of DESCENT. Genealogies are important in LINEAGE or descent-based kinship systems, since they provide the basis for membership in kin groups. In different societies with descent systems of varying types we may observe that there are degrees of importance attached to genealogies, in their time-depth and their detail. Some societies are more genealogically conscious than others, and there in addition may be genealogical specialists who retain specialist knowledge of ancestry in more detail than ordinary people. The possibilities of individuals or groups manipulating genealogies or shaping them selectively have been studied within lineage and descent theory as reflections of the characteristics of present day social and kinship structure.

generalized exchange. *See* ASYMMETRIC/ SYMMETRIC ALLIANCE.

generation. A term sometimes used loosely to refer to persons of roughly the same AGE or AGE GROUP, when speaking of intergenerational conflict or differences in society as a whole. More precisely, however, it refers to the relative position of persons within a genealogy or within the reproductive cycle of a family. Thus persons of the same age may be of different generations, and persons of the same generation may vary widely in age, due to the long period of time during which a person or a couple may continue to reproduce.

generational terminology. In the study of KINSHIP TERMINOLOGY, this refers to a system where LINEAL and COLLATERAL relatives are not distinguished, all same-sex relatives of the same generation being referred to by the same term. MORGAN called this the 'Hawaiian' system and postulated that it originated in the practice of GROUP MARRIAGE.

generative grammar. *See* TRANSFORMA-TIONAL LINGUISTICS.

genetrix. Following the distinction originally made between GENITOR and *pater* some anthropologists have similarly distinguished the 'sociological mother' or *mater*, who is the woman through whom the child is linked to other kin, from the biological mother or *genetrix*. In most cases, however, the biological and sociological mother are the same person.

genitor. The biological father of a child, as opposed to the sociological father or *pater*. The distinction derives from Roman law, where the *pater* was considered to be the mother's husband, regardless of the physiological paternity of the child. (*See* SOCIOLOGICAL PATERNITY; CONCEPTION.)

genocide. The policy or practice of systematic extermination of a people or ETHNIC GROUP. The term was first applied to the Nazi persecution of Jews and other ethnic minorities. Genocidal policies have also been applied to indigenous groups in many parts of the world, especially where they have stood in the way of DEVELOPMENT and colonization projects of a dominant national or foreign interest. The cultural extermination of minority or ethnic groups, as opposed to their physical extermination, is called ETHNOCIDE.

genotype. The genetic or hereditary potential of an organism. In interaction with the environment, this produces the 'phenotype' or observable manifestation.

gens. US anthropology follows MORGAN in generally adopting this term to refer to a patrilineal SIB, or 'patrisib', which is a group of two or more patrilineages related by common descent from a mythological ancestor. In British anthropology such a unit is conventionally termed CLAN, but US anthropology reserves this term for the 'matrisib' or group of related matrilineages.

gerontocracy. A system of social STRATIFICATION marked by the dominance of the old, generally the old men of a group, over the young. This dominance may be based on control over MEANS OF PRODUCTION such as

land and property, on control over access to wives and sexual partners, and/or on symbolic and religious systems which allot important functions to the elderly on the basis of their superior knowledge or position. Such age-based stratification is egalitarian in the sense that all members of society have access to superior status with the passing of time. But the degree of subordination of younger to older people may be considerable, as in certain Australian aboriginal groups where old men control access to women and keep for themselves the young girls as wives, while young men are unable to marry. Similarly, in some LINEAGE-based societies, the power and authority of lineage elders is considerable, and their control over younger generations may be based on ties of authority between individuals within the lineage, or on the collective relationship of elders to younger AGE GRADES or AGE SETS.

Gesellschaft. *See* GEMEINSCHAFT/GESELLSCHAFT.

Gestalt theory. A psychological theory of perception which emphasizes the tendency to register thoughts or experience as 'wholes' or CONFIGURATIONS. Gestalt theory places importance on the type of perception which 'completes' a slightly incomplete figure, operating automatically to supply the missing elements of the total configuration. This approach was influential in the development of CULTURE AND PERSONALITY theories.

gift. The subject of the gift has been central to anthropology since MAUSS' classic study (1954). Inspired among other material by MALINOWSKI's account of the KULA, by accounts of the POTLATCH and so on, Mauss developed a theory of the gift which he intended to be applicable to all 'primitive' or 'archaic' societies. He pointed to the existence of a kind of elementary morality of RECIPROCITY, a theme developed by LEVI-STRAUSS in his theories of ALLIANCE, and which has also been extremely influential in ECONOMIC ANTHROPOLOGY. Mauss points to three fields of obligation: to give, to recieve and to repay. Gifts, according to Mauss, create relationships not only between individuals but between groups, relationships which take the form of total

PRESTATIONS. The obligation to repay is linked to the belief that the gift retains a spiritual relationship to the giver in systems where things are 'parts of persons' and social identity, status and prestige are thus at stake in gift exchange. Elements of this morality are present in modern gift exchange, but they are largely eclipsed by the MARKET type of exchange which dominates the modern economy.

glottochronology. See LEXICOSTATISTICS.

Gluckman, Max (1911–75). British social anthropologist who made important contributions in the fields of African anthropology, the ANTHROPOLOGY OF LAW and the study of RITUAL. Gluckman is often associated with what is loosely termed the FUNCTIONAL or STRUCTURAL FUNCTIONAL school of British social anthropology, though in fact there are many discrepancies between his theories and those of FORTES or other anthropologists considered to form part of this school. Gluckman advocated a Marxist approach which stressed the existence of conflict within social structures, as opposed to the emphasis on consensus and norm convergence in functionalist social theory. However many would argue that Gluckman modified the functionalist model rather than radically opposing it, since for example in his studies of RITUAL REBELLION and CONFLICT resolution he tends to conclude that ritual expressions of conflict ultimately reinforce the existing social structure. Major works include *Essays on Lozi Land and Royal Property* (1943); *Rituals of Rebellion in SE Africa* (1954); *Custom and Conflict in Africa* (1955); (ed.) *Essays in the Ritual of Social Relations* (1962); *Order and Rebellion in Tribal Africa* (1963); *Politics, Law and Religion in Tribal Society* (1965).

godparents. See COMPADRAZGO; FICTIVE KINSHIP; RITUAL KINSHIP.

Goodenough, Ward Hunt (1919–). US cultural anthropologist who is well-known generally for his contributions to the study of KINSHIP systems and particularly for his development of the methodology of COMPONENTIAL ANALYSIS. Goodenough is an important figure in COGNITIVE ANTHROPOLOGY. Major works include: 'Componential

Analysis and the Study of Meaning', *Language* (1956); *Description and Comparison in Cultural Anthropology* (1970); *Culture, Language and Society* (1971).

gossip. The interchange of information within social groups about people and their behaviour. The term implies that the information may be either distorted or transmitted with malicious intent. However it is impossible to separate gossip as such from the transmission of other kinds of information among networks of social relationships. It is often stated that gossip is one of the mechanisms of SOCIAL CONTROL, because it is believed that one of the sanctions of great importance in small-scale societies is exposure to the censure of public opinion (*see* LAW, ANTHROPOLOGY OF). However this emphasis on the positive function of gossip should be weighed against the tremendous potential for CONFLICT which gossip generates. In both small-scale societies and restricted social groups within large-scale societies it may in itself constitute a major social problem as far as the perceptions of members of the group are concerned. Gossip as an anti-social activity is part of the configurations of values and attitudes which have been observed in certain small-scale or PEASANT communities, which some anthropologists have tried to relate to a dominant or prevailing set of values such as the LIMITED GOOD or the notion of AMORAL FAMILISM. It is an important element of ethnographic exploration of social and group relationships, because it reveals and reinforces social boundaries and sociopolitical or FACTIONAL divisions.

government. A set of public OFFICES concerned with the administration of the internal and external affairs of a social group. (*See* POLITICAL ANTHROPOLOGY.)

grammar. In its traditional sense, this term was defined by Bloomfield (1933) as 'the meaningful arrangements of forms in a language'. This essentially static view of grammar as a set of rules for the arrangement of forms has given way in recent years to a more dynamic conception in terms of the concepts of TRANSFORMATION and generative grammar. (*See* DEEP AND SURFACE STRUCTURE.)

great and little tradition. Terms employed by REDFIELD (1956) in his studies of PEASANT society and culture, in order to contrast the formal literate tradition of an urban elite with the largely oral and informal tradition of the peasant community. Thus great and little traditions are complementary aspects of a single CIVILIZATION. Elements of the little tradition are constantly taken up into and reinterpreted by the great tradition, and elements of the great tradition similarly filter down to the little tradition where they are reinterpreted or transformed in accordance with local customs and values. The contrast between great and little traditions corresponds in large part with the urban/rural division, since the great tradition is maintained by an urban-based elite and the little tradition by rural peasant communities. The conception of the dialectical relationship between elite and popular culture is of course applicable not only to peasant societies, and a similar relationship pertains in all class-based societies, which may be analysed from the point of view of the interrelationship between politico-economic dominance and ideological systems (*see* HEGEMONY). While Redfield regarded the culture of tribal peoples as autonomous, it is also now widely recognized in modern anthropology that the vast majority of tribal peoples too exist within the context of continuing interaction with dominant regional and national societies. (*See* FOLK-URBAN CONTINUUM; RELIGION.)

green revolution. A series of technological innovations permitting an increased yield of grain crops for each plant. The high cost of green revolution technology has meant that it has paradoxically further impoverished the rural and peasant populations of the Third World instead of benefiting them. (*See* AGRIBUSINESS; DEVELOPMENT.)

group marriage. This concept, which is related to that of PRIMITIVE PROMISCUITY, refers to a type of MARRIAGE rule in which the sexual and economic rights and obligations of the marriage relationship are held in common among a group of men and women. In 19th- and early 20th-century kinship theory the debate regarding group marriage was of central importance. MORGAN, for example, held that this was the earliest form of marriage, while others argued for the primacy of PATRIARCHAL, monogamous, or MATRIARCHAL forms. Later, interest in this controversy declined as both US cultural and British social anthropology devoted themselves instead to the exploration and documentation of the variety of existing systems of kinship and marriage. With the works of LEVI-STRAUSS, however, interest in the evolution of structures of kinship and ALLIANCE was revived, but the notion of group marriage is foreign to the Levi-Straussian conception of a human society ordered even from its very origin by principles of communication and reciprocity between groups.

gypsies. Nomadic or semi-nomadic peoples found throughout the world. The term derives from the English word 'Egyptians'. The Romany language spoken by gypsies is of Hindu origin. Gypsies and their mode of life have attracted the attention of ethnographers to a limited extent, particularly the processes of isolation and self-isolation which maintain them at the margin of the wider community, and the symbolization by both gypsy and non-gypsy groups of their relationships in terms of stereotypical social, moral and supernatural attributes.

H

hallucinogens. Substances which induce hallucinations, or the perception of objects when no objects are present. The visual aspect of hallucinations ('visions') is usually stressed in reports of the effects of hallucinogenic DRUGS, though hallucinations may in fact involve other senses as well as the visual. Many authors, following the lead of Eliade, have stressed the central role played by hallucinatory experiences in the complex of curing practices and religious beliefs associated with SHAMANISM. Hallucinations are part of ALTERED STATES OF CONSCIOUSNESS, which may be induced by a variety of means including fasting and other physical ordeals, but in cultures where hallucinations are accorded importance there is generally a well-developed native pharmacopeia of hallucinogenic plants which are prepared in order to induce hallucinations with greater facility. The use and preparation of these plants is the specialized area of skill of the shaman, who is an expert in the techniques of achieving altered states of consciousness as well as in channelling the experiences obtained in these states towards socially acceptable ends. In cultures where shamanism is competitive and aggressive, such as those of many Amazonian groups, the shaman may also seek support through 'visions' in order to attack other persons or groups. Michael Harner's descriptions of the complex of beliefs and practices surrounding Jivaro shamanism are a well-known example of this type (1973).

Various substances are employed in order to induce hallucinations, ranging from tobacco to species of vines, mushrooms and plants indigenous to the region concerned. P. Furst (1972) surveys some of the better-known hallucinogenic substances employed in different historical and geographical contexts. One of the recurring themes in the studies of the application of hallucinogens within shamanistic cultures is the profound spiritual and philosophical significance which many authors attach to the hallucinatory experience. Harner claims that the Jivaro believe that everyday reality is an illusion, while hallucinatory experience is 'real'. Similarly Carlos Castaneda's (1970) famous accounts of Yaqui shamanism attribute profound significance to the shaman's visionary experiences and the development of his knowledge and understanding through the progressive exploration of the reality they reveal.

In shamanistic cultures, there is generally great emphasis on the shaman or initiate learning to control the hallucinatory experience, and progressively becoming able to cope with more and more powerful doses of hallucinogens. The hallucinatory experience within shamanistic cultures is thus carefully structured, and subject to a series of culturally patterned interpretations which permit the initiate to incorporate the experience into a universe of cultural and personal meanings. Thus studies of the effects of hallucinogens have revealed that while there are certain common elements because of similarities in chemical action, there are also strong components of cultural tradition and interpretation which condition the response of the subject. In modern Western society hallucinogenic drugs, whether natural or chemically synthesized, are used for recreational purposes to a certain extent. Thus, like alcohol, tobacco, cannabis, cocaine and other substances which were originally employed in sacred or religious contexts, hallucinogens are divested of their religious significance when they are taken up into Western cultural or subcultural patterns.

harmonic/disharmonic. A distinction made by LEVI-STRAUSS in his theory of KINSHIP systems (1949). Harmonic regimes are those where locality (residence) and DESCENT follow the same principle: that is, they are

134

matrilineal and matrilocal or patrilineal and patrilocal. Disharmonic regimes are therefore those where residence and descent rules do not coincide: that is to say, they are matrilineal and patrilocal or patrilineal and matrilocal. Levi-Strauss suggests that restricted EXCHANGE occurs with disharmonic regimes and generalized exchange with harmonic ones.

Hawaiian system. The name given by MORGAN to the GENERATIONAL type of kinship terminology, where LINEAL and COLLATERAL relatives are not distinguished, all same-sex relatives of the same generation being referred to by a single term. Morgan linked this terminology to the existence of the practice of GROUP MARRIAGE.

headman. A term employed to refer to a local political leader within a small-scale community. The term may be used to refer to the leader of a BAND or local group within a HUNTING AND GATHERING or non-centralized TRIBAL society. In this case the headman is the maximal authority within an independent local group, though there may be FACTIONAL alliances or loose agglomerations of local communities, or both, without the existence of any overall political authority beyond the level of the local group. However, many anthropologists reserve the term for a local leader within a centralized political system: that is to say, within a CHIEFDOM or a state society, where he is characterized by his limited local authority and his subordination to a wider system of political offices. (See POLITICAL ANTHROPOLOGY; LEADERSHIP; BIG MAN.)

health. The concept of health is of course variable from culture to culture, and the study of what is considered in each context to be the absence of disease or the state of positive well-being whether physical, psychological, or both, involves not only the study of definitions and theories of disease but also that of all those cultural and social conditions and elements which contribute to the concept of the person and his or her development and relationship to the world and to others (see ETHNOMEDICINE). The subdiscipline of MEDICAL ANTHROPOLOGY has been criticized by some anthropologists and those from other disciplines for focu-

sing, like conventional medicine, on disease rather than on health. If the focus is predominantly on health however, the entire person and his or her social context may be treated, instead of just his or her current physiological condition, and the prevention rather than the treatment of disease can be emphasized.

Standards and concepts of health are not only geographically and culturally but also historically variable, as they change over time in response to changing socioeconomic and cultural patterns and also to prevailing systems and levels of health care. In societies with highly developed systems of conventional medicine, new definitions of disease develop along with new patterns of disease. It is well known that the types of disease and patterns of morbi-mortality have changed with the process of economic development: in developing countries INFANT MORTALITY rates are comparatively high, life expectancy is comparatively short, and the diseases which are the most frequent cause of morbidity and mortality are intestinal and respiratory infections. In developed countries, there are lower rates of infant mortality overall, as well as longer life expectancy, and the emergence of new types of disease such as cancer and heart or circulatory conditions as the main causes of death. In developed countries a separation emerges, which does not as a rule apply to developing countries, between causes of morbidity and causes of mortality. Common diseases which cause mortality in the Third World occur in the developed countries, but are no longer fatal in the majority of cases. This is due to a combination of factors including higher standards of nutrition and the greater availability of medical care. However in those countries with highly-developed systems of medical care, the original expectation that the demand for medical services would decline as higher standards of health for the population were achieved has not been fulfilled. For reasons involving partly the development of ever more sophisticated medical treatments, and partly changing public awareness and definitions of disease and health, the demand for health care is constantly increasing, absorbing more rather than less of national budgets. This is one of the important factors which is stimulating health planners in developed as well as developing countries to rethink the conventional disease-oriented approach to health care.

hegemony. A term sometimes used in a general sense to indicate the political control exercised by one state or nation over others. In Marxist thought the term has been developed in a different sense, following the writings of Gramsci (1971), who employed the term to refer to relations of class dominance. His use of the term encompasses not only political and economic dominance but also the ideological preponderance of the ruling class. Educational, religious and other institutions contribute to the imposition of the attitudes, norms, values and world-view of the ruling class upon society as a whole. There is thus an over-determination or redundancy of class dominance, extending beyond political and economic structures into other social institutions and cultural fields. Hegemony in Gramsci's usage therefore refers to the complex modes by which the ruling class extend their domination and influence throughout society and culture. (*See* CLASS; IDEOLOGY.)

heliocentrism. Applied to the DIFFUSIONIST theory of Eliot Smith and Perry, who held that civilization originated in ancient Egypt from whence it diffused to the rest of the world.

hermeneutics. The original meaning of this term is the interpretation of sacred texts. It has been extended within philosophy and the social sciences to mean the interpretation of or the search for meaning in texts, in human existence, in society, and so on. The philosopher Martin Heidegger employed the term to mean the understanding of the world as the object of human thought and action. Hans-Georg Gadamer (1979) proposed hermeneutics as a method for the social sciences, in opposition to scientism. (*See* CRITICAL THEORY.)

Herskovits, Melville Jean (1895–1963). US anthropologist well known for his African and Afro-American studies. Herskovits was a student of Boas, and was associated throughout his career with Northwestern University. Apart from his contributions to studies of BLACK culture and as a founder of Afro-American anthropology, Herskovits made important contributions to ECONOMIC ANTHROPOLOGY and the theory of ACCULTURATION.

historical materialism. The application of DIALECTICAL MATERIALISM to the specific field of human history.

historical method. *See* HISTORY AND ANTHROPOLOGY.

historical particularism. Anthropological approach associated with BOAS and the CULTURE HISTORICAL school. Boas argued against the general *a priori* evolutionary schemes of 19th-century anthropology and in favour of a detailed examination of the historical and cultural particularities of each ethnographic situation. (*See* CULTURAL RELATIVISM.)

historicism. This term has two distinct senses. It may be used to refer to 'historical relativism'. In anthropology, historical relativism is associated with CULTURAL RELATIVISM and with the CULTURE HISTORY approach of BOAS and others. In the second sense, that employed by POPPER (1957), the term refers to the doctrine or belief that history obeys 'laws' which can be discovered by the social sciences, and that the future development of society can therefore be predicted. Popper thus diverges from earlier usage of the term, and he refers to the doctrines of historical relativism as 'historicism'. Popper's use of the term 'historicism' as a pejorative epithet for Marxist theory has been widely adopted, though it leads to a certain confusion because of its divergence from earlier usage of the term. Historicism in its original sense refers to the thesis that each historical epoch is unique and must be studied and judged on its own terms, contradicting theories which tend to assume that the laws governing human institutions, behaviour and values are unchanging and universally fixed. Marxist theory on the other hand differs from both these positions, for while it argues for relativism in the sense that it rejects the attempt to universalize 'laws' which are in fact historical products of a specific regime of class dominance (for example, it rejects the 'laws' of the market economy enshrined as universal in bourgeois economics), it maintains that the overall evolution of human society may be understood by exploring the laws of development of productive systems. The Marxist position is thus not 'historical relativist', in the sense meant when labelling it 'historicist'.

historicity. In Marxist theory, the historical nature or aspect of phenomena. Historicity, as distinct from HISTORICISM, implies historical relativism less than the need to appreciate phenomena in relation to their historical context.

history and anthropology. The links between history and anthropology have been the subject of considerable debate and discussion. This debate is revealing and productive as far as anthropology is concerned, since many theoretical, methodological and philosophical difficulties are shared by the two disciplines. The relationship between them has been differently defined by different anthropologists, depending upon their conception of the philosophy of history and that of anthropology. LEVI-STRAUSS for example (1963) states that history and anthropology are basically similar in their approaches and in their aims, except that, while history devotes itself to the study of contexts remote in time, anthropology devotes itself to the study of contexts remote in space ('the exotic'). Levi-Strauss locates the fundamental difference between history and anthropology in the fact that while history always focuses on the particular and the individual, anthropology attempts to elucidate the general laws of social organization. He says: 'history organizes its data in relation to conscious expressions of social life, while anthropology proceeds by examining its. unconscious foundations'. He contrasts history with EVOLUTIONARY and DIFFUSIONIST theories, which have proposed cycles or processes which are conjectural and 'ideological' rather than empirical.

Levi-Strauss' views however leave much room for debate, and there are many anthropologists who see the relationship between history and anthropology in different terms. EVANS-PRITCHARD for example (1962) argued for the fundamental affinity of the two disciplines, in the sense that both history and anthropology are humanistic and interpretative, which do not aim at a 'scientific' or lawlike understanding of human social life, but rather at an interpretation and TRANSLATION of social and cultural phenomena. The HISTORICAL PARTICULARISM of BOAS on the other hand postulated the link between the two disciplines in terms of microhistorical study, which as it has been pointed out tends to become so absorbed in the detail of specific local processes that it loses sight of overall historical trends.

Another reaction to the conjectural history of evolutionism was that of MALINOWSKI and of FUNCTIONALIST and STRUCTURAL FUNCTIONALIST anthropology, which rejected history altogether in favour of synchronic analysis of social structure and function. This perspective has been amply criticized for its failure to take into account the dynamics and processual aspect of social life, whether the microprocesses studied within ACTION THEORY or the macroprocesses of historical CHANGE and social DEVELOPMENT.

The contradiction or opposition between evolutionary theory and history presented by Levi-Strauss is also controversial, pointing as it does to a major problem in evolutionary theory, the reconciling of general schemes with local and specific realities. Evolutionary anthropology and MARXIST ANTHROPOLOGY contain within their ranks many different interpretations of this problem, which also raises many philosophical difficulties in terms of the consequences of the different determinisms which are invoked as explanations of general evolution (ecological determinism, historical determinism etc.).

Another aspect of the relationship between the two disciplines is the use of historical materials and historical methods in anthropology. Modern fieldwork has increasingly moved away from exclusive reliance on synchronic analysis and PARTICIPANT OBSERVATION as anthropologists have come to recognize the need to include historical information, both ethnohistory and the historical background to the regional, national and international context of the fieldwork setting. The fieldworker today must therefore be prepared to evaluate documentary, testimonial and other historical sources critically and employ them usefully. The use of these materials is an essential part of modern research, since developments within CRITICAL ANTHROPOLOGY, Marxist anthropology and other theoretical trends have shown the manner in which conventional fieldwork in the past artificially isolated the 'primitive' SOCIETY or CULTURE from its historical, geographical and politico-economic context.

Hobbes, Thomas (1588–1679). English philosopher and social theorist, whose famous dictum regarding human life in the state of nature – 'solitary, poor, nasty, brutish and short' – is often contrasted with ROUSSEAU's image of the 'noble savage' (*see* ENLIGHTENMENT). Hobbes in his *Leviathan*, 1651, argued that the state is a refuge from the natural order of 'war of every man against every man'. The emergence of the state, in which each person abdicates his right to use force in favour of one centralized controlling force, permits the evolution of culture and society within the context of peaceful relations. Thus Hobbes' 'first and fundamental Law of Nature' is 'to seek Peace, and follow it'.

holism. A term used to describe doctrines or tendencies which emphasize that social or historical phenomena must be understood and interpreted in terms of the total context which encompasses them. It may be contrasted with INDIVIDUALISM or METHODOLOGICAL INDIVIDUALISM which holds that explanations of social phenomena must be reducible to explanations of individual behaviour. Anthropology is generally characterized as a holistic discipline which emphasizes the total social and cultural context in the explanation of the structure and patterning of human groups and their behaviour. However modern critiques of the theory, both of the US cultural anthropological tradition and British structural functionalism, have focused more closely on the need to study the dialectical relationship between individual and society/culture. Within ACTION THEORY and PSYCHOLOGICAL ANTHROPOLOGY among other areas, attempts are being made to develop a more sophisticated theoretical apparatus for the study of the relationship between the individual and the whole in anthropology.

hominid. The class of HOMINOID forms including *Homo sapiens* and his nearest evolutionary ancestors. (*See* EVOLUTION, HUMAN.)

hominoid. The living and extinct species of ape and human. (*See* EVOLUTION, HUMAN.)

homosexuality. Homosexuality, or sexual behaviour between persons of the same sex, is a phenomenon which exists universally but is subject to wide variations in its incidence and in the way that society and the culture 'frame' homosexual acts or relationships. The few anthropological studies of this topic have had male homosexuality as their principal focus, with little or no mention of female homosexuality, and have focused especially on ritual homosexuality, which is a feature of INITIATION rites in certain societies. However it is clear that we should distinguish between acts of ritual homosexuality, which are marked off as special and 'abnormal' acts, from homosexual acts and relationships occurring normally in non-ritual contexts. The latter are subject to a wide variety of responses, which range from tolerance and acceptance to severe criticism and punishment. Attitudes towards, and occurrence of, homosexual relationships should be studied as part of the total complex of attitudes towards sex and GENDER in the society under study.

horticulture. A system of cultivation distinguished from AGRICULTURE, although agriculture is indeed sometimes employed to refer to systems of cultivation in general, including horticulture. Horticulture relies on the use of the hoe or digging-stick, while agriculture is distinguished with the use of the plough and draft animals.

household. *See* DOMESTIC GROUP.

housing. *See* ARCHITECTURE AND ANTHROPOLOGY.

Human Relations Area Files (HRAF). The Human Relations Area Files began with the work of MURDOCK in the field of CROSS-CULTURAL COMPARISON. The Cross-Cultural Survey, as it was originally called, set out to compile a database of descriptive information on human cultures worldwide, and grew to a large-scale research organization devoted to the recompilation of information which facilitates cross-cultural comparative study.

Human Relations Movement. A school of thought which originated with Mayo and his famous Hawthorne Studies of industrial relations. Mayo, whose ideas were later developed by Chicago sociologists and applied anthropologists (notably W.F. Whyte), pointed to the frustration of human and social needs within the industrial workplace. These ideas were important in the development of INDUSTRIAL ANTHROPOLOGY.

Hume, David (1711-76). An important figure in the Scottish ENLIGHTENMENT. Hume was a historian and philosopher who argued for empirical observation as the basis for the 'moral sciences', rejecting metaphysical arguments.

hunting. The pursuit and capture of wild animals, including land animals, birds and sea mammals. Pre-agricultural societies have often been characterized as 'hunting societies', though it has been noted that this reflects the prestige and importance attached to hunting by the people themselves rather than an objective assessment of their economy, which in nearly all cases is more dependent on other activities than it is on hunting. Thus the term HUNTING AND GATHERING societies is preferred by modern anthropologists.

hunting and gathering. The hunting and gathering mode of subsistence characterized over 99 per cent of human history, and the domestication of plants and animals is a relatively recent development when the total timespan of human existence on earth is considered. As Lee and Devore have pointed out in their survey of this topic (1968), the hunting and gathering mode of subsistence is the most stable and persistent adaptation to the environment which humans have discovered to date, bearing in mind the apparently uncertain future of agricultural and industrial societies and the threats of an ecological crisis or massive destruction in war. Anthropologists who study the hunting and gathering mode of life thus perform the important task of redres-

sing the 'neolithic bias' of modern anthropology, which has devoted itself almost entirely to the study of organizational forms (tribe, chiefdom, state) which have emerged in comparatively recent times. But it would of course be wrong to suppose that in studying a modern surviving population of hunters and gatherers we are studying an equivalent to a pre-Neolithic hunting and gathering group. Nowhere in the world today do hunters and gatherers live in complete isolation from agricultural peoples or from regional and national societies which encapsulate the pre-agricultural minority and condition its existence. Outside technological, social, politico-economic and cultural influences and pressures have in every case radically transformed the conditions of existence of hunters and gatherers, and such peoples must always be studied within the historical and sociocultural contexts of the wider societies and states which encompass them. The influences and effects of the wider context on hunting and gathering peoples range from obvious examples such as the introduction of metal tools which revolutionizes productive techniques or the pressure on land and other resources which forces the hunter-gatherers to practice their traditional subsistence patterns in ever more reduced spaces, to the complex relations of exchange and interdependence which certain hunter-gatherers have developed with agricultural peoples (for example, the Pygmy–Bantu relationship described by Turnbull). ETHNOCIDAL processes and tendencies also continue to reduce the numbers of hunter-gatherers throughout the world. However, in spite of the growing awareness that contemporary hunter-gatherers are just as subject as other social types to the processes of historical development and inter-ethnic influence, there is a persistent interest in the comparison of contemporary and prehistoric hunting and gathering societies and in the study of the archaeological evidence of the evolution of the hunting and gathering mode of life. Modern studies are however aware of the need to exercise caution in the use of contemporary ethnographic data as evidence of prehistoric conditions.

In the modern world, societies representative of the hunting and gathering mode of subsistence are widely distributed, though in general they are reduced to marginal environments and constitute a tiny fraction of the world's total population. MURDOCK, in a summary of the current status of hunters and gatherers (excluding groups of mounted hunters, sedentary fishermen and incipient tillers, who possess special characteristics of their own) cites the following populations: (a) Africa: Bushmen, Koroca, Pygmies, East African hunters, Ethiopian hunters; (b) Asia: Siberian hunters, Indian hunters, Veddoid hunters, Southeast Asian hunters, Negritos; (c) Oceania: Australian Aborigines; (d) North America: Eskimo, Northeastern Algonquians, Northwestern Athapaskans, Plateau Indians, California Indians, The Great Basin, Gulf Indians, Apache, Seri; (e) South America: Warrau, interior marginal tribes of Southern Venezuela, Amazonian hunters, East Brazilian hunters, Gran Chaco, Ona, Fuegians. Many of the groups mentioned by Murdock are already extinct, and are known only from early ethnographic reports.

The hunting and gathering mode of subsistence has generally been equated within an evolutionary perspective with the BAND level of social organization, since hunting and gathering societies are generally characterized by the existence of small nomadic local groups, but it should be noted that this is not a perfect equation. There are a number of societies for which we have historical, ethnographic or archaeological evidence, which subsisted without agriculture but nevertheless achieved more advanced levels of social organization: this is particularly true of the societies of the Northwest coast region. On the other hand, it has been noted that many contemporary hunter-gatherer peoples are not survivors of pre-agricultural times, but former agriculturalists who have reverted to hunting and gathering for specific historical reasons. This is the case of many of the Amazonian native groups, among whom we find many combinations of subsistence techniques, from groups depending solely on hunting and gathering, to those combining hunting and gathering with varying degrees of HORTICULTURE. Similarly, many of the environments occupied by modern hunting and gathering populations are not typical of the habitats they occupied before the rise of agriculture. Richer environments which were formerly favoured by hunter-gatherers

have been taken over by agriculturalists, leaving the hunter-gatherer populations for the most part only the most isolated and unfavourable environments. The hunting and gathering peoples who survived long enough to be studied by modern anthropology are largely marginal and peripheral groups reduced to such difficult environments. This has contributed to the portrayal of the 'classic' hunter-gatherer population as one in precarious equilibrium with its environment, constantly poised on the verge of destruction by famine and in constant struggle for survival in extreme conditions. It is this image of the hunting and gathering adaptation which M. Sahlins attacks in his well-known definition of the 'original affluent society' (1972). Here he points out that the 'neolithic prejudice' against hunters and gatherers has led to a distortion of the evidence about both prehistoric and contemporary peoples of this type.

Sahlins reviews historical and ethnographic data in order to demonstrate that hunter-gatherers do not in fact work very many hours per day in order to meet their basic subsistence needs. Groups such as the Aborigines of Arnhem Land, the Bushmen, the Hadza of Tanzania, and others, spend comparatively little time in subsistence activities, which are generally sporadic and interspersed with long periods of leisure. Sahlins argues that among these hunting and gathering peoples who are nomadic and thus have few personal possessions, little importance is attached to possessions or to the notion of property in general. Similarly, the idea of accumulation or storage is absent, since the pattern of life is essentially nomadic and opportunistic. He concludes that hunters and gatherers are the original affluent society because they have very few wants, which are easily and simply satisfied using the materials and techniques which are freely available to all.

Ethnographic studies of contemporary hunter-gatherers tend to confirm Sahlins' contention that the working hours of these populations are generally short. Thus many ethnographers report that even the 'marginal' hunter-gatherers often subsist on an average of two to four hours' labour per day and exploit abundant food resources. However it should not be forgotten that many hunter-gatherers today are living in a state of ecological crisis and pressure, often due to the encroachment of agricultural populations and state society on their traditional habitats. The image of the 'original affluent society' would not be applicable to all hunter-gatherers, but this does not detract from the theoretical importance of Sahlins' contribution, which lies in his critique of concepts derived from the economics of scarcity which are applied to pre-agricultural societies whose economy must be understood in terms of radically different premises.

Modern hunter-gatherer studies have been persistently preoccupied with redressing the early male bias which characterized these societies as 'hunters', to the neglect of the real subsistence base which generally includes wild plants, and in some cases fish, in greater proportions than meat. Lee, reviewing the evidence from societies other than the arctic and subarctic areas, concludes that in general hunting of mammals provides only 20 to 40 per cent of the total diet. It is certainly true to say that hunting is surrounded by great prestige and magical importance, while gathering, typically a female activity, is accorded little ritual or weight. So some authors view such prestige and ritual importance when attached to hunting as part of cults of male dominance, while others view them as reflections of the important part that protein plays in the diet of such peoples. Authors who emphasize the role of protein argue that while meat may be a small proportion of the total diet, it is the most important constituent part, and that the scarcity of, access to and distribution of these protein resources is an important factor in the social organization and also in the geographical distribution and political structure of hunting and gathering groups. We may thus contrast SYMBOLIC and ecological interpretations of hunting, magic, and related male dominance, though in fact it is necessary to combine both these approaches and unite them to a careful examination of the ethnographic data in order to arrive at a satisfactory interpretation of the phenomena concerned. (*See* GENDER; WOMEN AND ANTHROPOLOGY.)

Most authors who discuss the social organization of hunter-gatherers stress the fluidity or flexibility of social forms in contemporary hunter-gatherer groups,

linking this to their nomadic way of life. SERVICE claimed that the basic form of organization in hunting and gathering societies was the PATRILINEAL PATRILOCAL band (Radcliffe-Brown's 'horde') which occupied a given territory and exchanged wives with similar territorial groups. Recent evidence summarized in Lee and Devore shows that while such patrilocal bands are in existence, they are certainly not the universal form of hunter-gatherer social organization. Many authors indicate the existence of composite and flexible band structures, which have been observed to be highly adaptive to the hunting and gathering subsistence pattern, permitting the ready adjustment of group size to available resources and their distribution. In many cases, instead of attempting to apply the notions of residence or descent 'rules', a more fruitful approach to the study of band composition would be via analysis of the interaction of bilateral kinship and patterns of MARRIAGE alliance within a flexible local group structure. It is difficult in most cases to conceive of the hunting and gathering band as a CORPORATE GROUP, since the clear definition of territory, resources and the persons with the right to use them is often lacking. In accordance with the lack of corporate property, and the nomadic lifestyle, the most common mechanism of dispute settlement in hunting and gathering societies is group FISSION, and these societies are characterized by the lack of coercive force vested in political authority and the lack of developed systems of litigation or dispute settlement.

Another central area of concern has been the study of DEMOGRAPHY and population ecology among hunter-gatherers. Several authors have devoted their attention to the processes which maintain these populations in equilibrium with their environment, and especially to the maintenance of low population densities. Attention has been paid to the susceptibility of hunter-gatherer populations to disease, to mechanisms of population control (*see* CONTRACEPTION AND ABORTION; INFANTICIDE), and to the effects of marriage alliance strategies.

husband/wife. *See* MARRIAGE.

hydraulic civilization. A concept related to the theory of Asiatic or ORIENTAL DESPO-

TISM. The hydraulic or irrigation civilization is one in which state power is based on control over systems of irrigation and water supply.

hypergamy. The norm that a man should marry his daughter into a family of higher status than his own. In such a MARRIAGE system, a woman should preferably marry a superior but may marry an equal, and a man should not marry a woman of higher status than himself. Hypergamy is encountered in India, although it is not universal there. Hypergamous marriages accord well with the notion of hierarchy pervading CASTE systems (*see* POLLUTION). In classical Hindu ideology the perfect marriage is conceptualized as a kind of gift or *dan*. This type of gift is also offered to brahmins (priests) in other circumstances, and its offering conveys a relationship of rank in which the receiver is considered as superior. Ideally the gift offered in marriage should be that of a virgin girl or *kanya dan* and this gift is meritorious provided that no payment is received by the bride's family. In fact payment, often in the form of extravagant dowries, always accompanies the bride. In return the wife-givers do not expect wives for themselves or for future generations but they may hope to improve or maintain their rank and prestige. The hierarchical relationship between wife-givers and wife-receivers may be expressed in COMMENSAL activities, in the pattern of PRESTATIONS and in the terminological system of kin classification. Hypergamous marriages may be strategies by which castes, subcastes or families improve their rank. They tend to occur against a background of competitive 'one-upmanship' characteristic of such high-ranking castes as the various types of Rajputs found in North India. In communities where high-ranking castes practise hypergamy, castes of lower status may exchange wives and pay brideprice to their wife-givers (*see* MARRIAGE PAYMENTS) without earning themselves either merit or prestige.

Repeated hypergamous intermarriage between wife-givers and wife-receivers may consolidate the affinal relationships and create a system of ASYMMETRICAL marriage alliances in which three or more groups are ranked. Women will accumulate at the top of the hierarchy where infanticide, POLY-GYNY, enforced spinsterhood and marriages far away ensure a demand for women from below. At the bottom, therefore, there will not be enough wives to go around. As J.P. Parry has shown (1979) this system is unstable. The status of both spouses is linked to the status of their offspring, and superiors as well as inferiors may decide that, temporarily at least, it is safer to marry equals. There is therefore a tendency for the system to break into ENDOGAMOUS circles of intermarrying groups who agree to boycott their superior and inferior affines in future marriages. The existence of such an ISOGAMOUS phase is also precarious because every marriage may itself, after the event, be conceptualized as hypergamous, and the system tends to revert to its original form. These cycles of transformation indicate that hypergamy and isogamy cannot be sharply distinguished. As an idea hypergamy, accompanied by unidirectional prestations and terminological distinctions between affines may exist either in a situation where there is a statistical prevalence of hypergamous marriages, or with the practice of isogamous exchange marriages.

hypogamy. A form of MARRIAGE norm in which a man should marry a woman of higher status than himself: in other words, wife-givers should be of higher status than wife-receivers. This type of marriage has been described by E. Leach (1961) for the Kachin of Burma, where marriages may be between spouses of equal status or alternatively men who are commoners may marry women of aristocratic lineages, and aristocratic men women of chiefly lineages. The asymmetric relationship between wife-givers and wife-receivers is present also in the terminology of KINSHIP and affinal relationships, which is predicated upon the norm of MATRILATERAL CROSS-COUSIN MARRIAGE. Considerable MARRIAGE PAYMENTS flow from the wife-receivers to the wife-givers, in which cattle are the predominant currency. The accumulation of cattle by higher-status men and the redistribution of meat in the form of FEASTS contribute to the maintenance and reinforcement of the superior status of the wife-giver.

Leach cites examples of the matrilateral cross-cousin marriage rule occurring also with hypergamous marriage patterns, and he suggests that this rule is likely to be associated with the accumulation of permanent status differences between wife-givers and wife-receivers, whether the resulting structure is hypergamous or hypogamous. The relationship between matrilateral cross-cousin marriage, ANISOGAMY and class structure was the subject of a debate between Leach and LEVI-STRAUSS, with the result that both authors modified their views to a considerable extent, Leach in his 1954 ethnography *Political Systems of Highland Burma* and Levi-Strauss in his revised edition of *The Elementary Structures of Kinship* (1969). In his book, Levi-Strauss argues that hypogamy represents 'the maternal aspect of anisogamy', since it privileges the female line, while hypergamy privileges the male line. He links these forms of anisogamy to his overall theory of HARMONIC/DISHARMONIC regimes, claiming that hypogamy is a sign of instability within a patrilineal system, since it employs cognatic relations, while hypergamy by employing solely AGNATIC ties is relatively stable. He thus suggests that hypogamy is a structural phenomenon which represents the tension between paternal and maternal lines, while hypergamy represents the triumph of the paternal over the maternal lineage.

hysteria. A type of mental disturbance, characterized by the onset of violent or extreme physical reactions not explicable as the result of normal physiological conditions or disease. In psychiatry, these reactions are considered to be a product of psychological stress in certain types of personality. Anthropological studies have shown that hysteria is subject to considerable cultural and social patterning, and may be channelled or encouraged in certain circumstances within some cultures. It has been suggested that states of POSSESSION and TRANCE are at base hysterical reactions which are culturally acceptable and culturally learned by persons taking part in certain types of religious or magical ceremonies. (*See* PSYCHOLOGICAL ANTHROPOLOGY.)

I

iatrogenesis. A term employed by Ivan Illich to refer to the direct and indirect pathological effects of medical practice on individual health and social organization. The most obvious examples of iatrogenesis are the diseases and suffering directly produced by medical treatments, many of which may be unnecessary or may result from a resort to aggressive 'high-technology' treatments which do not take into account the patient's general condition. But Illich extends the term to encompass a much wider range of the social and cultural consequences of medical practice, centring his critique on the manner in which the medical profession, by monopolizing and attempting to control the universal human experiences of disease, pain and death, progressively erodes and destroys normal cultural, social and community-based mechanisms for coping with these experiences. This critique is part of Illich's overall attack on centralized bureaucratic institutions in industrial society. (*See* ETHNOMEDICINE; MEDICAL ANTHROPOLOGY.)

iconicity. In SEMIOTICS this term refers to a type of relationship between signifier and signified. In an iconic relationship, signifier and signified are connected by their similarity: the sign is modelled on, or similar to, its referent. Examples of iconic signs include onomatopeia ('bow-wow' to indicate 'dog'), or gestures which indicate desired or intended actions by their similarity to the action (raising the hand to threaten a blow, beckoning to indicate the direction of movement of another, and so on). (*See* INDEX; SIGN; SYMBOL; SYMBOLIC ANTHROPOLOGY.)

id. According to the PSYCHOANALYTIC theories of FREUD, the id is part of the unconscious personality structure. It is the reservoir of Eros, the sex or life drive, and Thanatos, the death or aggressive instinct. The functioning of the id is governed by the pleasure principle, and takes the form of reflex or instinctual reactions. The ego is that part of the personality structure which represents the reality principle and which diverts or 'sublimates' instinctual drives which derive from the id.

idealism. A philosophical tendency opposed to MATERIALISM, which holds that mental phenomena or 'ideas' determine or create material reality, human existence, or social and historical phenomena. In the social sciences the term is broadly applied to those theories which are considered to give priority to mental or nonmaterial phenomena in the explanation of sociocultural or historical forms and processes.

ideal type. A methodological device or aid which is commonly employed in the social sciences, whether implicitly or with explicit purpose. According to WEBER (1949), who devoted considerable attention to this concept, the ideal type is an abstraction or exaggeration of certain features which tend to be present in reality. Not all of the features of an ideal type will therefore be present in any one concrete situation, nor will they all be equally developed in every case. However, once the ideal type has been constructed it becomes an aid for the interpretation of a variety of concrete situations, and in the formulation of hypotheses to explain them. Ideal types can however lead in many cases to the distortion of reality, because the features arbitrarily selected to compose them acquire a spurious importance or concreteness, and lead to the neglect of other features of equal or greater empirical significance. As Weber argues, the ideal type is not a hypothesis but rather should be seen as an aid to the formulation of hypotheses. But the use of ideal types involves risk: once we have constructed them, it is often easier to talk about the neat and selected model of reality that the type presents than it is to discuss reality itself, with its contradictory and changing characteristics. Social scientific discourse can take refuge all too easily in the debate over its own arbitrary models of reality or of history, models which become obstacles rather than aids to the understanding and analysis of historical and sociocultural phenomena.

identity. The psychological self-conception of the person. In the social sciences, the term has also been extended to encompass social identity, cultural identity and ethnic identity, terms which refer to the identification of self with a specific social position, cultural tradition, or ETHNIC GROUP. We may also speak of group identity, in the sense of the identification or self-conception held in common by a group of people. The use of the term 'identity' has been questioned by some recent writers because it can imply a fixed or stable quality of a person or group. Such writers suggest we should focus on the process of identification rather than seek a fixed 'identity'.

ideology. A term with at least two rather distinct, though related, senses. On the one hand, it is often employed to express false consciousness, or a set of misapprehensions regarding reality. On the other, it can be used more neutrally to refer to a 'system of ideas', without the necessary implication that these ideas are false. In the sense of a set of misapprehensions or false notions of reality, 'ideology' is used to refer disparagingly to a specific political or party political position, and to depict a set of beliefs or ideas which is specific to a certain social class and which tends to reinforce and justify its political and economic interests. This is its most commonly employed usage in modern social science, and is associated with the works of MARX and ENGELS. According to Marxist theory, the dominant ideology in a society is the ideology of its dominant class, and ideological positions generally are a function of class positions. In contrast, 'false consciousness' (a term first employed by Engels) is consciousness which does not accord with the objective class position of the person or group concerned. It is seen as a result of the emulation of dominant class values by subordinate classes, and of the penetration of dominant class ideology in society as a whole (see HEGEMONY).

Marxist MATERIALIST social theory has as a key element the contention that ideologies or belief systems are the product of material conditions, or their transformation into the realm of ideas or consciousness. It is a central tenet of Marxist theory that, contrary to the IDEALIST theory of Hegel and other philosophers of history and society, 'it is not man's consciousness that determines his being, but rather his being in the world that determines his consciousness'. The relationship between the material conditions of existence and consciousness or ideology is one of the most controversial and debated issues within Marxist theory. Marx is himself ambiguous on this point, and his ambiguity has given rise to a number of different 'Marxisms', each interpreting differently the extent to which ideology is determined by material reality. Some writers interpret this determination as direct and unilineal, while others stress the dialectical relationship between material reality and ideas, emphasizing ideas are only affected by the concrete is 'in the last instance'. At the other extreme, opponents of Marxist and materialist theories contend that ideas, attitudes, values, norms and ideal goals may generate and govern social action and social change (see MARXIST ANTHROPOLOGY).

In its original sense of 'the science of ideas' ideology encompasses all of the senses mentioned above, and it is, indeed, one of anthropology's central concerns to study the formation and transformation of systems of ideas, including the analysis of systematic distortions or misrepresentations of natural or social reality which serve to reinforce the dominant position of one social group or social class. The Marxist notion of ideology has therefore been extended within anthropology to the study of ideologies in pre-class as well as class-based societies: for example, in the study of ideologies of male dominance (see FEMINIST ANTHROPOLOGY; GENDER; WOMEN AND ANTHROPOLOGY) or of systems of social STRATIFICATION based on criteria such as AGE. In the anthropological study of RELIGION and RITUAL several modern theorists apply Marxist notions of ideology, often in opposition to earlier FUNCTIONALIST theories of religion and ritual which stressed the cohesive properties of religious systems and neglected the possibility of their use as part of an apparatus of social control or social stratification.

illocution. In the theory of SPEECH acts originated by J.L. Austin (1962) and developed by J.R. Searle (1985), the concept of illocutionary acts describes the performative aspect of speech (i.e. speech which 'does something'). Thus a statement such as 'I name this ship the Queen Mary' cannot be evaluated in terms of its truth value, but must be interpreted as an act in itself. (*See* LINGUISTICS AND ANTHROPOLOGY.)

imperialism. The foreign policy of a state which seeks to extend its political and economic control or its sovereignty over one or more other states. The classic form of imperialism is the military conquest of new territories by an expanding empire. In the ancient world, newly conquered territories provided human resources to perpetuate SLAVERY, but territories which had been conquered tended to become assimilated to the empire. Imperialism in its broad sense is a phenomenon which may be observed throughout human history, but the term also has a more limited sense, that developed in the works of Lenin and other Marxist thinkers, who reserve the term for a specific phase of CAPITALISM. According to Lenin's theory, imperialism is the highest stage of development of monopoly capitalism (1915). In this stage, the imperialist nations establish colonies in all available parts of the undeveloped or partially developed world, colonies which serve the purpose of sustaining the capitalist system at home. These colonies act to supply raw materials at low prices and as markets for finished goods as well as becoming important areas for the export of capital. Colonial exploitation enables the capitalist class in the imperialist nations to sustain their position at home, since the high levels of profit obtained by colonial exploitation effectively permit them to subsidize the working class of the industrialized nations, thereby delaying the development of their revolutionary potential. Imperialism may also bring about struggles between powers attempting to extend or maintain their control over colonized territories.

An important element in imperialism is RACISM, which defines subordinate populations as inferior or subhuman, and so justifying their exploitation under conditions which would not be acceptable at home. Systems of slavery and other forms of extreme economic exploitation have been consistently justified by recourse to racist ideologies. In the case of European capitalist imperialism, the Christian religion has also played an important part in the subjugation of colonial populations and in the justification of the imperial enterprise. Thus MISSIONARIES have played a vital role in preparing conquered peoples to adjust to colonial domination, in organizing them in ways more amenable to the colonial system, and in the introduction of new ideological elements conducive to the acceptance of European domination.

Since the vast majority of Third World nations have gained at least nominal independence from the former colonial powers, the study of neo-imperialism and neo-colonialism has devoted itself to demonstrating the way in which political and economic control is still exercised over them by the industrialized nations. (*See* CAPITALISM; COLONIALISM; CRITICAL ANTHROPOLOGY; DEVELOPMENT; DEPENDENCY; WORLD SYSTEMS.)

import substitution. A strategy for protecting home industries by prohibiting imports of foreign consumer goods, or raising tariff barriers which tax these imports to the point where they are out of the reach of the home market. It is adopted periodically by certain Third World nations in order to promote INDUSTRIALIZATION and DEVELOPMENT by allowing the home industries a protected environment. The success of this strategy is mixed, for while it may have the effect of stimulating home industries to a certain extent it also tends to make them uncompetitive in the export market where they enjoy no such protection. In addition, it has been observed that when tariff barriers prohibit the import of consumer goods, the importation by industry of producer goods rises, and DEPENDENCY is simply transferred from one sector of the economy to another. MULTINATIONAL CORPORATIONS can also escape the effects of import substitution policies because they have locally-based subsidiaries.

incest. Sexual relationships between prohibited categories of kin. The definition of incestuous relations varies from society to society, but the existence of some prohibition on sexual relations between kin is universal. In order to avoid confusion when dealing with the topic of incest, we should be careful to clarify the distinction between sexual relations and MARRIAGE; the range of relations defined as incestuous is not necessarily coterminous with the range of persons who are prohibited marriage partners. Similarly we may distinguish incest from 'mismating', which refers to sexual relations which are prohibited or inappropriate for reasons other than their classification as incestuous. The problem of incest or of the incest TABOO has attracted much attention from anthropologists, and has been the subject of widely varying and contradictory attempts at explanation. However most would agree that no entirely satisfactory explanation of the phenomenon has been arrived at, and perhaps it is impossible to arrive at a universal definition which would satisfactorily account for all the variations in incest prohibitions which we encounter in the ethnographic and historical record. It is often assumed, for example, that certain prohibitions on sexual unions between close relatives (mother and son, brother and sister, father and daughter) are universal, though in fact it has been shown that there are exceptions even to these prohibitions. The prohibition on sexual relations between biological mother and son is perhaps the only truly universal example. The most commonly cited exceptions to the prohibition on sexual relations between nuclear family members are those of Ancient Egypt, Peru at the time of the Inca Empire, and Hawaii. LEVI-STRAUSS (1949) mentions the additional examples of the Azande and other African peoples, and also Madagascar and Burma. It has however been pointed out that these exceptions are limited in the sense that the consanguineous marriages involved are generally either temporary and ritual in nature, or else limited to the highest social class or ruling families. In addition, there are always some prohibited categories: for example, the half, but not the full, sister may

be a permitted spouse, or the older sister but not the younger. At the other extreme, certain cultures are characterized by the wide extension of the category of incestuous relations, defining large groups of people as prohibited sexual and marriage partners.

Probably the most popular explanation of incest prohibitions is that which relates them to the supposed negative genetic consequences of consanguineous unions. This argument is in accordance with folk beliefs in some societies, which predict illness or death as the result of transgression of rules (not only of the incest prohibitions but also of many other types of social norms). However, this explanation is problematic in the sense that it does not account for the 'eugenic second-sight' (Levi-Strauss) by which human groups could be assumed to be aware of the long-term genetic consequences of intermarriage between kin. Neither does it explain the existence of many societies where consanguineous unions such as those between certain categories of cousin are prescribed, in spite of the supposed evolutionary disadvantages. Parallel cousins may in fact be defined as prohibited partners while cross cousins are prescribed spouses, and the genetic argument could not account for the differential treatment of these two categories which are biologically equally close. In fact the biological or genetic evidence about the long-term consequences of consanguineous unions seems to be inconclusive, though recent advances in DEMOGRAPHIC method and population genetics may be able to supply more exact information. In spite of the absence of scientific data, the eugenic explanation of incest prohibitions has been popular since the 19th century, when it was proposed among others by MORGAN and MAINE. Other explanations proposed by 19th-century writers include the theories of SPENCER and Lubbock, who contended that the prohibition of incest was related to the institutionalization of the practice of bride capture by warlike tribes, and those of DURKHEIM, who related the incest taboo to the more generalized taboo on menstrual blood, arguing that fear of contact with blood of the same clan or TOTEM was the origin of the taboo.

Incest prohibitions have also been explained in the light of psychological factors and mechanisms. The theories associated with Havelock Ellis and WESTER-MARCK attribute incest prohibitions to the expression of 'natural aversion' towards sexual relations between persons brought up together or living in close contact from childhood. Several criticisms have been levelled at this type of theory. Firstly, it is noted that the prohibition itself or the existence of a rule would not be necessary if it were true that people would automatically and instinctively avoid incestuous relations. Secondly, the theory of natural aversion cannot account for the range of incest prohibitions and marriage practices found in different societies, some of which extend prohibitions to many persons who have never had close contact with Ego, others favouring or permitting marriage between persons who have been brought up together, as in the custom of very early betrothal.

Similar objections could be raised against an opposing type of psychological theory about incest prohibitions, which relies on the notion of 'natural desire'. This theory is based on the argument that the need for the incest prohibition stems from the fact that humans naturally tend toward incestuous relations, a tendency which must be prohibited in order to avoid the disruptive consequences of such relations. FREUD in fact postulated that there is a universal human tendency towards incestuous relations, and he argued that the institution of the incest taboo was a result of man's guilt at the primeval act of parricide committed in order to gain sexual access to the mother.

In modern anthropology the tendency has been to seek sociological explanations of incest prohibitions, though not necessarily to the exclusion of the consideration of biological, evolutionary and psychological factors. Thus MALINOWSKI (1927) and others relate the need for incest prohibitions to the necessity of avoiding the disruption of nuclear family relations (particularly of relations of authority) or of avoiding the kinship categories and relations which incestuous unions would produce. This type of explanation has however been widely criticized as begging the question, since it is predicated upon the prior existence of an authority and affective structure based on the exclusion of sexual unions within the nuclear family.

In *The Elementary Structures of Kinship*, 1969, Levi-Strauss takes as his starting point the well-known dictum of TYLOR, who related the incest taboo to the need to 'marry out or be killed out' in primitive society. Like Tylor, Levi-Strauss – though he is careful to distinguish between incest prohibitions and rules of EXOGAMY – believes the former to be fundamentally related to the need for the latter. He points out that the incest prohibition is at the same time a natural phenomenon (because it is universal) and a cultural one (since it is a 'rule', and since it displays cross-cultural variability). He argues that in this rule is to be found the key to the origin of human society and culture, in the sense that it embodies, in the form of a prohibition, the positive injunction to 'marry out': that is to say, to exchange women with other groups. He sees this change as fundamental in that it establishes a system of RECIPROCITY between human families or groups, thus marking the emergence of culture and society which are based on principles of communication and exchange. For Levi-Strauss, 'the incest prohibition expresses the transition from the natural fact of consanguinity to the cultural fact of alliance'. His discussion of the problem of incest thus leads him directly into his discussion of the different forms of ALLIANCE pattern characteristic of human societies. But his theory has been criticized because it fails to take sufficient account of the fact that sexual relations are not identical to marriage, and that since incest prohibitions and exogamous rules are not necessarily coterminous the latter cannot fully explain the former. Similarly, empiricist criticism of Levi-Strauss by Leach and others has argued that rather than seeking a universal explanation of the incest prohibition we should concentrate on the elucidation of individual incest prohibitions and their range and functions in each ethnographic context.

index. In SEMIOTICS, indexality refers to an existential relationship between signifier and signified: for example, smoke is an index of fire.

Indian. This term was applied to the indigenous populations of the Americas by the first European explorers, under the erroneous impression that they had reached India. Subsequently the term persisted and is still in general use, though it has been rejected in certain countries and in certain contexts due to the racist overtones it has acquired. The terms 'American Indian', 'Amerindian' or 'Amerind' are sometimes employed to distinguish the indigenous population of the Americas from the population of India, especially in areas such as the Caribbean where there is a significant community of persons from the Indian subcontinent. In Spanish-speaking Latin America the term 'indio' is frequently regarded as a racial insult, and the terms 'nativo' (native), 'indigena' (indigene) or 'campesino' (peasant) may be substituted. In Brazil however the term 'indio' is generally employed. (*See* ETHNICITY.)

indigenous. When applied to populations this term refers to the original inhabitants of an area which has subsequently been occupied by migrants. It is thus synonymous with the term native, to which it is sometimes preferred where the latter has acquired pejorative connotations.

indirect exchange. *See* ASYMMETRIC/ SYMMETRIC ALLIANCE.

individualism. A term applied to a series of loosely related political, social and/or historical theories and tendencies, which give the individual priority to the exclusion of groups or aggregates of persons, or to the exclusion of HOLISTIC constructs and theoretical models. As a political and economic philosophy, it gives priority to the pursuit of individual interests and liberty above collective interests or demands. Methodological individualism in the social sciences argues that all explanations of social phenomena must be reducible to explanations in terms of individual motivations or behaviour, thus denying the validity of explanations in terms of social groups or institutions, social structure, or theoretical constructs such as social CLASS. (*See* ACTION THEORY; PSYCHOLOGICAL ANTHROPOLOGY.)

industrial anthropology. The field of industrial anthropology is generally considered to have originated with the classic studies of Elton Mayo, whose analysis of industrial work organization pioneered the HUMAN RELATIONS MOVEMENT. Mayo's school, with

its focus on the human dimension of labour, emphasized the subjective experience of work and not the objective constraints which determine its nature, and viewed the workplace in isolation from its wider social and economic context, considering conflict as a pathological phenomenon. Later industrial anthropology has focused on the political and economic context of the workplace, and the way in which the historical development of industrial structures influences conflict or co-operation in the labour process. These developments were prefigured in the work of Whyte, who pointed out that to concentrate exclusively on psychological and other aspects of worker management relations an insufficient means of resolving conflict: it was necessary instead to observe the social structure of the workplace and the position which the worker occupies in the system of social relations. Following the Hawthorne studies conducted by the Human Relations Movement, later anthropologists began to focus on the investigation of specific industrial contexts, though often with an uncritical view of the industrial phenomenon itself, which they took as given. Thus we have an anthropology of industry in the narrow sense of ethnographic descriptions of industrial workplaces, but not in the broader sense of an anthropology of industrial society as a type. Recent developments in industrial anthropology have included the study of cognitive aspects of industrial work, and the analysis of how overall historical trends in WORLD SYSTEMS affect industrial work. Attention has also been paid to the role of WOMEN, and how structures of male dominance as well as class affect their participation in industry.

industrialization. The transition to large-scale factory production as an economic type, an economic process with many social and cultural consequences and concomitants. Researchers attempting to delineate the necessary conditions for industrialization have often focused on psychological factors affecting socioeconomic changes (*see* ACHIEVEMENT MOTIVATION). Many have also stressed the importance of the entrepreneurial role. But a number of these theories, apart from their tendency to neglect overall structural process and change in favour of the consideration of individual psychology or behaviour, fall into the trap of ethnocentrically assuming that all industrialization must necessarily follow the pattern established by Europe or the United States. It is therefore assumed that the Third World can only industrialize by imitating a Western personality, social organization and commercial habits. Analysts like Geertz (1963) who argue against this imposition of Western models, have defended historically and culturally specific alternative models of industrialization and advocated careful examination of the relationship between values, cognitive patterns, social organization and the industrialization process, rather than a crude opposition of 'traditional' and 'modern'. Some traditional patterns of social or group organization may facilitate the development of new economic activities while others obstruct it, and in each case the specific characteristics of the community concerned must be considered. The cross-cultural and ethnohistorical analysis of industrial phenomena aims both to dispel ethnocentric theories of industrial economy and to reveal the conditions of industrialization which seem culturally and historically variable, and those which appear to be universal or invariable.

Anthropologists who adopt a Marxist perspective analyse the industrial phenomenon in terms of the concept of MODE OF PRODUCTION. They stress the social relations of production (control over the MEANS OF PRODUCTION and over labour power) which determine industrial structures and processes on local, national and international levels. The relations of economic DEPENDENCY which condition local industrialization processes in the Third World are viewed as products of the evolution of CAPITALISM, which is in its turn seen as a historically specific mode of production which extends its political and economic boundaries in order to amass SURPLUS value. Thus Nash (1981) in her study of Bolivian tin mines focuses on the miners' experience of class contradiction within an industry which is an extreme example of Third World dependency and class exploitation. Marxist studies also examine the relationship between capitalist and pre-capitalist modes of production in specific instances of industrialization. For example, Meillassoux (1972) sees the persistence of rural allegiances and lineage structures in an urban industrial setting in Africa as a result of the ARTICULATION of capitalist and pre-capitalist modes of production. In this case the capitalist system employs the pre-capitalist agricultural system in order to provide the reproduction of labour power for the industrial economy.

The theory of WORLD SYSTEMS approaches the industrialization process rather differently, considering that rather than a series of lineally ordered modes of production there is only one capitalist world system which creates 'core', 'periphery' and 'semi-periphery' zones. (*See* DEVELOPMENT.)

inequality. Social inequality is a concomitant of human classification according to differential STATUS, POWER and PRESTIGE. G.D. Berreman suggests that inequality originates as a social phenomenon in the instinctive perception and evaluation of people as differentiated (1981). He terms the behavioural expression of inequality 'dominance', and the dual phenomenon of inequality and dominance is generally termed 'social inequality'. Some authors would reserve the term STRATIFICATION for class-based or state societies, speaking only of inequality or 'ranking' in pre-state societies. In the so-called egalitarian societies, the division of labour and the distribution of status and relations of social inequality are based on criteria such as age, sex and personal attributes, and do not constitute permanent ranked categories. In inegalitarian societies, there is institutionalized inequality based on a series of hierarchical statuses, which may be linked to kin groups or to specific occupational roles such as warrior or priest. In state societies, inequality is based on social stratification, where all members of society are ranked in terms of broad strata not based on age, sex or kin classification. Types of social stratification include CLASS, CASTE and ETHNIC GROUP.

infant mortality. Infant mortality is usually defined as the death of children between birth and the age of 2 years, as opposed to neo-natal mortality, or the death of babies between birth and the age of 28 days. The infant mortality rate is an important element in the measurement of overall health standards in a nation or region and is often taken as an indicator of levels of overall socioeconomic DEVELOPMENT. In the Third World, such rates are generally high, indicating the poor levels of health and health care and the manner in which this particularly affects the most vulnerable sector of the population. Strategies of primary health care are directed primarily towards the reduction of infant mortality rates. One of the important aspects of the rates and their social scientific interpretation is the differential distribution of infant mortality in both developed and developing nations according to such factors as social class, occupational group, race or ethnic group, and urban or rural areas. For example, it is well known in the United States that overall infant mortality rates among blacks are nearly double those among whites. In Third World nations, too, the dramatic differences between infant mortality rates among the urban and rural poor and among the middle or upper classes reveal mechanisms of poverty, deprivation and denial of access to basic health care.

infanticide. The practice of killing newborn babies is generally attributed to the need for population control, especially in HUNTING AND GATHERING and NOMADIC societies where it may be impossible for a mother to carry around more than one small child and perform the necessary tasks for the subsistence of her family. In some cases female infanticide is preferentially or exclusively practised because the higher value placed on male offspring, and this has led to the formulation of hypotheses within ecological anthropology which link warfare, cults of male dominance and female infanticide to protein supply and population distribution. Infanticide may also be practised in the case of sickly or deformed infants, or for ritual or religious motives, as in the case of certain African peoples who left TWIN babies to die because of the supernatural significance of twin births. (*See* CONTRACEPTION AND ABORTION; DEMOGRAPHY.)

informant. The informant supplies the anthropologist with data, and the relationship between informant and ethnographer is one which has come under closer scrutiny as modern anthropology has moved away from uncritical assumptions of the homogeneity of 'primitive society'. In carrying out and reporting ethnographic fieldwork, the anthropologist must take into account the purposiveness both of ethnographer and informant when evaluating the information which results from their relationship. In other words, it is essential to examine critically both the relationship which the ethnographer establishes with the community and with his or her informants, and the manner in which the social status, position and relationships of individual informants affect the data they supply. In modern ethnography, it is no longer usual to read global statements of 'what such-and-such a people believe', since it is recognized that attitudes, beliefs and values vary considerably from person to person and according to each person's status and position in the network of social relationships of the community.

Among the attempts to develop more systematic, publicly observable and testable methods of anthropological fieldwork, some studies have proposed methodologies for the testing of concordance between informants and fieldworker. Such techniques are of especial importance when hypotheses or conclusions depend upon the assumption that events or situations perceived as having a certain significance by the observer have the same significance for the informants involved. (*See* CRITICAL ANTHROPOLOGY; ETHNOGRAPHIC WRITING; FIELDWORK; RESEARCH METHODS.)

infrastructure. In Marxist and other materialist theories of society, a division is made between the infrastructure or economic base of society and the SUPERSTRUCTURE which is believed to be dependent on, or determined by, the former. Different Marxist and neo-Marxist writers interpret the infrastructure's determination of the superstructure in different ways. Godelier (1978), for example, points out that a crude economic determinism is clearly not applicable to many of the societies studied by anthropologists, where it is kinship or religious, and not economic, systems *per se* which are the dominant organizational axes of society. However, as Marx himself noted, economic determinism applies only 'in the last instance', and does not imply that in every society economic relations are dominant. Instead, Marxist analysis should seek to explain why in each case kinship, religious or legal institutions dominate in a particular society by defining the role which these institutions play in the organization of relations of production and other aspects of the economy. Thus, inasmuch as kinship systems or religous beliefs serve to organize the relations of production and distribution in society, we may account for the domination of these relationships within specific social formations.

inheritance. The transmission of PROPERTY following the death of its owner. In its strictest sense it should not be considered in isolation from other forms of property transmission and distribution, including MARRIAGE PAYMENTS, GIFTS etc. which may transmit property to the succeeding generation before the death of the owner. Patterns of inheritance and transfer of property between the generations constitute an important element in social organization in those societies where there is considerable accumulation of property, which may take the form of land rights, cattle or animals, or money and other valuables. Such property may be held and transmitted by kin corporations, by family or kin groups, or by individuals, and it is common for different types of property to be subject to different forms of ownership and inheritance. We should not forget that inheritable property is not limited to material goods in the sense in which we conventionally understand them in Western society. Names, titles, ceremonial and ritual knowledge and paraphernalia etc. may also be inherited, and may constitute important valuables even in those societies which are generally characterized by the inconsiderable development of property.

initiation. Rites of initiation have attracted considerable anthropological interest, much of which may be traced to the influence and inspiration of VAN GENNEP's celebrated analysis of RITES OF PASSAGE, where he suggests that the pattern of initiation rites provides a conceptual model upon which many ritual forms are based. Van Gennep noted that in initiation rituals, the initiates are separated or secluded from ordinary life and social relations, entering a phase of LIMINALITY and RITUAL REVERSAL. Subsequently, they are reincorporated into society

in their new status, and this reincorporation constitutes a symbolic rebirth. The initiation rites which have most commonly been studied by anthropologists are those which are performed for boys or girls to mark their change of status from children to mature members of society capable of sexual activity and/or marriage. In some cases these rituals involve physical operations upon the body such as CIRCUMCISION or other forms of MUTILATION, SCARIFICATION etc. Apart from the initiation rites held to mark physical maturity or marriageability, other types of initiation rites may be held by secret societies or to mark the transition between AGE GRADES or AGE SETS. Similarly, elements akin to initiation ritual may be perceived in the process of admission to any ASSOCIATION and in any process of status transition.

Many analyses of initiation rituals, like those of RITUAL in general, have been influenced by psychological or psychoanalytical theory. Thus Bettelheim (1954) suggests that male initiation rites involving circumcision in Australia may be explained in terms of male envy of female reproductive powers. Circumcision, he argues, represents the attempt to induce a male 'menstruation' (bleeding) and thus symbolically usurp female powers. Many analysts have disagreed with Bettelheim's psychoanalytic interpretation, and have rejected the parallel which he draws between initiation rites in tribal society and the fantasies of disturbed children in Western culture. However the theme of male usurpation or imitation of female natural reproductive power is common to many anthropological interpretations of initiation ritual. Several authors have argued that initiation and certain other LIFE CRISIS rites represent the symbolic assertion of male cultural superiority and domination over the natural female power of reproduction. The ritual rebirth, in the hands of men, accordingly asserts that the natural child created by the woman is made social or cultural by the symbolic and spiritual powers controlled by men.

Analyses of female initiation rites have also shown that these rites assert male control over key aspects of female reproductivity and behaviour. Thus La Fontaine's analysis of female initiation rites among the patrilineal Gisu (1972) shows how these rites, which take place at first menstruation, marriage and first childbirth, emphasize the control exercised by agnates over a woman's reproductive activity, and the transfer of rights and control over her from her lineage to her husband's lineage. The Gisu also hold elaborate male initiation rites, which employ much of the symbolism of female physiology: explicitly comparing male circumcision to female childbirth as the mark of having attained maturity. Among the matrilineal Bemba studied by Audrey Richards (1956), the transmission of status and inheritance is through women, and the initiation of women is the occasion for a major ceremony which does not coincide with any specific physiological event. This ritual, *Chisungu*, is an essential prerequisite for marriage and childbirth, and the ritual itself, rather than the physiological fact of menstruation or childbirth, is what makes the woman. The ritual emphasizes the dangers of sexual contact between husband and wife, and serves to protect women and their children (the matrilineage) against the dangers of contact with symbolically and socially powerful men. As La Fontaine points out, different forms of male and female initiation rites represent variations upon 'a universal theme: the nature of men and women, their opposition and conjunction in procreation'. In common with other rituals, initiation rites also lend themselves to the LEGITIMATION of relations of authority and/or dominance, whether they are structured along the lines of GENDER, AGE or kinship relations.

innovation. The mechanism of creation of new ideas, new techniques, or new behaviours which makes social and cultural CHANGE and EVOLUTION possible. An important feature of adaptive ability is the human tendency to go beyond the problems of immediate subsistence, and to devote considerable time and energy to RITUAL, PLAY and other activities whose immediate necessity is not apparent, but which nevertheless contribute to the creation of a total human culture capable of reflection, transformation and innovation. Innovation is thus dependent upon human CREATIVITY, and upon the receptiveness of the community to accept or adopt the products of this creativity. The balance between TRADITION and innovation, and the significance or profundity of innovations, depend upon the historical conditions which influence the development of ADAPTIVE STRATEGIES in human populations.

instinct. Behaviour patterns which are not learned, but genetically programmed or encoded in all members of a given species, with the result that an identical behaviour pattern will be elicited in any member of the species given the appropriate stimulus. The concept of instinct is less broadly applied in modern science than in former times, as it has been shown that it is in many cases an oversimplification of the complex process of interaction between genetic programming, environment and learned behaviour. Most modern students of human behaviour would refrain particularly from applying the term to human beings. ETHOLOGY has tended towards the demonstration that most behaviours formerly held to be instinctive in animals are in fact modifiable to some extent by learning, and the concept of 'ethogram' (the psychobiological pattern characteristic of each species) and that of 'species characteristic behaviour' are proving to be more satisfactory than that of instinct.

institution. A term widely used in the social sciences, in spite of the fact that there are frequent ambiguities in its scope and reference. When we refer to a 'social institution' we usually imply, as Leeds points out (1976), forms of standardized action or behaviour linked to a set of complex and interdependent NORMS and ROLES and applying to a relatively large proportion of persons within a society or territory. In FUNCTIONALIST theory, the concept of institution is linked to that of human NEEDS or the functional prerequisites of social systems: Malinowski (1944) lists seven basic social institutions which respond to biological or psychobiological needs. Other functionalist theories relate social institutions in a similar way to the basic functions necessary for the survival and maintenance of a sociocultural system. However there is a looser usage of the term, which refers to the rule-bound or patterned nature of behaviour, without the necessary implication of a functionalist theory of society.

insults. Insults may have considerable social and even RITUAL significance when they are systematically directed between certain categories of persons or when they are channelled into specific cultural contexts. The Eskimo, for example, traditionally practised 'song duels' involving competitive exchanges of insults. Insults are also a feature of JOKING RELATIONSHIPS. In addition, the content of insults provides the ethnographer with an important key to the significant categories of acceptable or unacceptable behaviour, or personal characteristics, in a given culture. (*See* CONFLICT).

integration. A term used in two rather different though related senses. On the one hand, within FUNCTIONALIST theory, it refers to the observation that all aspects of a sociocultural system tend to operate in close interrelation to one another and to the whole. This sense of social integration is sometimes referred to as 'functional interrelatedness' or 'pattern maintenance'. On the other hand, integration or 'cultural integration' and its converse, disintegration, are sometimes used to refer to the degree of COHESION or of disorganization of social relations and cultural systems within a given ethnographic context. Thus the first use refers to a general theoretical postulate about the nature of sociocultural systems, while the second use refers to the belief that specific sociocultural systems may possess greater or lesser degrees of integration, especially under the influence of situations of ACCULTURATION and CHANGE.

interaction theory. A type of social theory which assumes that individual behaviour is to be described and/or explained in terms of the interaction between persons engaged in the construction of social events. This perspective has links to ACTION THEORY, ETHNOMETHODOLOGY and COGNITIVE ANTHROPOLOGY.

interethnic relations. *See* ETHNICITY.

intermediate technology. This field, which was pioneered by E.F. Schumacher (1973), seeks to develop and disseminate technology which lies in an intermediate position between the Western capital-intensive pattern and the indigenous one. (*See* APPROPRIATE TECHNOLOGY; DEVELOPMENT.)

internal colonialism. This refers to COLONIAL-type social systems occurring within complex multi-ethnic states. It has been applied after independence to former colonial nations where national elites have to some extent taken over the dominant position of former colonial elites where subordinate ethnic groups are concerned. It has also been applied to situations of systematic racial discrimination, such as the relations between whites and blacks and other ethnic groups in the United States.

international division of labour. *See* WORLD SYSTEM.

invention. A technological INNOVATION. In 19th- and early 20th-century anthropology, the debate between proponents of DIFFUSIONISM and those who proposed the importance of independent invention of culture TRAITS was an important one, but in modern anthropology this controversy has subsided to a large extent.

Iroquois. A type of KINSHIP TERMINOLOGY found among the Iroquois Indians and which has come to be used as a general term for similar systems found in other parts of the world. The Iroquois system is of the BIFURCATE merging type, equating parallel cousins with siblings and distinguishing cross-cousins from both. It is often found in conjunction with symmetric alliance or DUAL ORGANIZATION.

irrigation. The artificial use of water in order to exploit land which would otherwise be unsuitable for AGRICULTURE. Irrigation systems may involve the construction of systems of terracing, canals or aqueducts of varying degrees of technological complexity. The theory of Asiatic or ORIENTAL DESPOTISM draws attention to the potential political consequences of centralized control over irrigation systems and water supply.

isogamy. The practice or norm of MARRIAGE between partners of equal status. (*See* ANISOGAMY.)

itinerant agriculture. *See* SHIFTING AGRICULTURE.

J

jajmani. It has become common practice to refer to the DIVISION OF LABOUR which exists within Indian villages as the *jajmani* system. In this system landowning and occupational CASTES exchange goods and services in a manner which is held to be incompatible with modern MARKET economies. Each caste is associated with a set of appropriate occupations. Agriculture is the largest occupational category, and may be practised with varying degrees of involvement by castes who specialize in non-agricultural work such as priests, potters and blacksmiths. In traditional accounts of the *jajmani* system landowning families (sometimes called *jajmans*) are provided with services which they themselves consider to be defiling by lower castes and with ritually pure services by the Brahman priest. Landowning castes pay the servicing castes in kind with grain or other products. The redistribution often takes place on the threshing floor and shares may be defined as a proportion of the grain heap. The relationships are hereditary and personal and tinged with PATRONAGE.

In the 1950s and 1960s the nature of this system was intensely debated. W.H. Wiser (1958), who was first to offer a detailed description, saw these relationships as forming an integrative, almost egalitarian, system. This was challenged by T.O. Beidelman (1959) who considered the system exploitative. L. Dumont (1970) pointed out that the Hindi term *yajman* derives from Sanskrit and means the person who has the sacrifice performed, and this is fundamental to his argument that the *jajmani* system is one manifestation of hierarchy.

Although specifically associated with northern India, *jajmani* has become the model applied to Indian villages generally. Most anthropologists have ignored the existence of other variations. The *baluta* system is one such variation. This system has been described by many older sources and its variation in modern western India has been described by H. Orenstein (1966). In it service castes and hereditary officials such as the headman, accountant and watchman, serve a village as a whole. The close association between landholding households and clients who are farm labourers and often remunerated in kind has been described for southern India by D. Kumar (1965) and for Gujerat by J. Breman (1974) and may be another variation. Finally, *jajmani* relations exist in towns as well.

The systematic integrated character of *jajmani* is also doubtful. D. Pocock (1972) has made the distinction between *jajmani* relationships, by which he means relations between patrons and properly religious specialists such as priests and washermen, and relationships with artisans and unskilled agricultural labourers. These latter, he argues, are only *jajmani* by extension. Such distinctions have been widely recorded by ethnographers, as have distinctions in the manner by which remunerations are made (either as gifts or payments) and in the nature of the intercaste economic relationships (long or short term, personal or detached). Some writers, like T.S. Epstein (1967), have considered variations on the traditional *jajmani* model as a result of the impact of Western values on caste systems. Implicit in this approach has been the assumption that traditionally caste systems were largely unchanging and static. The prevalence of this view has been strengthened by the scant attention in comparative terms devoted to political and economic processes in pre-British India by social anthropologists.

In pre-British India, the shares redistributed from the grain heap included the share due to the ruler as revenue. The collection of revenue in kind was a cumbersome affair and already in Mughal India a revenue

155

system had been designed to fix revenue rates in cash. Such a system presupposed the existence of coinage and markets in which cultivators could sell their produce. It also presupposed the possibility of converting means of production such as land, labour and rights to collect revenue into cash. Although unevenly developed, the existence of these factors in India is beyond dispute. Far from being diametrically opposed to market systems, Indian village economic relationships were in part integrated into larger political units through such systems.

Contrary to what is generally believed 'the *jajmani* system' is not a pan-Indian phenomenon, nor does it refer to a systematic set of relationships which may be isolated from all others. The term obstructs rather than facilitates the development of a comparative framework. It is to be hoped that it is not too late to replace it.

joint family. This term may be used with the same meaning as EXTENDED FAMILY, or it may be reserved for special forms of extended family. In the latter case it is sometimes employed to refer to extended family forms composed of nuclear families linked by sibling ties (married brothers and/or sisters and their families), or may refer to other special arrangements of combinations of nuclear families.

joking relationship. Joking relationships, or ritualized joking between certain categories of persons, are widespread in the ethnographic record, and have been especially reported for North American Indian and certain African peoples. Joking relationships (usually defined according to specific KINSHIP or AFFINAL relationships, though they may also exist between larger categories or groups such as entire clans) have been the subject of different types of anthropological explanation. RADCLIFFE-BROWN (1940) interpreted joking relationships as the equivalent to relationships of avoidance, in the sense that they function in order to maintain the distance between persons in a potentially conflictful relationship. Thus according to Radcliffe-Brown the relationship reflects a combination of social conjunction and disjunction which reveals a feature of the social structure. Others, however, have viewed the relationship rather as one of ritual license or privileged familiarity, and not as an expression of strain or potential conflict. They thus place joking relationships and avoidance relationships in diametric opposition. Goody (1977) points out that we should distinguish asymmetrical joking relationships from symmetrical ones. The former occur between persons of different rank or status, and may take the form of a superior teasing an inferior or of an inferior having license to joke with a superior. Symmetrical joking relations occur between status equals, and contrary to Radcliffe-Brown's thesis they may characterize close and equal relations. Goody suggests that joking relationships and 'joking partnerships' between groups should be placed within the wider context of the social functions of humour. These include its expressive or cathartic value, and its functions relating to social control and the management of CONFLICT. It is probable that joking relationships perform different functions in different ethnographic contexts, but have in common the manner in which they mark out relationships in some way special or different from others, whether this special difference be the possibility of conflict, the possibility of marriage alliance, and so on. (*See* RITUAL; RITUAL REBELLION.)

jural. The domain of LAW or prescription in social organization. FORTES and other social anthropologists employed the distinction between moral and jural relations, using 'jural' to refer to the rules and obligations attached to structural principles of social organization (such as patrilineal descent, for example), while 'moral' is used to refer to the moral order which both supports and transcends these jural principles.

jurisprudence. *See* LAW, ANTHROPOLOGY OF.

justice. *See* LAW, ANTHROPOLOGY OF.

K

killing, ritual. *See* SACRIFICE.

kin group. A social group in which membership is defined by relationships of KINSHIP.

kindred. A culturally recognized category of BILATERAL kinsmen, which may extend only to a certain degree of relationship from Ego, or may be conceptualized as the total universe of Ego's kin. The social significance of the kindred varies according to the nature of the kinship system, because different kinship systems employ different principles of selection or closure which limit or channel Ego's social relations with certain members of the kindred. Thus unilineal DESCENT systems privilege links through one sex only for the purposes of many important areas of social organization, while systems of NON-UNILINEAL DESCENT and bilateral kinship systems may employ other criteria such as residence, marriage alliance or property inheritance in order to create CORPORATE kindred-based groups. In societies which do not possess corporate descent or kindred-based groups, the kindred is then termed a 'personal kindred' since it is different for every individual. (*See* NODAL KINDRED; STEM KINDRED.)

kingship. *See* MONARCHY.

kinship. Kinship, which in its broadest sense includes MARRIAGE alliance and relations of AFFINITY, has been central to anthropology since its origin, and perhaps especially so since the publication of MORGAN's *Systems of Consanguinity and Affinity* (1870). Indeed it is often regarded as the most specialized and in some senses privileged area of anthropological enquiry. Following Morgan, the dominant emphasis in early kinship studies was on KINSHIP TERMINOLOGY, so that studies of kinship systems were organized around contrasting and explaining different terminological systems. MALINOWSKI and the STRUCTURAL FUNCTIONALISTS, breaking away from this 'kinship algebra', strengthened the study of kinship in its sociological context. Within the structural functionalist school, the burgeoning of sociologically-oriented kinship studies was indivisibly linked to the development of LINEAGE THEORY. J.A. Barnes (1980) suggests that this development of functionally oriented approaches produced a rupture in kinship studies, reducing kinship within mainstream anthropology to an aspect of other topics, while technical kinship studies continued to develop but in isolation from other areas of anthropological theory.

In spite of an early anthropological interest in forms of marriage alliance, the field of kinship studies in the 20th century both in the USA and in Britain was dominated for a long period by the almost exclusive emphasis on DESCENT to the exclusion of alliance. The 'underlying spell of descent', as Dumont has termed it, was broken by the publication of LEVI-STRAUSS' *The Elementary Structures of Kinship* (first published in French in 1949, revised edition in 1967, translated into English 1969). The work of Levi-Strauss and anthropologists inspired by his method established the school of ALLIANCE THEORY, which redressed the balance in the study of systems of kinship and marriage alliance. (*See* ELEMENTARY STRUCTURES; COMPLEX STRUCTURES; PRESCRIPTION/PREFERENCE.)

Kinship as an isolatable category came under attack from anthropologists such as LEACH and Needham (1971), who argued, as Needham states, that 'there is no such thing as kinship, and it follows that there can be no such thing as kinship studies'. This 'rethinking' of kinship studies was influenced to a great extent by the development of STRUCTURAL ANTHROPOLOGY and by the rejection of the traditional assumptions of functionalist social and cultural anthropology. Thus in the 1960s and 1970s there was much debate between 'alliance and descent theory', sometimes confused with the quite separate debate between empiricist and structuralist orientations in social science.

US kinship studies during the same period tended to turn away from the study of kinship's sociological aspects and concentrate on the analysis of the cognitive dimensions of kinship as a cultural domain (*see* COMPONENTIAL ANALYSIS; FORMAL SEMANTIC ANALYSIS). This poses one of the central problems of modern kinship studies, that of relating such FORMAL ANALYSES to the reality of social events and interaction. On the one hand, methods for the formal analysis of kinship systems become ever more sophisticated, while on the other the sociological study of kinship tends to reaffirm the flexibility and modifiable nature of these systems in their social context.

Another central problem in kinship studies has been the relationship between the natural facts of genetics and biology, and kinship systems as cultural or sociocultural constructs. While on one hand the intuitive definition of kinship is based on some connection to 'blood' or biology, on the other, as the sociological or cultural determinist analysts of kinship have pointed out, kin classifications are social and cultural constructions which do not necessarily refer to the biological facts. Thus the considerable debate about the EXTENSION OF KINSHIP TERMS revolves precisely around the question of whether the 'basic' or 'core' meaning of kin terms is in fact a limited set of universal family relations, or a category of persons grouped together by a single term without necessarily privileging the biologically closest member. Most anthropologists today would agree that kinship relations involve some kind of modelling on 'natural' or 'biological' ties, but would recognize too that such natural ties are conceived of in many different ways in different cultural contexts, and do not necessarily correspond to our own intuitive definitions (*see* CONCEPTION). The refinement of techniques in cognitive anthropology has been a breakthrough, permitting accurate mapping of the cognitive and referential domains which are related in specific cultures to kinship terms (*see* COMPONENTIAL ANALYSIS; FORMAL SEMANTIC ANALYSIS).

The importance of kinship studies in anthropology is due in large part to the great importance attached to kinship relations in the societies typically studied by anthropologists. It has frequently been noted that the significance of kinship in pre-industrial society is more far-reaching and systematic than in modern industrial society. Thus it is often stated that kinship (and/or marriage alliance, which is sometimes included under the general rubric of kinship) constitutes the basic organizational principle of a pre-industrial or small-scale society. In many such societies the universe of kin and affines is the universe of significant social relationships, all persons who enter into relationship with Ego being defined in terms of some kinship status, whether or not their exact relationship to Ego is known. Thus many ethnographers have noted that the world is divided, for members of a small-scale society, into kinsmen and enemies (with affines or potential affines sometimes occupying an ambiguous position intermediate between these two categories).

Marxist analyses of pre-capitalist modes of production relate the importance of kinship ties in small-scale or pre-industrial societies to the role played by kinship in the organization of economic relations and particularly relations of production. However Marxist analyses of kinship have not been especially developed as yet, and there are interesting possibilities for future studies in this field, elaborating and specifying the relations between productive systems and kinship IDEOLOGY in different ethnographic contexts.

kinship terminology. Since its origin, generally traced back to the pioneering works of MORGAN the study of KINSHIP and ALLIANCE has been closely linked to the study of kinship terminology. Thus to a large extent theories of kinship have addressed themselves to analysis and explanation of the properties of kinship systems, and opposing theories within different theoretical schools (alliance and DESCENT theory, FORMAL SEMANTIC ANALYSIS and SOCIAL LEARNING theories etc.) have often shared in common the stated or unstated presupposition that kinship terminologies are in some way identical to, or the key to, kinship systems. We tend to assume therefore that those relatives grouped together under a single term share some common characteristic, be this conceived of in COGNITIVE, psychological or sociological terms.

However, it has been pointed out that we should exercise caution in equating kinship systems with kinship terminologies, particularly when we employ formal or structural analyses to construct abstract models of kinship systems based on terminological evidence alone. Analyses which focus solely on kinship terminologies tend to neglect the dynamic integration of kinship terms, ATTITUDES and behaviour, and the fact that kinship terms are often strategically and tactically employed in social situations in order to achieve desired communicative or other ends. Kinship terminologies are often employed by social actors in flexible and variable ways, as they choose among a number of possible terms in order to communicate a given attitude towards another person. Similarly it is erroneous to assume that all persons classed together by a kinship term are fundamentally similar in their relationship to Ego, since the use of a common term may mask considerable differences of role and attitude. Some of these tactical aspects of kinship terms are revealed by the study of contrasts between terms of address (used by Ego in directly addressing relatives) and terms of reference. In modern anthropology it has also become customary to include in accounts of kinship terminology the terms employed by female Ego apart from those employed by male Ego. Nevertheless there is still to be found a degree of ANDROCENTRISM or male bias in many kinship studies which continue to privilege the male viewpoint over and above that of women (*see* FEMINIST ANTHROPOLOGY; GENDER; WOMEN AND ANTHROPOLOGY).

Typologies of kinship terminology began with the work of Morgan, who formulated the distinction between CLASSIFICATORY AND DESCRIPTIVE systems. This distinction is however no longer employed, as it is recognized that all kinship terminologies have both descriptive and classificatory aspects, and in many cases there exist alternative descriptive and classificatory terms for the same relationship. The formal properties of kinship systems are generally described in terms of the dimensions of sex, GENERATION, LINEAL, COLLATERALITY and sex of linking relative(s) (*see* BIFURCATION). In

addition, in some terminologies the criterion of relative age (older/younger than Ego) is significant. It is common to classify kinship terminologies according to cousin terms. Typical classifications of kinship terminologies include CROW, ESKIMO, HAWAIIAN, IROQUOIS and OMAHA. These have become IDEAL TYPES in kinship studies, but we should not forget that any actual kinship system will display important modifications or variations from the type, especially when we take into account the unique characteristics of its embeddedness within a concrete sociocultural system.

Kluckhohn, Clyde Kay Maben (1905–60). Major US cultural anthropologist whose contributions to CULTURE AND PERSONALITY theory and to the study of North American Indians were especially influential. Kluckhohn was trained in classical studies before entering anthropology, and his continuing interests throughout his career included the study of VALUES, personality and RELIGION (e.g. 1950; 1952).

knowledge. The study of knowledge is one of the central concerns of anthropology, which since the pioneering studies of DURKHEIM and MARX in particular has paid especial attention to the social and cultural origins and functions of ideas, thought and knowledge. Some of the principal areas of anthropological enquiry which have devoted themselves to the study of knowledge in human culture and society are COGNITIVE ANTHROPOLOGY, the study of systems of CLASSIFICATION, and SYMBOLIC ANTHROPOLOGY. (*See* IDEOLOGY; MARXIST ANTHROPOLOGY; LINGUISTICS AND ANTHROPOLOGY.)

Kroeber, Alfred Lewis (1876–1960). US cultural anthropologist associated with BOAS and with the CULTURE HISTORY school. Kroeber's broad range of interests included a special concern for the historical aspect of anthropology, and his work is characterized by its tendency to study cultures as configurations and to attempt a global understanding of these configurations and their historical development. Kroeber built up the Anthropology Department at the University of California, and also carried out extensive ethnographic studies of Californian Indians. He is often accused of being a CULTURAL DETERMINIST since he adopted the SUPERORGANIC view of culture. His studies of the environmental correlations of CULTURE AREAS gave impetus to CULTURAL ECOLOGY, and he pioneered the use of the concept of CONFIGURATIONS or basic cultural patterns identifiable by dominant cultural aspects and 'style'. Major works include *Anthropology* (1923), *Handbook of the Indians of California* (1925) and *Configurations of Culture Growth* (1944).

Kula Ring. A system of ceremonial exchange decribed by MALINOWSKI (1922) for the Trobriand Islands and other islands off the coast of New Guinea. The inhabitants of these islands, though diverse in their linguistic and cultural affiliations, share a common system of ceremonial exchange characterized by the circulation of two kinds of ceremonial object: shell necklaces and shell armbands. Necklaces flow one way along the circuit of exchange partners, armbands the other way. Transactions vary from informal 'inland' ones to overseas visits accompanied by much ceremony and magical activity. Kula is accompanied by other kinds of exchange, and is an important element in the negotiation and maintenance of prestige, status and rank. In addition, it performs important functions of regional integration. The integrative properties of Kula exchange have been compared to the model of generalized EXCHANGE in LEVI-STRAUSS' theory of systems of kinship and marriage. (*See* RECIPROCITY).

Kulturkreis. This term, meaning 'culture circle' was one of the key concepts of German DIFFUSIONIST and CULTURE HISTORICAL theories. The culture circle was conceived of as a historical-geographical stratum representing a distinct phase of the diffusion of sets of related culture traits.

L

labour. The labour process is the organized process of the activities which support human societies, and it includes not only work or the purposive expenditure of human energy but also the use of the MEANS OF PRODUCTION, the social relations of production, and the organization of DISTRIBUTION and consumption of the product. In societies characterized by an advanced DIVISION OF LABOUR there may exist a labour MARKET, which reaches its maximum level of development in CAPITALISM, where labour is often conceptualized as a COMMODITY which may be bought and sold on the open market. In pre-capitalist societies labour markets are nonexistent or incipient in form, and labour in these societies is generally embedded in social and kin contexts, or attached to territorial, kin or personal allegiances.

labour aristocracy. The term 'labour aristocracy' denotes the concept of a sector of highly paid or privileged workers in contrast to the general level of wages and conditions of the mass of the working class. The term originated in Marxist discussions of the history of labour in Britain, and has also been applied to Third World nations. In the Third World context, the labour aristocracy is generally the small sector of persons employed in foreign-dominated capital-intensive sectors of the economy, and who enjoy wages, stability and conditions far above those attainable by the population in general. (*See* DEVELOPMENT.)

labour theory of value. In Marxist economic theory, labour is considered the true or objective measure of value. In CAPITALISM, however, the existence of COMMODITY FETISHISM and the dominance of EXCHANGE VALUE enables the capitalist to extract surplus VALUE from the producer, which is the difference between the cost of maintaining labour and the exchange value obtained for the product. Objections to labour as the measure of value have been raised on the grounds that different levels of capital intensivity, of technological involvement, and of social usefulness or demand for the product should also be taken into account in determining the value of commodities.

land. In economics 'land' refers in a very general sense to all natural resources, and as such constitutes one of the factors of production. In its limited sense of physical TERRITORY, land is of course a vital resource in agricultural societies, where its distribution and transmission constitute important features of social organization. In nomadic societies of the HUNTING AND GATHERING or pastoralist types, it is not land *per se* which is valued but the resources it contains: thus territories and their exploitation are often conceived of and defined in terms of the availability and distribution of vital resources such as vegetable or animal resources and water. Similarly in traditional systems of SHIFTING AGRICULTURE which relied on the availability of virtually unlimited areas of fresh land for exploitation, such as in the Amazon region, land tenure tended to be temporary and *de facto* by nature.

Agricultural societies with a scarcity of suitable land for cultivation have achieved the highest development of social mechanisms for land tenure and transmission. Thus in tribal and peasant societies of this type land is often the most valued form of PROPERTY, and is held in common by the community, by kin-based CORPORATE GROUPS (unilineal or otherwise) or by the FAMILY. In the FEUDAL type of social system, political authority and economic dominance was closely linked to land ownership, which carried with it a series of rights and relationships between the landholder and the tenants or serfs who occupied the land. With the advent of CAPITALISM individual ownership of land and the exploitation of land using paid agricultural labour become the predominant forms.

land reform. The deliberate reform by government of systems of land ownership and tenure, often accompanied by broader reforms in agricultural technology and techniques. Land reform is designed in most cases to reduce social inequalities and to eliminate forms of semi-feudal land ownership regarded as obsolete or politically undesirable. Thus such reform may involve the redistribution of large estates in the form of smallholdings to their tenants, or the formation of agricultural CO-OPERATIVES. Land reform policies have met with varying degrees of success, such success being dependent upon a number of factors, including the suitability of the proposed reforms in terms of pre-existing patterns of social and productive organization. It has for example been frequently argued that the failure of co-operatives after land reform is due to an 'individualistic' mentality among PEASANTS which makes smallholdings or family firms a more appropriate model for economic development. Other factors which should be taken into account, however, include the lack of availability of technical support and supplies such as fertilizer and seed to the co-operative, as well as the failure to develop systems of transport and market conditions for their produce. In some cases, land reform has even accelerated processes of proletarianization and rural-urban migration among the peasant population, due to the superficial nature of the reforms and the perpetuation by other means of the dominant position of the former estate-holding elite.

land tenure. A concept broader than that of 'ownership', referring to the rightful holding of land by a person or group, whether or not this holding involves ownership. Thus land owned by one person or group may be held by another, or the concept of land ownership may be absent.

language. A term often used to refer to the unique verbal communication system employed by humans, and which is characterized, amongst other features, by its highly specialized and independent development, its complexity of symbolic use and its arbitrary nature. The term is also applied frequently to other types of communicative system which possess SYMBOLIC or SEMIOTIC and grammatical features. Thus we may speak of artificial 'languages' employed by computers, or of other human and non-human systems of signs as 'languages'. In linguistics, the term is employed also with a limited technical sense, referring to the total set of possible utterances which can be generated by a given grammar. (*See* LINGUISTICS AND ANTHROPOLOGY.)

langue/parole. This distinction was formulated by Saussure (1916), and may be translated as 'language/speech'. Language is a set of rules and the possible utterances which may be generated by these rules, while speech is the set of actually observable utterances or linguistic behaviour. This distinction has sometimes been applied to the study of culture, where some authors have proposed that we should similarly distinguish between culture as a set of rules or possible choices on the one hand, and observable actions or behaviour on the other.

latent function. FUNCTIONALIST theory follows Merton (1949) in drawing a distinction between latent and manifest functions. Manifest functions are those which are intended and recognized by actors, while latent functions are unintended and unrecognized. This distinction plays an important part in Merton's critique of earlier functionalist theory, and in pointing to the unintended consequences of social action Merton addresses one of the central problems in functionalism, that of connecting global theories of functional prerequisites to the actions and motivations of individuals and groups in society.

latifundia. This term derives from the Latin and may be translated as 'large estates'. It is employed to refer to a system of LAND TENURE in which land is divided into large holdings owned and/or managed by an elite group and worked by a labour force. The labour force may be paid, or may consist of SLAVES or other forms of bound or dependent labour as in FEUDAL or semi-feudal systems. The contrasted term *minifundia* refers to the pattern of landholding in which land is divided into smallholdings.

law, anthropology of. Many of the anthropologists and social theorists of the 19th century began as lawyers or were drawn into anthropological study by their interest in primitive law and the history of legal institutions. Prominent among them were BACHOFEN, MCLENNAN, MAINE and MORGAN. The interest in law, often combined with a background in classics, was an important stimulus to the formulation of 19th-century theories of society and social evolution. Thus Maine, for example, traced the evolution of society via the evolution of legal regimes. The field of legal anthropology is concerned with the management of CONFLICT in human society, and theories of law are closely connected to theories (and political philosophies) of conflict. As Collier points out in his review of this topic (1975), if humans are seen as basically evil and society as the organized defence against human nature, then law is assigned a positive role in conflict management and regulation. However, if humans are considered basically good and conflict as inherent in society then the role of law is seen rather as a repressive one. In fact there is always in any legal system an element of ambiguity or tension between these two aspects: the regulation or control of deviance and the maintenance of the status quo. Different theories of law and deviance reflect this ambiguity, some focusing on the individual deviant under the assumption that he or she is the product of an imperfect socialization process, others on the manner in which society itself is predicated upon and generates conflict between persons, groups and social classes.

Epstein (1974), writing on Melanesian customary law, draws the distinction between 'contention', which is the tension resulting from endemic stresses in the social fabric, and 'dispute', which is a specific expression of contention. He points out that the resolution of a dispute does not solve the underlying problem which has been the source of contention. There is therefore a tendency, in Melanesian as in all other societies, to lay the blame for structural problems in society on the special characteristics or failings of individual persons. The legal process, by focusing on the individual 'victim of circumstance' and on the processing of the case, contributes to the perpetuation of the system which produced the problem. Legal systems may consequently be conceived of as safety valves, in the sense that they personalize problems which are in fact social, distracting attention from root causes and focusing it on specific events.

The theories of DURKHEIM have been important in social scientific approaches to law. Durkheim (1947) suggested that deviance is a collective creation of society, which in order to promote and preserve social SOLIDARITY must necessarily define its moral boundaries by creating outsiders or deviants. Durkheim's theories were the origin of the 'labelling theory' of deviance, which investigates the processes of selection and labelling of deviant persons and groups. Durkheim's ideas also influenced conflict models of deviance, which relate the selection and labelling of deviants to social STRATIFICATION and view crime and the legal process as products of the IDEOLOGY of the ruling class which act to perpetuate their dominant position. Conflict theories have also shown that law and legal process are themselves ARENAS for the expression of conflict and political manipulation, for example when litigation is pursued for political motives.

As many anthropologists and sociologists have pointed out, to focus on law as a set of rules or codes, or on legal philosophies and concepts as self-contained systems, leads us to ignore those aspects of the application and process of law which are not stated within the law itself, but form part of its total sociocultural context. Many social scientific theories of law focus not on legal codes *per se* but rather on the disputing process, which includes the formation, expression, management and resolution of disputes. The focus on dispute settlement is linked to the CASE STUDY method which reveals the operation of legal processes and principles through the study of their application to specific cases. Anthropological studies of law have explored the social organizational correlates of different forms of dispute settlement such as AVOIDANCE, DIVINATION, ORDEALS, MEDIATION, NEGOTIATION, ARBITRATION, and ADJUDICATION. Avoidance, for example, is a typical mode of dispute settlement where social space is relatively unlimited and formal mechanisms of social control are relatively undeveloped, as in HUNTING AND GATHERING societies. Adjudication, on the other hand, is the formal legal mode of social control which develops with increasing division of labour, social differentiation and the growth of BUREAUCRACY. Thus WEBER (1958) argued that implicit in the growth of capitalism and a necessary condition for such growth, was the development of a complex system of formal legal RATIONALITY. It has been argued by GLUCKMAN (1965) that in tribal society, on the other hand, the low level of technology and of permanent or durable private property sets limits on political centralization and leads to the predominance of RITUAL forms of social control.

Considerable debate has been generated over the question of the definition of law in anthropological perspective, and whether the term should be extended to societies where formal specialized legal institutions are underdeveloped or non-existent. Thus MALINOWSKI (1926) viewed 'primitive law' as 'the rules which curb human inclinations', thereby equating law with social obligation and social control. REDFIELD (1956) and others argued however that this definition is too broad, and would restrict the term 'law' to proto-legal institutions or codes of conduct relating to conflict. These include conventions relating to dispute settlement and mediation, codes of compensation, customary sanctions, and so on. According to this view, the anthropological study of law is not the study of social control or obligation in general, but rather of the specific codes of conventional procedures and sanctions, which include ceremonial expressions of disapproval, punishment following the consensus of public opinion, and the processes of COURTS in those societies where they exist. The range of settings in which conflicts or disputes may be resolved varies from formal courts with legal specialists to informal meetings of neighbours, peers or kin. Such informally-constituted gatherings may be referred to as moots, which are characterized by the attempt to reach a consensus among persons who must continue to live together following the dispute, and thus tend towards the search for social harmony and acceptable compromise rather than abstract principles of law or justice.

Pospisil (1974) defines law as 'rules or modes of conduct made obligatory by some sanction imposed and enforced for their violation by a controlling authority'. He points to four basic characteristics of law: the existence of AUTHORITY, the principle of universal application (a legal decision applies to all similar cases, unlike a political one), the principle of *obligatio*, under which a decision or statement becomes law inasmuch as it implies rights and duties, and the existence of sanctions, which may be physical or moral (ostracism, ridicule, and so on).

Bohannan (1967) argues that law, as distinct from CUSTOM and rules of conduct, is distinguished by the fact that it is 'doubly institutionalized'. All societies, he states, have some form of legal institutions whereby disputes are settled and breaches of NORMS are sanctioned. Legal institutions for Bohannan are part of the political framework. They are distinguished by the fact that they 'reinstitutionalize' or restate customs or rules derived from other institutions. Thus he says that a law is 'a custom that has been restated in order to make it amenable to the activities of the legal institutions'. Further, there are established procedures whereby these legal institutions themselves are conducted. Laws are thus doubly institutionalized norms, not just norms as in Malinowski's view. In pre-state societies, no one centralized authority can impose a consistent code of law, so law itself is less codified and less consistent than in state society. But roles of legal authority may nonetheless be well-defined, as in the case of the Nuer 'leopard-skin chief' who creates a compromise solution between parties to a dispute. More common than formal courts in pre-state societies are other procedures such as moots, oracles and divination, contests or ordeals and self-help. Courts form an organized body which represents a political authority, acting in the name of the state or the group as a whole, and thus exist only in politically complex or centralized systems.

Another area of importance within the anthropology of law has been the study of legal systems and legal process where these are highly developed, especially in traditional African kingdoms which have been the particular focus of studies of customary law. Bohannan shows that the judicial process among the Barotse, a traditional African monarchy, is similar to Western law in aspects such as the assessment of evidence, the concept of justice, and the manipulation of precedent, custom and legal code. But the lack of LITERACY and the relatively undifferentiated nature of social relations influence the operation of law in other ways. Notable differences between Barotse and Western law thus include the tendency to pursue social equilibrium, the tendency not to separate the case in question from the overall conduct of the parties, and the performamce by the courts of administrative and political as well as legal roles. Bohannan also points out the flexibility or ambiguity of key legal concepts, due to their unwritten nature, thus permitting strategic decisions with greater facility.

An important aspect of the anthropological study of legal systems is the plurality of such systems, which often coexist within a single national or regional framework. Thus, within multiethnic and multicultural contexts, subsystems such as criminal, civil and commercial law may coexist with other legal codes of a different type. These other codes have varying degrees of formality and elaboration, and are observed by different sectors of the population. The application of a legal system by a colonial or national dominant elite to an ethnic minority or colonized population is one of the means by which political dominance is asserted, and the resulting conflicts and contradictions between traditional and imposed law are an important field for anthropological enquiry. The specialized application of anthropological knowledge to the resolution of individual legal cases within the system of Western law is termed 'forensic anthropology', but the possible applications of the anthropological perspective in law are much broader than the giving of 'expert evidence' in specific cases affecting members of ethnic minorities. The anthropological comparative perspective on legal systems is of great theoretical and practical importance in such fields as the formulation of laws relating to native populations, defence and advocacy of the rights of ethnic minorities, advisory functions for native federations or community development organizations, and many other areas within the field of APPLIED ANTHROPOLOGY.

The study of the theory or philosophy of law is termed 'jurisprudence' and the field of comparative jurisprudence, or the comparative study of legal theories, is another area of important potential for the application of anthropology. An area which has been little developed is the application of the anthropological perspective to the study of modern Western legal systems. While the sociology of law has explored fields such as the roles of lawyers and legal institutions, the operation of law in relation to different social classes, and so forth, the comparative perspective of anthropology has been little applied in the context of modern industrial society.

Leach, Sir **Edmund R.** (1910–). British social anthropologist who has influenced, and in many ways shaped, the development of modern social anthropology. His *Political Systems of Highland Burma* (1954) was profoundly influential in the development of POLITICAL ANTHROPOLOGY, and demonstrates the complex interrelationship of ideal models and political action within a historical context. Leach has been a principal interpreter of the works of Levi-Strauss to an English-speaking public, and has developed approaches influenced by structuralism in the fields of KINSHIP, SYMBOLIC ANTHROPOLOGY, MYTH, and the study of culture and communication. His *Rethinking Anthropology* (1962) was an important challenge to the received orthodoxy of STRUCTURAL FUNCTIONALISM in British anthropology, and was influenced in part by his interpretations of the work of Levi-Strauss and in part by his own more empirically inclined stance. Other major works include *Pul Eliya* (1961); *Genesis as Myth, and Other Essays* (1969); *Levi-Strauss* (1970) and *Culture and Communication* (1976).

leadership. Leadership is an important aspect of political systems, and in POLITICAL ANTHROPOLOGY the analysis of the cultural definition and social enactment of leadership roles is an important area of enquiry. Leadership should be distinguished from AUTHORITY, as persons who exercise effective leadership are not necessarily those who occupy political OFFICE or positions of authority. Leadership is generally measured by the taking of decisions, the leader being regarded as the person who either takes decisions himself or herself or is the focal point of decision-making by the group. Thus leadership occurs in a multiplicity of contexts of social action (including, for example, in work groups, family or kin groups) and is not always part of a political system. Political leadership – or the existence of a leadership role which plays a part in the political system – also takes a variety of forms, and analysis of the definition and functions of political leaders is part of the analysis of the total system of political roles of the group. (*See* BIG MAN; CHIEF; HEADMAN; MONARCHY; POWER; STATUS.)

legal anthropology. *See* LAW, ANTHROPOLOGY OF.

legitimacy. In political theory and POLITICAL ANTHROPOLOGY, 'legitimacy' denotes ideas or beliefs which justify the exercise of POWER or the existence of superior STATUS, privilege, and so on. The term may also be applied more broadly to the justifiability of any action: an action is legitimate if it is performed by a person who has the moral and/or legal right to do so. The legitimate exercise of power is thus termed AUTHORITY, since authority is distinguished by a generally accepted right to take decisions affecting others. Legitimacy is a necessary condition of political systems, which cannot exist by coercion alone. Yet paradoxically it is never fully achieved, since there are always divergent viewpoints or dissenting individuals or groups who challenge the legitimacy of existing political LEADERSHIPS or of dominant elites. The balance between legitimacy and coercion is one which manifests itself in many different ways, and the study of this balance is related to the study of IDEOLOGY, or of the social concomitants of ideas and beliefs. Legitimacy is a double-edged weapon, for not only does it justify the position of a dominant group or political leader, it also sets limits – by its moral and normative nature – on the exercise of power or the conduct of those who are in a dominant position. In addition there may be different ideologies and different criteria of legitimacy which coexist within a complex political system which is based on divergent class interests and class conflict. Anthropological studies have shown that in pre-class societies too divergent models of legitimacy, and not just competing claims to legitimacy may exist, which may be revealed in moments of fission or political tension.

legitimation. The process whereby POWER gains LEGITIMACY. In Marxist theory, legitimation is a function of IDEOLOGY.

levelling mechanism. In the anthropological study of PEASANTS and other COMMUNITY STUDIES some use has been made of the concept of levelling mechanisms, which are presumed to inhibit the accumulation of wealth by specific individuals or families, encouraging its redistribution or consumption whether in RITUAL or other forms. (*See* CARGO SYSTEM; ECONOMIC ANTHROPOLOGY; LIMITED GOOD; POTLATCH.)

levels of sociocultural integration. A concept formulated by STEWARD (1951), which he proposed in order to conceptualize sociocultural systems better in a comparative and EVOLUTIONARY perspective. Given that not all people live in homogeneous tribal societies, the anthropologist must analyse different levels. The family, the FOLK society and the state each constitute a distinct level of integration of social relations and cultural phenomena. Steward's formulation of the concept introduces a confusion however in the sense that the levels are seen both as evolutionary stages (FAMILY; BAND; TRIBE; CHIEFDOM; STATE) and as levels within a context of cultural change, or within a complex society, which are all interacting at one and the same time. (*See* ARTICULATION OF MODES OF PRODUCTION.)

levirate. A form of MARRIAGE rule in which upon the death of a married man his widow is required to marry one of his brothers. This rule is often interpreted as an expression of patrilineality, since it is predicated upon the notion that the woman once married becomes in some sense property of or indissolubly attached to her husband's patrikin. However the rule is not found in all patrilineal societies, and it is found in some societies which are not patrilineal. The practice of leviratic marriage should be interpreted not only in terms of lineality but also in terms of the system of GENDER relations and concepts of female subordination in the society concerned.

Levi-Strauss, Claude (1908–). Leading French anthropologist whose influence as one of the foremost STRUCTURALIST theorists extends not only to cultural and social anthropology but also throughout the social sciences and humanities. After studying law and philosophy in Paris Levi-Strauss travelled to Brazil, and recorded his experiences among the Brazilian Indians in his *Tristes Tropiques* (1955; trans.). *World on the Wane,* 1968) which is an important and enduring document of the anthropological vocation. In his *The Elementary Structures of Kinship* (1949; trans. 1969) Levi-Strauss presented major theoretical advances in the study of KINSHIP and MARRIAGE. In subsequent works Levi-Strauss turned to the further explication of structuralist method, its links to LINGUISTIC theory, and its applications to a variety of domains, with an increasing emphasis on the study of thought and symbolism. In consequence, he produced *Structural Anthropology* (1958; trans. 1968); *Totemism* (1962; trans. 1963); and *The Savage Mind* (1962; trans. 1969) in fairly rapid succession (*see* PRIMITIVE MENTALITY; TOTEMISM). There followed the four volumes of *Mythologiques* (1964–72) which apply structuralist analysis to a vast body of MYTHS, and the second volume of *Structural Anthropology* in 1973 (trans. 1977).

Levy-Bruhl, Lucien (1857–1939). French philosopher whose interest in ethnological and sociological theory was stimulated by his concern to analyse the nature of PRIMITIVE MENTALITY. Levy-Bruhl argued (1923) that primitive thought was qualitatively different and pre-logical (not, as he has often been interpreted, 'illogical') in that it did not separate cause from effect. His theories have been much criticized, by DURKHEIM and MALINOWSKI among others, though some anthropologists have come to his defence, claiming that he does point to important differences in RATIONALITY between different types of society.

Lewis, Oscar (1914–70). American cultural anthropologist whose studies of Mexican and other communities led him to formulate the concept of the CULTURE OF POVERTY. The extensive criticism of this concept does not detract from the enduring impact of Lewis' portraits of family and community

life among the poor. Major works include *The Children of Sanchez* (1961) and *La Vida* (1966).

lexicostatistics. A method for measuring the relationship between languages. By comparing standard vocabulary lists in two languages and recording the number of cognate forms, lexicostatistics (or glottochronology) attempts to measure how far the two languages have diverged from a common base over time. The main drawback of the approach is the failure to clarify and investigate the interaction between the independent evolution of languages and other factors such as diffusion and contact.

liberation. This term, originally applied in contexts of political REVOLUTION to refer to the liberation of a subordinate group, nation or class from a dominant power, has also been applied both by Marxist and socialist thinkers and by certain sectors of the Catholic church to refer in a broader sense to the search by minority or oppressed groups and populations for social justice and self-determination. The 'theology of liberation' associated with thinkers such as Paolo Freire and Gustavo Gutierrez represents a combination of Christian and socialist thought which has had a mixed reception among leaders of the Catholic Church, who advocate the search for justice and harmony in social relations while at the same time condemning party political involvement of priests and counselling against Marxist philosophies which they regard as fomenters of hatred, violence and class antagonism. Freire's ideas on education and social action among oppressed groups have been profoundly influential, especially in Latin America where considerable sectors of the Catholic Church today are associated with 'progressive' and liberation oriented work in education, communication and community development. Gutierrez' works include *Teologia de la liberacion*, which advocates the active and revolutionary imitation of Christ's 'option for the poor', but many have detected a softening recently in his change of emphasis towards theological questions in the theology of liberation, and away from political or social ones. The continuing debate within the Catholic Church about its political role, and the involvement of certain sectors of the Church with progressive social and communal projects is of great interest and importance in Latin American and other largely Catholic countries, where the political potential of an alliance between Catholicism and Marxism is incalculable.

license. *See* RITUAL REBELLION; JOKING RELATIONSHIP.

life crisis. The life crisis is a specific moment of especial importance in the LIFE CYCLE of the person. Such moments include birth, illness and death among others, but may be defined differently in different sociocultural contexts, as life crises are not only naturally occurring events but also may be socially and culturally created and defined. Life crises which exist in Western industrial society but not necessarily in other cultures include divorce and unemployment, for example. Other cultures similarly have specific life crises defined and interpreted in terms of the categories and roles within each culture. Life crises may be accompanied by RITUAL observances (*see* RITES OF PASSAGE) which are of psychological and social importance in defining and interpreting the nature, course and outcome of such events.

life cycle. The phases of the individual life cycle, though universally bounded by the experiences of BIRTH and DEATH, are differentially perceived and defined in different cultures (*see* AGE, ANTHROPOLOGY OF). Indeed even the experiences of birth and death are not necessarily limits of the individual life cycle, since it may be believed that persons exist as ANCESTORS, SPIRITS, names, and so on, after their death or before their birth. The study of RITUAL is in large part concerned with the manner in which sociocultural systems act upon, interpret and employ the natural life cycle in ritual statements and actions. (*See* SOCIALIZATION; INITIATION; MARRIAGE; RITES OF PASSAGE.) The concept of the individual life cycle has been extended and enriched by the consideration of the DEVELOPMENTAL CYCLE OF THE DOMESTIC GROUP.

life history. Social scientific research and writing focusing on life histories or biographies of individual persons is a valuable adjunct to other research methods. Biographical data is often used to give realism to or to illustrate social scientific theories and approaches. This use of life histories is often anecdotal or literary in style, and like any other ethnographic approach lends itself to selective or distorted presentation of events and behaviour. The use of life histories and their interpretation has not as yet been the subject of widespread theoretical and methodological scrutiny in anthropology.

liminality. In the theory of RITES OF PASSAGE formulated by VAN GENNEP and extensively developed in the anthropological study of RITUAL, one of the stages of ritual is referred to as the 'liminal' stage because the initiate or the person undergoing the ritual process is regarded as in a special state apart from society and normal life, a state regarded as SACRED, ritually dangerous, vulnerable, polluting or subject to pollution. The liminal stage follows the stage of separation from normal social life and from the community, and is followed by the stage of reincorporation.

limited good. A concept formulated by FOSTER in his attempt to explain the behaviour and value orientation of PEASANT communities in Mesoamerica (1965). Foster argued that the cognitive orientation of Mexican peasants was basically CONSERVATIVE, and that 'peasants see their universe as one in which the good things in life are limited...and hence personal gain must be at the expense of others...social institutions, personal behaviour, values and personality will all display patterns that can be seen as a function of this'. Peasants were consequently held to display extreme individualism, competitiveness, personal envy and only sporadic co-operative relationships. This formulation was challenged in terms of its ethnographic validity (for Mexican or other peasant groups) by REDFIELD and others, who stressed the positive aspects of peasant social and cultural organization and world view (*see* FOLK/URBAN CONTINUUM). The ethnographic validity of Foster's construct has been repeatedly challenged, and it has been pointed out that notions of 'limited good' and the sociocultural role of envy should be related to the specific MODES OF PRODUCTION in which peasants are involved.

Thus Dow argues (1981) that the image of limited good applies only to peasant attitudes in the face of the capitalist mode of production, while in relation to the DOMESTIC MODE OF PRODUCTION they display a different set of attitudes which recognize the fact that the labour and accumulation of each household contributes to the wealth of the community as a whole. In addition, like the concept of the CULTURE OF POVERTY advanced by LEWIS, Foster's theory was heavily criticized for locating in the community itself and its value or cognitive orientations the roots of resistance to change and DEVELOPMENT, rather than focusing on the external power structures maintaining peasant communities in a subordinate position with regard to national society. Thus critics argued that the failure of peasant communities to develop economically was the result not of conservative peasants refusing to take advantage of opportunities, but rather of structures of domination and exploitation beyond the control of the local community.

lineage. A DESCENT group which is generally defined as a group of persons who trace descent from a known common ancestor: PATRILINEAL if descent is traced through males only, and MATRILINEAL, if through females only. Larger units within a descent system are termed CLANS, SIBS or GENS, the definition of these larger groups varying according to the author concerned.

lineage theory. Lineage theory or DESCENT theory dominated British social anthropology from the 1940s to the 1960s, and was also influential in US cultural anthropology during the same period. It developed out of earlier anthropological theories which, as shown by Kuper in his review of this topic (1983), had as their central concerns the relationship between KINSHIP and territory on the one hand, and on the other that between the FAMILY and larger social units such as CLAN, GENS or SIB. Maine's *Ancient Law* (1861) expounded the PATRIARCHAL theory of the origin of society, arguing that the first social units were patriarchal families under the authority of the senior male. The aggregation of such family units constituted the next stage of social EVOLUTION. On the death of the senior male, Maine argued, his sons and their families would stay together, thus forming a larger unit based on extended consanguineal kinship ties. Maine contrasted these 'blood' ties with the relationships based on territorial attachment or 'local contiguity' which become the basis of more advanced stages of social evolution. Later theories preserved Maine's distinction between kinship and territory (see, for example, MORGAN's distinction between *societas* and *civitas*) though differing from Maine in the details of the evolution of family- and kin-based groups. Thus Morgan and MCLENNAN argued that the original state of society was not patriarchy but PRIMITIVE PROMISCUITY, which was superceded first by matriliny and later by patriliny.

In the USA, BOAS and his followers began to develop a critique of these theories, based on their tests and comparisons with ethnographic data from a wide range of cultures, data which was only then becoming available as a result of the new emphasis on the importance of field research in anthropology. This empiricist critique culminated, according to Kuper, in the work of LOWIE (1937), who reached three important conclusions: that historically the family is present at every stage of culture, that there is no fixed evolutionary order of matriliny and patriliny, and that both the bilateral family group and the unilineal kin group are based on territorial as well as consanguineal principles.

While the unilinear model of social organization continued to dominate US evolutionary and later CULTURAL ECOLOGICAL schools in anthropology, it was in Britain that lineage theory became such a dominant theme that it seemed for a time to become synonymous almost with social anthropology itself. With the new emphasis in British anthropology on the importance of fieldwork and the study of FUNCTIONAL interrelations of social institutions rather than their evolutionary development, the lineage came to the forefront as a major unit of social organization. The unilineal corporate localized exogamous descent group came to dominate the ethnographic record, especially under the influence of those studying specific regions of Africa who found characteristics there (later recognized to be specific to these regions rather than universal) which they thought shaped the theory of lineage systems.

The works of RADCLIFFE-BROWN were important in influencing these developments. In his essay on 'Patrilineal and Matrilineal Succession' (1952) Radcliffe-Brown argued that kin-based CORPORATE GROUPS were necessarily unilineal, since only unilineal descent could provide fixed and unambiguous group membership. Thus unilineal descent groups were the natural solution to the problems of social stability and continuity in kin-based societies. The 'ethnographic paradigms' for lineage theory were provided however by FORTES and EVANS-PRÌTCHARD with their research in Africa, which was influenced both by Radcliffe-Brown and by MALINOWSKI's functionalist theories. Thus the two classic monographs, Evans-Pritchard's *The Nuer* (1940) and Fortes' *The Dynamics of Clanship among the Tallensi* (1945) marked both the establishment of the functionalist and lineage theory perspectives as the dominant paradigms in British social anthropology. In *The Nuer* Evans-Pritchard postulated a model of SOCIAL STRUCTURE based on the interaction of territorial and descent principles. The SEGMENTARY lineage system, he claimed, functioned in such a way as to define territorial-political units contextually, according to specific situations of opposition and unity and processes of FISSION and fusion. At the same time, the lineage system provided a language in terms of which political relations were expressed and articulated.

Evans-Pritchard's model of the segmentary lineage system has been widely criticized, both in terms of contradictions with the empirical evidence and in terms of its theoretical presuppositions. He himself came increasingly to stress that the model was not intended to account for actual social organization or group structure on the ground, but rather as an approximation to Nuer values or ideal models of social structure, in terms of which actual social relations could be expressed and interpreted. However Kuper claims that the model is not relevant to either Nuer values or their social structure, while others such as Holy (1981) have pointed out that the segmentary lineage model relates only to one aspect of Nuer values or social organization, and that other sets of values and other domains of social life should also be taken into account.

Fortes' study of the Tallensi is the other pioneering ethnography in the development of lineage theory and kinship studies. Fortes defined Tallensi clans as localized associations containing lineages. Unlike Evans-Pritchard's neat and hierarchical model, Fortes described the sometimes ambiguous 'fields of clanship' created by cross-cutting and overlapping ties between clans and their segments. These clan ties consisted of a variety of social and SYMBOLIC elements, including RITUAL relations and also relations of MARRIAGE as well as genealogical connections. Neither clans nor lineages were conceptualized by Fortes as necessarily constituting corporate economic or dominant political groups. Nevertheless Fortes did argue that unilineal descent was primary to group structure and Tallensi values. In order to account for the importance of matrilateral ties in this patrilineal system, Fortes distinguished the domain of family and kinship relations (which are bilateral) from that of clanship, which is unilineal and where jural priority is given to patrilineal descent as a principle regulating inter-group relations. He later elaborated this model in his study of the matrilineal Ashanti (1953) and developed it into his theory of COMPLEMENTARY FILIATION which accounted for the existence of matrilateral ties in patrilineal systems and patrilateral ties in matrilineal ones.

The 'Africanist' descent model established by these pioneering ethnographies and the many which followed came under increasing attack during the 1960s on a number of fronts. On the one hand the influence of STRUCTURALISM led to critiques of 'typologizing' pioneered by LEACH, who argued that rather than prejudge the content of social relations by employing the labels 'patriliny' or 'matriliny' we should seek more value-free or 'mathematical' ways of expressing the relations between structural elements. The strongest challenge to descent theory was the development of ALLIANCE THEORY by LEVI-STRAUSS and his followers who, while at first not questioning the exogamous unilineal descent group as the basic unit of social structure, argued that the articulation of the social system was given by the marriage alliances between such groups.

Another strand of criticism focused on the relationship between the ideal model of lineage structure and the reality of social action on the ground (*see* ACTION THEORY). The attempt to apply or adapt the Africanist model to other ethnographic regions has resulted at times in its modification or its rejection in favour of models stressing social interaction in the determination of group composition. Indeed it may be argued, as Kuper contends, that the whole of lineage theory rests on a fundamental confusion between ideal models and actual group relations and organization on the ground. By privileging one aspect of a specific native model the work of Fortes and Evans-Pritchard led many ethnographers either to ignore or else explain away the existence of non-unilineal principles such as COGNATIC and AFFINAL ones, and to misconceive the nature of the relationship between social organization and anthropological model-making. At the same time the development of alliance theory and the study of NON-UNILINEAL DESCENT have shown that it is not only unilineal principles which can be employed to create corporate groups: other principles such as marriage alliance and residence rules may also be employed (*see* ENDOGAMY; KINDRED).

New models derived from other ethnographic regions have been applied to African societies as part of the attempt to demonstrate the bias introduced by classic lineage theory. Attempts to refine lineage theory itself have been rendered difficult by the fact that it is hard to find an ethnographic example of a 'pure' lineage system, since even classic cases such as the Nuer and Tallensi may be successfully reanalysed using cognatic models. Hence lineage theory is no longer generally regarded as the privileged perspective for the study of tribal society or kinship systems, and principles of unilineal descent are studies, alongside other types of kinship and alliance relation, which enter into the determination of group structure and group composition.

linguistic relativism. The hypothesis associated with SAPIR and WHORF, who argued that each language expressed and created a distinct and autonomous system of thought. This view influenced US CULTURAL RELATIVISM and later came to be challenged within COGNITIVE ANTHROPOLOGY.

linguistics and anthropology. The relationship between linguistics and anthropology has always been a close one, though the form which this relationship has taken has changed considerably over time. 19th- and early 20th-century anthropology was closely linked to comparative linguistics which studied exotic languages and attempted to trace the genetic relations and historical development of languages and language families. Because of the revolution in linguistics brought about by the advent of TRANSFORMATIONAL and generative theories the relationship between the two disciplines took on a new dimension. In the new linguistics the empirical focus tended to be on European rather than non-European languages, but the relationship with anthropology took the form of theoretical and conceptual influence. Linguistic models were extensively adopted as models for cultural and social behaviour, notably in the fields of STRUCTURALISM and COGNITIVE ANTHROPOLOGY.

The adoption of linguistic models for the interpretation and analysis of sociocultural systems naturally raises philosophical and methodological difficulties. Some anthropologists have questioned whether it is legitimate to regard language as the basic model upon which all thought or CLASSIFICATION is structured, on the one hand, and on the other whether it is accurate to regard culture and social organization as purely COMMUNICATIVE systems to be analysed in the same fashion as linguistic codes. Thus linguistically-inspired theories such as structuralism and approaches within cognitive anthropology have been criticized as 'idealist' and for concentrating on mental or communicative phenomena to the exclusion of the material conditions and historical development of society. Behind these differences are fundamentally different views of the nature of social 'reality', which some anthropologists see as a product of objective or material conditions (*see* CULTURAL ECOLOGY; MARXIST ANTHROPOLOGY) while others see it rather as a conceptual or SYMBOLIC construction. Perhaps the most productive anthropological approaches are those which recognize that society and culture are in fact both of these things: a material reality and a conceptual construction, and which examine the interplay between these dimensions.

Modern linguistics and SOCIOLINGUISTICS have moved away from the exclusive concentration on formal models and towards the

172   **Linton, Ralph**

study of the social use of language (*see* ILLOCUTION). These developments have been paralleled in anthropology and sociology by ETHNOMETHODOLOGY and the ethnography of speaking.

Linton, Ralph (1893–1953). US cultural anthropologist who entered anthropology from archaeology and who was an important influence on the development of the CULTURE AND PERSONALITY school. Linton pioneered the use of the terms STATUS and ROLE in anthropology, and was also concerned with the need to synthesize different areas of anthropological enquiry and socio-cultural data. Major works include *The Study of Man* (1936), *The Cultural Background of Personality* (1945) and *The Tree of Culture* (1955).

literacy. The distinction between literate and pre-literate cultures has been the focus of considerable anthropological interest. Among cultures where some form or degree of literacy exists, we should distinguish those where literacy is a majority phenomenon from those where it is a privilege or attribute of a specialist group or ruling elite. 'Specialist literacy' as Goody (1977) terms it, is limited to a ruling class or a specialist group of 'scribes', thus creating a division into two cultures, the literate and the oral. 'Restricted literacy' in Goody's terminology is special purpose literacy which is limited to specific fields such as religion on the one hand or administrative purposes such as tax-collecting on the other.

The development of literacy is often cited as one of the defining characteristics of a CIVILIZATION, though in the case of the ancient Inca empire of Peru most of the features commonly associated with the concept of civilization were present in the absence of a system of writing. In Egypt, India and China and to a lesser extent in Mesoamerica the rise of URBAN civilization was however accompanied by the growth of a literate tradition which was typically employed in its initial phase for religious and/or administrative purposes.

As Goody has pointed out, the tendency to dichotomize cultures into 'literate and pre-literate', 'logical and pre-logical', or 'scientific and pre-scientific' results in an over-simplification of how modes of thought

and of communication develop over time. Thus, he argues, we should examine more carefully the ways in which the means of communication (oral or written) change over time, as do the persons and classes of persons who control the use of such means. He argues that literacy and the mechanisms of written language are indeed the key to many of the changes and contrasts between 'primitive' and 'advanced' societies. Literacy increases the pool of available knowledge and thus the possibility of innovation, as opposed to the ORAL TRADITION which has no reservoir for items it does not immediately incorporate. Literacy favours historical consciousness by the creation of texts with an independent existence, thus permitting the confrontation of different viewpoints and different texts more readily than in oral history. It also facilitates the development of impersonal and abstract codes for the purposes of administration, LAW or BUREAUCRACY. By 'freezing' data at a particular point in time, literacy also contributes to the standardization of cultural and craft techniques and tradition, and to the development of specialized educational institutions.

The question of who controls the means of communication, and which sectors of the population have access to literate skills, is of importance for the anthropological study of IDEOLOGY and structures of class dominance. Since literate skills and the different levels of mastery of written language are invariably linked to different social roles, the study of differential levels and types of literacy enables us to grasp readily the mechanisms of control and distribution of knowledge in society as well as the ways in which access to privilege or POWER may be regulated according to the mastery of literate skills. The growth of mass media in modern industrial society and especially the growth of forms such as television, radio and cinema, which do not require literacy from their public, likewise has important consequences for the social control of knowledge. Just as it has been suggested that literacy itself changes cognition, so it may be argued that the dominance of audio-visual communicative technology changes cognitive orientations among the population, and possibly competes with literacy which according to some studies would seem to be in decline. The advent of computer technology on a massive scale has stimulated further speculations regarding the cognitive and social consequences of possible mass computerization, and like other technological innovations the uses and effects of computerization depend in large part upon who owns and controls the technology and directs the decisions regarding its application. The use of computers until the present has been largely controlled by commercial interests and placed at the service of large-scale capital enterprise, with experiments in socially appropriate or community-oriented computer projects being still in their infancy.

Another anthropologically important aspect of literacy is the process of contact and domination between literate and pre-literate cultures. The overall historical tendency resulting from IMPERIALIST and COLONIALIST policies has been the more or less gradual replacement of minority unwritten languages by the written languages of the dominant nations. The adaptive advantages of literacy as well as the ETHNOCIDAL tendencies implicit in colonial and neo-colonial power structures have contributed to the virtual elimination of many minority languages, and the linguistic factor is of such importance in the determination of ETHNICITY that the survival or destruction of the language is often taken as a measure (or indeed the measure) of ethnic persistence. In various parts of the world BILINGUAL education projects attempt to rescue or preserve minority languages by establishing for them a written form, and by advocating that native children be taught to read and write first in their own language. Such programmes have had some small measure of success, though they do not function in isolation from the overall political and socio-cultural climate, and are not sufficient by themselves to ensure the survival of a threatened ethnic group or language.

little tradition. *See* GREAT/LITTLE TRADITION.

Locke, John (1632–1704). This English liberal philosopher and social theorist is best known for his theory of social contract, according to which the function of the STATE is to defend the natural rights of persons to life, liberty and property. Locke's theories were influential in the development of INDI-VIDUALIST political philosophies. In his *Essay Concerning Human Understanding* (1690) he propounded that the origin of ideas is empirical rather than innate, the human mind being a *tabula rasa* to be written upon by learning and experience. (*See* ENLIGHTENMENT.)

Lomax, Alan (1915–). US cultural anthropologist who has pioneered the study of MUSIC and DANCE in cross-cultural perspective. Lomax has elaborated methods for the cross-cultural measurement and comparison of music (cantometrics) and dance (choreometrics). He has also postulated correlations between musical and dance forms and levels of societal complexity or evolution (e.g. 1968; 1977).

Lounsbury, Floyd Glenn (1914–). US linguistic anthropologist who is best known for his work in the field of FORMAL SEMANTIC ANALYSIS of kinship systems (e.g. 1971).

Lowie, Robert H. (1883–1957). An early student of BOAS, this US cultural anthropologist also worked with WISSLER during the early years of his career. His special ethnographic focus was the Plains Indian groups. His *Primitive Society* (1923) is a rebuttal of MORGAN's evolutionary theories, emphasizing the diversity of causes and historical processes leading to the current distribution pattern of culture traits. Like Boas, Lowie emphasized the importance of specific historical explanation and careful field research, avoiding evolutionary speculation. Other major works include *The Crow Indians* (1935) and *History of Ethnological Theory* (1937).

lumpenproletariat. This term was employed by Marx to refer to the most marginal or impoverished sector of the proletariat, those who had no fixed employment and who were the focus of criminal activity. The *lumpenproletariat*, unlike the industrial proletariat, was considered to be essentially apolitical or opportunistic in its political allegiances, unlike the industrial proletariat, the basis of working-class organization. In Third World nations where there is generally a small industrial proletariat with stable employment and a large sector of unemployed or underemployed, a great proportion of the population would fall into the category of *lumpenproletariat*. Nevertheless anthropological studies have shown that it is not correct to conceptualize this sector of the population in solely negative terms, because they do not participate in industrial work. The populations of SHANTY TOWNS in the Third World, for example, possess a series of socio-cultural characteristics and features of community organization which have been studied within URBAN ANTHROPOLOGY and MIGRATION studies and which demonstrate the potential for social and political organization among those sectors denied access to industrial employment.

M

magic. The study of magic is closely linked to the study of RELIGION and RITUAL in general. Indeed it is not always possible to sharply delimit the field of magic from that of ritual or religious belief. A definition often adopted is that magic is ritual which is motivated by a desire to obtain a specific effect, magic being seen as the attempt to manipulate supernatural or spiritual forces or agencies by ritualized means. The relationship between magic and science has attracted considerable anthropological attention and debate. TYLOR (1871) held that magic was a form of primitive science, with the function of explaining the nature and cause of phenomena which humans observe and experience. FRAZER (1890), following Tylor, postulated a three-stage development of human thought from magic through religion to science. Magic, he argued, was based on the false association of ideas, and he divided magic into two basic types: sympathetic, based on the idea that like influences like, and contagious, based on the idea that things which have been in contact may continue to influence one another even when separated.

Later anthropologists challenged this view of magic as primitive or erroneous science. MALINOWSKI (1948) in particular denied the validity of Frazer's and Tylor's views, arguing that magic was not a substitute for science but instead possessed distinctive social and psychological functions which were particularly important in societies with low levels of technological development. According to Malinowski, magic is resorted to when technology does not permit people to ensure the outcome of their actions, and it functions to allay anxiety and to allow the cathartic expression of emotion. RAD-CLIFFE-BROWN, following DURKHEIM, stressed the effects of magic on the social structure, arguing that it acted to reinforce social solidarity and group identity in mo-

ments of stress (1952). Many social and cultural anthropologists followed the lead of Malinowski and Radcliffe-Brown in analysing the symbolic, expressive and sociological functions of magic. However the 'neo-Tylorian' approach advocated by Robin Horton (1967) revived interest in Tylor's and Frazer's theories about the explanatory functions of magical beliefs.

The study of magic is beset by the difficulties inherent in attempting to delimit magical and scientific beliefs or world views. As has been noted, in modern 'scientific' cultures a large proportion of the population 'believe' in scientific or technological phenomena without understanding them, a belief which is perhaps as magical or as religious as that held by a member of a simple society in the knowledge which the ritual specialists of the group possess. The scientific knowledge for which we all tend to take credit is in fact only understood and created by a very small proportion of the population. Thus dichotomies of primitive and advanced or scientific cultures will inevitably oversimplify the real processes of development of knowledge in society.

In modern anthropology the tendency is not to separate 'magic' as a sharply defined field with ritual and religion on the one hand and technical activity on the other. The anthropologist consequently studies the interpenetration of the symbolic and scientific aspects of knowledge, as well as the techniques for its application. (*See* PRIMITIVE MENTALITY; SORCERY; WITCHCRAFT.)

Maine, Henry James Sumner (1822–88). This English jurist and social theorist is best known for his work *Ancient Law* (1861) which concentrated on the evolution of legal systems as the key to social evolution. Influenced by evidence from classical Rome and Greece, he argued that the most primitive societies were patrilineal and PATRIAR-CHAL, a theory which contrasts with the views of other evolutionary thinkers who put forward the primacy of PRIMITIVE PROMIS-CUITY or MATRIARCHY. Maine's broad evolutionary scheme was based on the development of society from systems based on kinship to those based on territoriality, from status to contract and from civil to criminal law. However Maine was not a rigid unilinear evolutionist, since he did not hold that all societies necessarily must follow an identical pattern in every detail.

male dominance. *See* ANDROCENTRISM; FEMINIST ANTHROPOLOGY; GENDER; WOMEN AND ANTHROPOLOGY.

Malinowski, Bronislaw Kaspar (1884–1942). Polish-born anthropologist who after training in mathematics and physics entered anthropology as a postgraduate student in England. After studying at the London School of Economics, Malinowski carried out his classic fieldwork in the Trobriand Islands, which was to be of immense significance in the establishment of anthropological fieldwork methods and particularly of the methodology of PARTICIPANT OBSERVATION. Malinowski opposed earlier EVOLUTIONARY theories in anthropology, and is considered one of the founders of the FUNCTIONALIST school. His functionalism emphasized the interrelations between all the parts or elements of a culture or social system, denying the validity of the concept of SURVIVALS and arguing for functional, rather than historical or evolutionary, explanations of sociocultural phenomena. For him culture and social institutions served needs which he divided into primary and secondary, or derived. Malinowski was also concerned with the psychological dimensions of culture, and was one of the first anthropologists to put psychoanalytic theories to the test in cross-cultural perspective. Major works include *Argonauts of the Western Pacific* (1922), *Crime and Custom in Savage Society* (1926), *Sex and Repression in Savage Society* (1927), *The Sexual Life of Savages* (1929), *Coral Gardens and Their Magic* (1935), *Magic, Science and Religion* (1948) and *A Diary in the Strict Sense of the Term* (1967).

Malthus, Thomas Robert (1766–1834). English economic and political theorist, whose *Essay on Population* (1798) pioneered DEMOGRAPHIC theories. Malthus argued that human populations naturally tend to increase and outstrip their food supply, and that this increase would inevitably tend towards the creation of poverty until the point where disease and hunger put a limit on the growth of the population. He thus introduced a note of pessimism into the 18th century intellectual atmosphere, with its beliefs in progress and the infinite perfectibility of society through rationality. It is interesting that in reaching his conclusions, Malthus sets aside the possibility of rational methods of fertility control, dismissing artificial methods as immoral and pointing to the improbability of the adoption of sexual restraint by the population as a whole. Some political and social theories and ideologies which might be termed neo-Malthusian retain Malthus' basic premise of the natural tendency of populations to increase towards poverty and starvation, but at the same time advocate the use of artificial methods of fertility control in order to contain the population explosion before negative checks come into operation. A prominent feature of aid and DEVELOPMENT programmes in many parts of the Third World is the promotion of population control methods.

Marx later challenged Malthus' theories, arguing that the creation of poverty was not a result of natural demographic trends but a specific consequence of the historical development of CAPITALISM. Marxist theorists have indeed argued that population control programmes based on neo-Malthusian premises merely serve to distract attention from the root causes of poverty and to reduce the revolutionary potential of the poorer classes by controlling their reproductive capacity, and it has been argued that under socialist regimes natural population increase can be absorbed without leading to poverty. However opinions and policies are somewhat divided and can be seen to have changed over time in socialist countries. China, for example, moved from an early position of encouraging population growth to a later policy of strict control of fertility. In the Third World and among ethnic minority groups within Western nations fertility control programmes often meet similarly with mixed or negative response since they are suspected in this case of genocidal intent.

mana. A term which from Polynesian and Melanesian ethnography has passed into general anthropological usage, and which refers to a type of spiritual POWER or energy which manifests intself in natural phenomena, places, persons etc. (*See* ANIMATISM.)

manifest function. *See* LATENT FUNCTION.

manners. *See* ETIQUETTE.

Mao Tse-Tung (1893–1976). Chinese political leader and Marxist theorist whose concepts of revolution and of the development of a socialist society have been of great influence in the Third World. This influence is due to the fact that Mao modified in great part Marxist theory, which was essentially biased towards industry, to suit better the reality of a predominantly PEASANT society based on agriculture. He thus revindicated the revolutionary potential of the peasant class, which in orthodox Marxism had been underestimated or dismissed. Other distinctive features of Maoist thought include the insistence on the continuing nature of the revolution and the need for profound and constant reform and renewal in order to avoid stagnation and arrest counter-revolutionary trends, the need for the interprenetration of the urban and rural domains and of intellectual and manual labour, and the importance of cultural and ideological reforms in order to sustain economic ones.

Marett, Robert Ranulph (1866–1943). British anthropologist whose special interest was the study of RELIGION and MAGIC. Marett was a student of TYLOR, whose theories of the origins of religion he developed in his works, including *The Threshold of Religion*.

marginality. Marginality in its economic, political and sociocultural dimensions is an important element in most contexts of anthropological research, and has varying dimensions which have been explored in ethnography and anthropological theory to varying extents. On the one hand, it has been pointed out that in the FIELDWORK experience the anthropologist is a kind of 'marginal native', who while not fully incorporated into the host community, is nevertheless somewhat detached from his or her 'native' culture. The consequences of this marginality have been explored within ethnographies influenced by CRITICAL ANTHROPOLOGY. On the other hand, the vast majority of the populations studied by anthropologists are to a certain extent marginal ones: often doubly marginal, as in the case of ethnic minority groups existing within Third World nations which are themselves marginal to the world capitalist system. Anthropological research within Western nations also tends to focus on groups which are in some way marginal to the dominant national society, whether they are ethnic minorities or groups that are in some other way set apart from the mainstream.

In spite of anthropologists' clear preference for marginal populations, the profession tends at times to shy away from the possible consequences of this choice, and few would define the discipline generally in terms of 'the study of marginal groups', though it has often been defined as the study of 'small-scale' or pre-industrial' societies, definitions which ignore the crucial common feature of marginality which unites the vast majority of anthropological host communities. In fact, as studies within diverse areas of critical anthropology, APPLIED ANTHROPOLOGY, MARXIST ANTHROPOLOGY and theories such as DEPENDENCY theory and WORLD SYSTEMS theory have shown, the processes and structures which create, define and maintain marginality are in themselves essential and legitimate areas of anthropological enquiry. It is the function of the ethnographer not only to document the distinctive sociocultural features which exist within the apparently closed universe of a marginal group, but also to document the experience and process of marginalization itself, thereby revealing the links between the marginal group and the wider socioeconomic and political system. When underlying power structures at a regional, national and supranational level are revealed, the illusion of a hermetic or self-contained culture or society vanishes, demonstrating that all human communities (whether bands, tribes, ethnic minorities or sectors of modern industrial society) exist within the context of evolving relationships with neighbouring groups, and with broader sociocultural systems whose historical development affects them either directly or indirectly.

market. In the anthropological discussion of this concept we must first distinguish clearly the market as 'marketplace' or physical setting for the exchange of goods, from the principle of market exchange, which is that of the exchange of goods at prices determined by forces of supply and demand. Thus markets as marketplaces may exist in societies where the market principle is not the dominant or exclusive mode of exchange, and similarly market exchange may take place without being localized in a specific marketplace. POLANYI (1968) and members of the substantivist school of ECONOMIC ANTHROPOLOGY who have followed his classificatory scheme, divide types of economy according to the predominant mode of exchange in each. The three types of exchange according to this classification are RECIPROCITY, REDISTRIBUTION and market exchange. Markets may exist in societies where the predominant mode of exchange is reciprocity or redistribution, but in these cases their functioning and socioeconomic context is different from that which we may observe in societies where the market principle is dominant.

The predominance of market exchange in the economy is related to growing specialization of occupational and productive roles, to an increase in food surpluses produced by the agricultural sector of the population, and to the correlated development of MONEY. In certain tribal economies money-like valuables are present, such as brass rods among the Tiv or shell money in parts of Melanesia. These are termed 'special purpose' money because their use is more limited and specific than the general purpose money of a market-dominated economy. Thus as Dalton points out (1965), the *tambu* shell valuables of the Tolai of Papua New Guinea could be said to resemble money in the sense that they were used in a wide range of transactions, could be used for the purchase or sale of all forms of property, and were interchangeable in standard denominations. On the other hand, their central significance as ceremonial valuables and the peripheral function of the traditional market with

relation to the economy as a whole mean that we cannot fully equate them with modern general purpose money.

In the peripheral markets of nonindustrial societies, market participation is limited to certain specific goals and is not central to the organization of production in the economy as a whole. Market prices have only a limited influence on the organization of labour and the movement of subsistence goods. Not all goods produced enter into the market – subsistence goods may never be marketed or only a small surplus portion may ever reach the market. At the same time, the 'non-market' functions of the market (ritual, social, political and ceremonial) are often of central importance: perhaps of more importance than the economic exchange itself.

Markets in PEASANT societies share some of the characteristics of traditional tribal markets, but at the same time display greater integration into the regional and national market economy. The peasant market, like peasant society as a whole, displays a double and sometimes contradictory orientation towards subsistence needs within family and community and the need or desire to participate in the wider market system. In peasant as in tribal society not all goods produced enter into the marketplace, much of what is produced being reserved for family use and for the discharge of obligations of reciprocity with kinsmen and neighbours. In peasant markets too social and ceremonial functions may similarly be very important. Thus in the Andes and in Mesoamerica markets are an important mechanism of regional integration, linking local communities which are often ecologically distinct, geographically separated, and specialized according to their technological or craft activities. The market system links these communities to one another and also to regional and urban centres. As well as serving the needs of the local communities, peasant markets also link these communities – by means of the actions and operations of BROKERS, PATRONS and middlemen – to the regional and national market economy.

The disadvantageous conditions under which the peasant producer participates in the market, due to the small scale of his or her production, the lack of access to credit and other factors related to the marginalization of the peasantry, mean that his or her integration into the regional and national market economy is necessarily on unequal terms. The low prices paid to the producer, together with a series of mechanisms of indebtedness invariably associated with the patron-client relationship, maintain the peasant producer in a dependent relationship and generally unable to produce or market enough to ensure the acquisition of the basic goods which he or she requires from the wider market system. However, this is not to say that peasant producers or those who participate as craftsmen in peasant markets may not under certain circumstances accumulate considerable wealth, and it has been suggested that the economic stability and wellbeing of certain peasant communities tends to be disguised by the fact that in these communities the conspicuous display of wealth is discouraged.

As Sahlins points out (1972), the integration of tribal hinterlands, like that of peasant communities, into a wider market-dominated economy leads to a contradiction between reciprocity and redistribution within the community, and market exchange outside it. Thus he says: 'The engagement with the market makes a key minimal demand: that internal community relations permit household accumulation...else the amounts required for external exchange will never be forthcoming. This stipulation must prevail in the face of limited and uncertain ...production. The fortunate households cannot be responsible for the unfortunate; if internal levelling is encouraged then the external trade relations are simply not sustained.' A topic of anthropological enquiry which has received less attention than peasant participation in market systems is the study of the integration of tribal peoples into wider regional and national market systems, under conditions of socioeconomic change and development.

Another characteristic of market systems in pre-industrial economies is the relative autonomy of local marketplaces, lacking an overall regional or national mechanism of co-ordination or fixing of prices from one locality to another. Prices thus depend either upon the vicissitudes of local supply and demand, which itinerant merchants may take advantage of in their travels from market to market, or else upon bureaucratic administration of prices by local authorities.

The modern market system within CAPITALISM possesses certain distinctive characteristics which set it apart from earlier market systems. One of the most important is its relative independence from other spheres: the market in capitalism functions in relative independence from ceremonial, political or social considerations, since it is a self-regulating mechanism which co-ordinates COMMODITIES (including labour) on a regional, national and worldwide basis. Thus the market in capitalism is much broader than the physical marketplace, embracing all aspects of economic activity. Price-fixing in the capitalist market system is likewise more systematic and sensitive to the forces of supply and demand on a large scale. As Sahlins shows, supply and demand mechanisms do affect prices in pre-capitalist and tribal economies, but in a more indirect and unsystematic fashion. The 'ideal type' market system within capitalism is one in which there exists perfect competition, so that supply and demand alone account for price variations. However the system of perfect competition does not occur in reality, though it is an important element of the ideological justification of the free market system. In fact the concentration of productive and distributive activities into the hands of relatively few firms leads to monopolistic tendencies which restrict competition and increase profit. At the same time, all modern governments intervene to some extent in the market, whether in the fixing of prices or wages (the price of labour) in the redistribution of income and wealth by means of taxation, in the control of monopolies, or in the provision of goods and services regarded as essential or socially beneficial.

marriage. There is no one universally applicable definition of marriage, because the cross-cultural variability in the social organization of GENDER relations and the existence of rare forms of marriage in specific societies render such definitions invalid. Some writers have attempted to define marriage, by indicating the universal core functions of the institution, which are usually related to control of or rights over sexual activity and the legitimation of children. Gough (1959) focuses on the legitimations, stating that marriage is a universal social institution which establishes the legitimacy of children. However there are societies where this is not a function of the marriage relationship. Goodenough (1970) focuses rather on the marriage relationship as a contractual one which establishes rights over a woman's sexuality. However these minimal definitions are perhaps of little utility in the development of the anthropological study of marriage, which has such complex and varied forms as the well-known Nuer 'ghost marriage' and woman-woman marriage. In 'ghost marriage', the children borne by a widow after she has remarried or taken lovers continue to be regarded as legitimate offspring of her dead husband. In another rare form of marriage among the Nuer a woman may be married to another senior woman, and the children borne by the wife are regarded as members of the 'husband's' patrilineage. Another famous 'limiting case' of the marriage institution in human societies is that of the matrilineal Nayar studied by Gough, where young girls are ceremonially 'married' but do not reside with their husbands, being permitted to take lovers by whom they bear children. Neither the ritual husband nor the recognized lovers have rights over the woman's children, who are simply members of the mother's lineage. Another form of marriage which may be observed not to fit conventional definitions would be marriage between male homosexuals, which however would appear to be modelled on the conventional male-female form. Similarly it should be remembered that the rights and relationships established by marriage are not always individual ones, but may be shared by corporate kin groups. This has been demonstrated both by LINEAGE THEORY which has emphasized the transfer of rights in women and their potential offspring to a unilineal kin corporation by marriage, and by ALLIANCE THEORY which stresses the marriage alliance as the creation of a relationship of exchange between groups and examines the sociological consequences of different types of exchange relationship. Within alliance theory the marriage relationship is considered principally from the point of view of the alliance which it creates (see ASYMMETRIC/SYMMETRIC ALLIANCE; ELEMENTARY STRUCTURES, PRESCRIPTION/PREFERENCE.) Leach, in his essay on the topic of the definition of marriage

(1962) takes as his starting point the *Notes and Queries* definition, which is: 'Marriage is a union between a man and a woman such that children born to the woman are the recognized legitimate offspring of both partners'. He questions whether the definition of marriage in terms of a single attribute is adequate, and points to the existence of a number of distinguishable classes of rights which may be allocated by the marriage relationship. These rights include the establishment of legitimacy of a man's or woman's children, the granting of rights of control over the spouse's sexuality, over domestic or labour services, or over the property of the spouse, the establishment of a joint property fund, and the establishment of a relationship of affinity between the husband and the wife's brothers. This list, he adds, is not complete, since in specific societies the marriage relationship may have other specific functions. Nor would it be possible, he adds, for all these features to be present in a single society. He suggests that we should expect instead to find at least one and probably several of these functions or classes of rights in any given society. Thus 'the institutions commonly described as marriage do not all have the same legal and social concomitants'. He suggests that the anthropological study of marriage should be directed towards elucidating the relationship which exists between the nature of the marriage relationship (that is, the peculiar constellation of rights it implies) and other features of social organization such as DESCENT and RESIDENCE. (*See* ADULTERY; DIVORCE; POLYGAMY.)

marriage classes. Used by LEVI-STRAUSS to establish a conceptual distinction between descent groups (clans) and groups related by marriage alliance (classes). Marriage classes are groups which 'permit a positive determination of the modalities of exchange.' (*See* ELEMENTARY STRUCTURES.)

marriage payments. The topic of marriage payments has been the focus of considerable anthropological discussion and debate, as several authors have attempted to establish and refine schemes of correlation between marriage payments and other features of social organization. Marriage payments may take the form of bridewealth when the payment flows from the husband or his group to the wife's group, or of dowry when the payment flows from the wife's group to the husband's group or typically to the couple themselves. The use of the term 'brideprice' was rejected in anthropological writings due to its connotation of 'buying and selling' a wife, and the term bridewealth was substituted to refer to the flow of goods or payments which compensate the wife's group for the loss or transfer of certain rights in the woman and her children. Where the payment is specifically for rights in the children born to the woman, the term 'childprice' has sometimes been employed. Common to most anthropological discussions of marriage payments are the agreement that these payments serve to legitimize marriage relationships at the same time that they signify or mark the transfer of rights in women and/or children. The STRUCTURAL FUNCTIONAL school in social anthropology produced several interpretations of marriage payments as 'compensation' for the transfer of a person or rights in that person from one kin group to another, for the granting of rights in offspring, and so on. It was suggested in consequence that bridewealth exists in patrilineal societies where marriage transfers the productivity and/or reproductive powers of a wife to her husband's group. Comaroff, in his intoduction to a volume dedicated to this topic (1980), points out that these early theories did not entirely fit the facts, since bridewealth exists in some societies where a woman is not alienated or 'transferred' from her natal group, and dowry also occurs in some patrilineal and virilocal systems.

Goody, in a volume of essays on bridewealth and dowry (1973), suggests that these should be analysed in terms of the wider context of property relations. He suggests that dowry is a form of premarital inheritance or 'diverging devolution' associated with bilateral kinship systems, while bridewealth is associated with unilineal (though not necessarily patrilineal) systems. Dowry in Europe and Asia, he argues, is associated with the hierarchy and HYPERGAMY of stratified societies. It is often associated too with positive marriage rules of varying kinds, whose consequences for the ultimate destination of property may be traced within each

system. African systems characterized by bridewealth are associated with egalitarian societies where status differentials in marriage are insignificant. Further, dowry, by endowing the couple with a conjugal fund at the expense of the kin group, makes the couple the focal point in property holding. Goody suggests that dowry is associated with a tendency to MONOGAMY as well as with systems of marriage alliance which stress 'status negotiation'. Bridewealth, on the other hand, is associated with unilineal descent corporations as the central property holding groups, with POLYGAMY and with the lack of status negotiation in marriage. He further argues that the degrees of social stratification in societies characterized by bridewealth and dowry may be correlated with the existence of hoe agriculture (horticulture) and plough agriculture respectively.

Comaroff notes that Goody's model is suggestive but perhaps too general, and points to the existence of exceptions to the association between marriage payment forms and forms of agriculture, as well as to significant regional variations within Africa and Eurasia in forms of marriage payment, types of agriculture and systems of descent and alliance. Comaroff's critique of Goody's theory is concerned mainly with the diversity of empirical forms of marriage payment and their function within specific social systems, and the need to examine marriage payments not as isolable institutions but rather as part of the total system of affinal relations in the society concerned.

Other approaches to marriage payments include that of Meillassoux (1972), who suggests that control over bridewealth permits elders to perpetuate the dependency of young men in age-stratified societies, since the elders who control the property of kin groups are thus enabled to negotiate and control marriage relationships. Levi-Strauss, on the other hand, argues that marriage payments are 'tokens' in systems of delayed reciprocity (1969). He seeks the significance of African bride-wealth, for example, in the fact that it provides a guarantee – in the form of special goods – that the wife-givers will themselves be able to find wives.

marriage rules. *See* ALLIANCE; INCEST; PRESCRIPTION/PREFERENCE.

Marx, Karl Heinrich (1818–83). German revolutionary thinker and one of the founding fathers of the social sciences, whose works cover the fields of political philosophy, sociology and economics. Marx was educated in Germany and was associated during his student days with the radical Young Hegelian movement. From Germany he moved to Paris and after brief periods in this city and in Brussels and Cologne he moved to London, where he was to stay for most of the rest of his life. In Paris, where he began his lifelong association with ENGELS, the two produced *The Holy Family* and *The German Ideology*. Another important work of this period was Marx's *The Poverty of Philosophy*. During the revolutionary period of 1848 and the years immediately following, Marx and Engels produced the *Communist Manifesto*, which was intended as a political programme for the revolutionary Communist Party.

In England, Marx devoted his attention to the studies of politics and economy which form the core of Marxist social theory. *Grundrisse*, the *Contribution to the Critique of Political Economy* and *Capital* (in three volumes) are the fruits of this period. During the period 1864–72 Marx was an important figure in the direction of the First Socialist International.

Marxist anthropology. Marx was a socialist and a revolutionary, but much more than any of his predecessors he based his politics on a study of society and of the mechanisms which made it change. As he got older he pushed back his study of society ever further, and as a result the fields which had traditionally been of interest to anthropologists increasingly came under his scrutiny.

Marx read very widely in anthropology, but was particularly powerfully struck by the work of MORGAN, which he read towards the end of his life. He felt that Morgan's theories could be made to dovetail with his and planned a book on the topic, but it was written only after his death by ENGELS, working in part from Marx's own notes. This book, *The Origin of the Family, Private Property and the State*, presented the idea, then very radical, that what was thought of as private – the family, moral rules regulating sexuality – as innate or the differences between men and women – were in fact all

interlinked and were connected also with the politico-economic system of the society, even with the nature and existence of the STATE. Engels made the point by adopting from a number of anthropologists the idea that mankind had gone through a number of stages, in this case PRIMITIVE COMMUNISM, SLAVE SOCIETY, FEUDALISM, CAPITALISM and COMMUNISM, and the passage from one of these stages to another implied a systematic transformation of all the factors at issue.

In many ways the adoption of a particular list of EVOLUTIONARY stages was quite problematic, and had very unfortunate effects – especially in the USSR, where the anthropological record was pushed willynilly into this scheme. Right from the start however a number of Marxists refused the straightjacket of the five stages. In particular many pointed out that in a number of his earlier writings, which came to light gradually during this century, Marx had suggested other stages or MODES OF PRODUCTION. In particular Marx had evoked the ASIATIC MODE OF PRODUCTION to explain the lack of development of capitalism in such places as India and China. As a result there has never been a fully-accepted Marxist anthropology in the USSR or elsewhere, and the field has always been one of theoretical controversy.

From the 1960s on two very different approaches began to develop. The first is largely derived on the one hand from the work of ALTHUSSER, who influenced a number of anthropologists such as E. Terray (1972), and of M. Godelier (1977), who combined the influences of LEVI-STRAUSS and Marx, creating what has sometimes been called 'structural Marxism'. Both schools share some fundamental ideas, just as they reject Marx's specific evolutionary scheme more or less completely, and instead seek to use the methods of analysis Marx had used for capitalism for non-capitalist systems. These writers pay particular attention to the notion of 'mode of production', which Marx had used to examine the interrelated social totality which organizes PRODUCTION and REPRODUCTION in society. Following Marx these writers emphasized the way LABOUR is organized usually by the exploitation of one CLASS by another. This is made possible by such things as the PROPERTY system, the political system, the kinship system, and the religious system. A study in terms of modes of production examines the related role of these various factors in enabling a specific system to continue, and tries to explain under what conditions it breaks down. It is not a study in terms of technological determinism.

The second tendency which has developed since the 1960s also derives from the ideas of Althusser, and is concerned with the ARTICULATION OF MODES OF PRODUCTION. 'Articulation' denotes the way different modes of production, for example the capitalist and the communal in a Mexican village, interact and affect the way both reproduce. The details of how this is examined are quite technical, but Marxist writers concerned with this question are continuing a tradition which goes back to the very origins of Marxism: a concern with the effects of the political and economic domination of one group of people by another, often taking the forms of COLONIALISM and IMPERIALISM. Among the earlier anthropological writers dealing with this question are E. Wolf (1969) and P. Worsley (1957), and among the more recent J. Suret-Canale (1971) and P.P. Rey (1971).

Another newer trend in Marxist anthropology has come from a re-examination of Marx's notion of ALIENATION and IDEOLOGY.

material culture. Material culture includes the sum or inventory of the TECHNOLOGY and material artefacts of a human group, including those elements related to subsistence activities as well as those which are produced for ornamental, artistic or ritual purposes. The study of material culture is linked on the one hand to ARCHAEOLOGY, where the material evidence of the existence of a population is often the only data available on their culture, and on the other to the anthropology of ART, MUSIC, DANCE, SYMBOLISM and RITUAL, and the anthropology of technological systems.

material forces of production. According to Marxist theory, these are the real foundations of economic systems and thus of society. The material forces of production and the social relations of production together constitute the MODE OF PRODUCTION.

materialism. This term refers to theories or schools of thought in philosophy and the social sciences which assert the primacy or determining role of matter, as opposed to IDEALISM. (*See* CULTURAL MATERIALISM; DIALECTICAL MATERIALISM; HISTORICAL MATERIALISM.)

mathematical models in sociocultural anthropology. Mathematical models are formal abstract representations which intentionally simplify complex reality. Their construction and manipulation enable analysts to examine possible consequences of interactions among important variables. Two well-known mathematical models in the natural sciences are Einstein's theory of relativity and Mendelian genetics. Anthropological models include representations of DEMOGRAPHIC processes, social organization (MARRIAGE systems, KINSHIP algebra, residence rules), resource use ('optimal foraging', ecological systems), decision-making and folk systems of CLASSIFICATION.

Many sociocultural anthropologists became quite enthusiastic about mathematical modelling during the 1960s and 1970s. The first COMPUTER simulations to construct and evaluate anthropological models were devised, and reviews of 'mathematical anthropology' (e.g. White, 1973) devoted many pages to model building. In recent years the use of mathematical models has levelled off as researchers have become more aware of certain limitations of the technique.

Well-constructed mathematical models can be great aids in theory-building since they force researchers to be explicit about the assumptions they make in their analyses. When mathematical models yield unrealistic results, anthropologists must either re-evaluate such assumptions or consider new variables in their analyses. Mathematical models also allow researchers to examine the possible future effects of changing conditions.

Despite these advantages, anthropologists' attempts to create mathematical models have sometimes been disappointing. Theorists have occasionally misunderstood the mathematical assumptions of formal methods such as GAME THEORY, operations research and SYSTEMS ANALYSIS, and computer simulation involves programming skills that few anthropologists have. The biggest problem, however, is that many researchers become so involved in the implications of their model that they forget the shaky nature of certain essential assumptions. (*See* FORMAL ANALYSIS.)

matriarchy. This concept originally gained importance in anthropology as a result of the theories of matriarchy developed by BACHOFEN (1967), who asserted that matriarchy was the earliest form of human society, preceding PATRIARCHY. Theorists who adopted Bachofen's notion of the evolutionary primacy of matriarchy included MORGAN, MCLENNAN and ENGELS. These writers associated matriarchy with MATRILINY and MATRILOCALITY, and with religious features such as cults to female goddesses. They argued that in these early human groups positions of power or dominance were held by women. Morgan and later Engels related the development of patriarchy to the origin of private PROPERTY in society. Other evolutionary theorists, notably MAINE, held that patriarchy was the original form of human society.

The concept of matriarchy fell into disrepute in 20th-century anthropology along with the general movement away from evolutionary speculation and towards functionalist theories of human society within both US cultural anthropology and British social anthropology. At the same time, the development of kinship studies and LINEAGE or DESCENT THEORY began to show clearly that matriliny, matrilocality (or UXORILO-CALITY) and the distribution of power between the sexes are separate though interrelated phenomena, to such an extent that the early association of matriarchy with matrilineal descent was proved to be an oversimplification of the ethnographic reality. Descent theorists showed that even in matrilineal societies power and positions of authority are generally held by men (though transmitted though women).

The concept of matriarchy enjoyed a revival, however, within FEMINIST ANTHRO-POLOGY, where it has been given more serious consideration by many authors. However the image of matriarchy in feminist thought is not identical to the 'mother-right' postulated by early theorists. In feminist anthropology matriarchy may imply gender equality rather than female dominance. There is an observable difference between those feminist writers who follow Marxist theory in asserting that male dominance or patriarchy did not exist in the earliest forms of communal society, and that therefore these earliest forms of society can be conceived of as in some sense matriarchal, and those feminists who argue that male domination and exploitation of women is a universal phenomena which predates all other forms of social inequality. These latter writers emphasize evidence for the universal existence of patriarchal values. (*See* WOMEN AND ANTHROPOLOGY.)

matrifocal. 'Mother-centred' family forms which are usually defined by the absence or weak role of the father and the corresponding emphasis on the female role in the domestic group. Black Caribbean family structure is a frequently cited example. Sometimes matrifocality is taken to refer to the physical absence of the father-husband, though it should be noted that the absent male may retain strong economic and authority ties with his family. At other times 'matrifocal' is used to denote that the female is the central figure of family and household identity and continuity, though this may be true in a wider range of societies. In the mother-children nucleus within a patrilineal system, or the British working-class family described by Bott (1971), for example, males have authority in the public sphere while the domestic sphere is focused upon women. In fact the concept of matrifocality lacks analytical value, firstly because it is ethnocentric to focus on matrifocality as problematic while 'patrifocality' is taken to be normal, and secondly because to lump societies together on the basis of a criterion such as domestic female role dominance produces an arbitrary classification which fails to do justice to the range of variations in marital and gender roles. However the notion of matrifocality does point to several interesting areas of enquiry, such as the extent to which patrifiliation may be unnecessary for the legitimation of children in certain societies, the existence of 'matrifocal' family forms as a stage in the developmental cycle of domestic groups, or as one of many possible forms of marriage and family. An important point raised in discussions of matrifocality is the extent to which female-centred households are regarded as entirely normal or ideal, and the extent to which they are capitulations to real economic and social problems in societies where the ultimate ideal is stable monogamous marriage and the father-centred family. Similarly, it has been suggested that mother-centred family forms are related to certain economic circumstances, in particular labour instability and unemployment among males. (*See* CONSENSUAL UNION.)

matrilateral. 'On the mother's side'. Refers to those relatives who are linked to Ego through Ego's mother.

matrilateral cross-cousin marriage. Marriage of male Ego with his MBD is a pattern which LEVI-STRAUSS, in his theory of the ELEMENTARY STRUCTURES of kinship and marriage, characterized as generating a system of 'indirect exchange' or 'generalized reciprocity' since if strictly observed this rule would give rise to the circulation of women between groups. Levi-Strauss points out that this system is less secure than SYMMETRIC ALLIANCE in the sense that a man or group *a* gives a woman to a man or group *b* without the immediate security of return, since *a* will receive his wife not directly from *b* but from another man or group *c*, *d* or *e*, and so on, depending on the number of groups involved in the system. On the other hand, argues Levi-Strauss, this system also integrates more local groups than direct exchange will, because it is open-ended and will not tend to break up into separate wife-exchanging dyads as a direct exchange system will.

In systems of matrilateral cross-cousin marriage the wife-exchanging circuit may be closed ('marrying in a circle') where the groups concerned are of equal status, or it may be open, as in HYPERGAMOUS and HYPOGAMOUS marriage systems which are associated with systems of status differential between wife-exchanging groups. Modern studies of this as of other types of marriage PRESCRIPTION have increasingly come to recognize the flexibility and situational variability of marriage norms, and thus to pay less attention to the hypothetical consequences of strict adherence to the rule and more to the dialectical relationship which exists between model and practice.

matrilineal. Matrilineal DESCENT is that which is traced through females: thus children are affiliated to the group of their mother, or, as it is sometimes expressed, of their mother's brother, since in matrilineal societies power and position are generally held by men, though transmitted through women. The kinship group formed by persons linked by matrilineal descent to a known common ancestress is termed a matrilineage. (*See* KINSHIP; LINEAGE THEORY.)

matrilocal. Matrilocal postmarital residence is residence of the couple with or close to the wife's family, or more specifically the wife's mother. Matrilocality is not necessarily associated with matrilineality, and in order to avoid the confusion of the two concepts many anthropologists prefer to use the term UXORILOCAL which simply refers to residence 'in the wife's place' and does not prejudge that the most important element of this residence pattern is coresidence with the wife's mother. The term 'matri-uxorilocal' has also been employed to mean residence with the wife's mother or matrilineal kin group.

Mauss, Marcel (1872–1950). Student and nephew of DURKHEIM, Mauss collaborated with him on *Primitive Forms of Classification* (1903). His major work is *The Gift* (1925; trans. 1954) which demonstrated the importance of GIFT exchange and structures of RECIPROCITY in social organization. This work has had a profound influence in ECONOMIC ANTHROPOLOGY, SYMBOLIC ANTHROPOLOGY and the study of KINSHIP and MARRIAGE. Mauss' theories have influenced many anthropologists, among them LEVI-STRAUSS.

McLennan, John F. (1827–81). A Scottish lawyer who was inspired by ethnographic accounts of BRIDE CAPTURE to formulate a theory of the evolution of MARRIAGE. Like BACHOFEN, McLennan postulated an original stage of PRIMITIVE PROMISCUITY in human evolution, followed by MATRIARCHY. He argued that early humans practised female INFANTICIDE since women were not valued as hunters or warriors, and then resolved the consequent shortage of women by the practice of bride capture and fraternal POLYANDRY. The practice of fraternal polyandry then gave rise to PATRILINEAL descent. In *Primitive Marriage* (1865) McLennan coined the terms ENDOGAMY and EXOGAMY.

Mead, Margaret. (1901–78). Margaret Mead was a student of BENEDICT, and from the start of her anthropological career her main interest was in CULTURE AND PERSONALITY. Mead carried out a number of well-known ethnographic studies including *Coming of Age in Samoa* (1928), *Growing Up in New Guinea* (1930), and *Sex and Temperament in Three Primitive Societies* (1935) whose main conclusions were that patterns of personality are culturally, and not biologically, determined. She set out to show that such phenomena as the adolescent phase of personal development and the roles and behaviour typical of men and women, were not products of biologically-determined or innate patterns but rather of culturally specific child-rearing practices. The extreme CULTURAL RELATIVIST position of Mead has been questioned by many, and the ethnographic accuracy of her fieldwork in Samoa came under attack from Derek Freeman (1983), who attempted to exploit the weaknesses of Mead's ethnographic data in order to argue a case for the biological determination of behaviour and social institutions.

Margaret Mead is most celebrated for her considerable success in disseminating anthropological ideas among a wide public, and as an advocate of change and reform in US society in the light of the results and insights afforded by an anthropological and cross-cultural perspective. In this sense, she was particularly active in advocating educational reform and the rethinking of established wisdom about age- and sex-linked roles and behaviour in US society. Major works apart from the early ethnographies include *Male and Female* (1956), *New Lives for Old* (1956) and *Culture and Commitment* (1970).

meaning. The question of meaning in anthropology is linked to the problem of interpretation or translation between different languages and cultures. There are several interlinked difficulties in the anthropological presentation of meaning. One of these is the overcoming of the anthropologist's own ethnocentric bias and/or the barriers which impede communication and understanding between anthropologist and informants, in order to arrive at a satisfactory understanding of the EMICS of an alien culture: that is to say, in order to capture the meaning of cultural elements for the actor within that cultural system. Another related difficulty is that meanings are by no means always well-defined, nor are they necessarily held in common by all members of a culture. We may adhere to common behavioural norms and participate in common social institutions yet lack a consensus of opinion as to the meaning of our acts.

Another major problem is that of the relationship between emic and etic understanding: the participant's viewpoint and the anthropological analysis. Different types of anthropological theory imply different levels and degrees of correspondence between the anthropological interpretation and the informant's meanings or psychological reality. STRUCTURALISM, for example, does not require that the anthropological model have psychological reality for the informant, since it is supposed that informants will not be conscious of the underlying or deep structure of culture. Marxist theory, on the other hand, examines the relationship between popular meanings and interpretations and objective analysis of social and historical phenomena in terms of the concept of IDEOLOGY. The term is used here to describe the imposition of beliefs and values by a dominant group or class, or by society as a whole; an imposition which systematically distorts the objective conditions of socio-economic life. Thus Marxism unlike structuralism argues that popular and social scientific models can coincide, by means of political education and organization of the subordinate groups in society, and as a concomitant of revolutionary praxis. (*See* CULTURAL RELATIVISM.)

means of production. In Marxist theory, all the elements which enter into the productive process in society. These include land and raw materials, technology, natural resources, and so on. The differential relationship to or control of the means of production is the defining factor in the structure of CLASS relations in society.

mechanical/organic solidarity. According to DURKHEIM's theory of the DIVISION OF LABOUR (1933), there is an evolutionary continuum from mechanical to organic solidarity. Mechanical solidarity refers to societies which are composed of a number of essentially similar units, where the division of labour is as yet little developed. Organic solidarity on the other hand refers to modern society, in which there is an advanced division of labour and the component parts of society therefore stand in a relationship of interdependence.

mechanical/statistical model. This distinction is employed by LEVI-STRAUSS in his theory of ELEMENTARY STRUCTURES of kinship (1969). A mechanical model preserves the relations among the phenomena it models and is thus a representation of the phenomenal world 'on the same scale' as the phenomena themselves. For example, an elementary structure of kinship with a PRESCRIPTIVE marriage system can be represented by such a model which is like a simplified version of reality. A statistical model on the other hand bears a more complex relationship to the reality it models or explains. Complex structures of kinship and marriage require statistical models for their explication.

mediation. Mediation, an important mechanism of conflict resolution or dispute settlement, is the intervention of a third party not involved in the dispute, who may be of a high status which gives him or her a certain moral authority, of equal status to the parties to the dispute, or perhaps a low status 'outsider' who may be regarded as a suitable neutral go-between. Mediation is a common mechanism of dispute settlement in societies with systems of formal legal authority which are not well-developed.

medical anthropology. The field of medical anthropology, which some prefer to call ETHNOMEDICINE, is one of the most highly developed areas of anthropology and APPLIED ANTHROPOLOGY, having almost acquired the status of a discipline apart. Some authors reject the term 'medical anthropology' because it implies that the sub-discipline subscribes to the 'medical model' of disease and health as presented by Western professional medicine, and since

one of the most important functions of this area of anthropological enquiry is precisely to question conventional medical wisdom they feel the term to be an inappropriate one. However it continues to be the most commonly used denomination, though the term ethnomedicine is gaining increasing currency. We may further distinguish the field of 'clinical anthropology', which is the application of anthropological knowledge to the resolution of specific clinical cases in medical practice.

Medical anthropology, or the anthropology of health, as we may also term it, is a field which has grown very rapidly – especially in the USA – over the past 20 years. This growth in interest in the field is due not only to the increasing sophistication of anthropological discourse about sickness, but also to the increasing openness of doctors and health planners to social scientific approaches. This latter trend is related to the growing legitimacy of and interest in ALTERNATIVE medical therapies and strategies of community-based health care. Ethnographies which were written before the development of medical anthropology as an independent sub-discipline tend to emphasize the social and symbolic aspects of sickness (*see* WITCHCRAFT). More recent studies however attempt to evolve what Young calls in his review of this topic (1982) a 'conceptual system centred on the social and experiential particularities of sickness and healing'. Ethnomedicine, on the other hand, focuses on non-Western medical systems and the study of beliefs and practices other than those embodied in conventional allopathic 'scientific' medicine.

Young, like other writers within this field, distinguishes between 'sickness', 'illness' and 'disease'. Sickness is a global term which refers to all events involving ill health, be these defined in terms of disease or of illness. Disease refers to pathological states of the organism, whether or not they are culturally or psychologically recognized (the medical definition of ill health). Illness refers to culturally and socially defined or conditioned perceptions and experiences of ill health, including some states which may be defined as disease and others which are not classifiable in terms of medical definitions of pathological states. The anthropology of illness, influenced by the anthropology of

SYMBOLISM and hermeneutically oriented, has focused on the cognitive and symbolic dimensions of illness. Good, for example, develops the notion of the 'semantic illness network' which he defines as the 'network of words, situations, symptoms and feelings which are associated with an illness and give it meaning for the sufferer'. Similarly Kleinman (1980) refers to 'explanatory models of illness', which are both models of reality and models for purposive action. The anthropology of sickness, on the other hand, focuses on the social relations which 'produce the forms and distribution of sickness in society' (Young). This approach concentrates not on the experience of illnes but on social systems, power structures, and the social meaning and outcome of sickness. Each society possesses its own set of rules for the translation of signs into symptoms, the definition of illness and the patterns of treatment. Social forces not only affect diagnosis but also the access to different kinds of treatment and therapists by different sectors of the population. At the same time, medical practices are also ideological practices, since, as Young notes, 'symbols of healing are simultaneously symbols of power'.

We may distinguish clinical anthropology, which aims principally to increase clinical efficiency, from the type of medical anthropology which is concerned with the analysis of social power relations and the production of medical knowledge. Clinical anthropology incorporates cross-cultural sensitivity into medical practice and encourages awareness of the patient's cognitive-symbolic organization of the experience of sickness and healing. The second type is concerned with showing how medical systems function as part of the ideological and power structure of society, and with the critique of the medical system as part of the apparatus of SOCIAL STRATIFICATION.

men's houses. Men's houses are found in a wide range of ethnographic areas, and may be associated with systems of AGE SETS or AGE GRADES, or with other types of ceremonial association or secret society. The function of men's houses varies according to the ethnographic context, but common to all these societies is some development of ritualized sex antagonism, especially in the Amazon and New Guinea areas where men's houses are found in conjunction with cults of male dominance. In societies where young men or all men reside in the men's house, the traditional definition of the DOMESTIC GROUP may be difficult to maintain, since the organization of domestic functions as well as of labour and co-operative relations in productive and other activities may cross-cut the boundaries of nuclear or extended family units and be organized on a community-wide GENDER-specific basis.

menstruation. A stage of the female physiological cycle, which occurs approximately at monthly intervals if the woman has not become pregnant. In many cultures considerable SYMBOLIC significance is attached to blood in general and menstrual blood in particular, which may be regarded as polluting and dangerous but is also regarded as especially powerful since it is the symbol of woman's potential (if unrealized) fertility. DURKHEIM based his theory of TOTEMISM on the universal fear or TABOO about menstrual blood, relying on ethnographic evidence which suggested that contact with menstrual blood was regarded as dangerous and polluting especially for males. However it should be noted that the fear of menstrual blood and the polluting nature of a menstruating woman are not universal phenomena. There are societies in which menstruation is subject to no special observances, just as there are others in which a menstruating woman is regarded as dangerous and polluting, and others where she should avoid contact with specific persons or specific activities (for instance, she should not have sexual relations, she should not go near a hunter or a particular type of food) in order to avoid possible negative consequences either for herself or for the activity concerned. The first menstruation of a girl may be the occasion for a RITE OF PASSAGE which signals her attainment of sexual and social maturity. The symbolism of male INITIATION rites also frequently borrows allusions to female reproductive powers including menstruation and childbirth, as part of the assertion of male social power (*see* RITUAL SEXUAL SYMMETRY). It has been noted that in many small-scale societies menstruation is likely to be a comparatively rare event for many women once they initiate sexual activity, due to frequent pregancies and pro-longed periods of lactation which suppress menstrual periods.

mentality. *See* PRIMITIVE MENTALITY.

Merton, Robert K. (1910–). This US sociologist both influenced and was influenced by anthropology, especially in his contributions to FUNCTIONALIST theory. Concepts associated with the work of Merton include those of LATENT and manifest function and DYSFUNCTION. He is also well known for his classification of different types of DEVIANCE, derived from the Durkheimian notion of ANOMIE. Major works include *Social Theory and Social Structure* (1949) and *The Sociology of Science* (1973).

messianism. A special category of relogious movement, often MILLENARIAN, distinguished by its centering around a cult of a saviour or Messiah who may be believed to be already living (the leader of the movement) or about to appear. The attribution of godlike qualities to a living leader of a religious movement is a not uncommon feature of REVITALIZATION and millenarian movements, though the term 'messianic' is generally reserved for those movements in which belief in a present or future leader as a reincarnation of God or the Messiah is a central feature. Such movements have been especially common in the Judaeo-Christian tradition, but have also occurred in parts of the Third World under the impact of violent processes of social and cultural CHANGE as a result of COLONIAL domination. In these cases the term is extended to movements where the 'Messiah' is regarded not as the Christian god but as a reincarnation of a native deity or deity-monarch.

As Kopytoff has pointed out in his study of the classification of religious movements (1964), we do not gain much in anthropological insight by attempting to define religious movements as members of unitary classes such as 'messianic' or 'revitalization'. He suggests instead that we should characterize each movement in terms of a cluster of dimensions, thus affording a more sophisticated analytical approach to the variation and association between different features of different religious movements. The category of 'messianic movements' according to this approach would not be retained as a separate one: instead we should seek to analyse how different types of leadership or kinds of belief in the role of a personal saviour or deity are held by religious movements in general. Thus messianism could be regarded as an aspect of many religious movements, rather than as an exclusive type of movement in itself.

mestizo. A term originally employed in the Spanish colonies to refer to the offspring of a Spanish parent (almost without exception the father) with a native. It was thus contrasted in the Americas with *indio* (Indian), Spanish (born in Spain) and *criollo* (pure blood descendants of Spanish families). In addition there existed locally variable terminologies to refer to blacks and the different racial mixtures produced by the intermarriage of blacks with other categories. Over time the categories of Spanish, *criollo* and *mestizo* have tended to blur, and the term *mestizo* has come to signify the 'mixed' population, product of many generations of intermarriage, which is now the majority in many Latin American nations. In parts of Latin America (mainly Guatemala) the term *ladino* is employed rather than *mestizo*. (*See* ETHNICITY.)

metacommunication. A term employed by BATESON to refer to the ability, especially highly developed in humans, to communicate about communication. Metacommunication consists in different types of 'framing' of messages which allow us to understand how these messages should be interpreted.

Metraux, Alfred (1902–63). Swiss anthropologist whose ethnographic accounts of native South American cultures are especially well-known. Metraux also carried out research in Haiti and on Easter Island (see e.g. 1940; 1959).

metropolis-satellite. A model developed by Frank which has influenced both DEPENDENCY theory and WORLD SYSTEMS theory. Frank argues that an international chain of metropolitan-satellite relationships stretches from world centres of capitalism to rural communities and the Third World. This is also a chain of exploitation and dependence, such that even the remotest populations are fully integrated into a hierarchical system whereby the metropolitan centres siphon off surplus wealth.

micro/macro. These prefixes are attached to a number of different terms with the meaning 'small, small-scale' and 'large, large-scale' respectively. Thus microeconomics is the study of economics from the perspective of decisions taken by individuals and firms, macroeconomics the study of the behaviour of the economy as a whole. Similarly microevolution is the study of small-scale evolutionary processes within limited timespans, macroevolution the study of the broad sweep of evolutionary development over a large timescale.

middle man. A term used to refer to an economic, cultural, social or political intermediary. In modern non-sexist terminology it would be 'middle person'. However, this term has not found favour and the neutral term intermediary or BROKER is more likely to be employed. (*See* PATRONAGE.)

migration. The large majority of rural communities studied by anthropologists are affected to some extent by processes of migration, and the urban settings which have been the subject of anthropological enquiry are very often likewise cities or towns formed by large proportions of migrant inhabitants. We generally think of migration as a one-way (usually rural–urban) process, since this is the most evident historical trend, and one which generates constant concern due to the demographic growth of cities which, especially in the Third World, continually outstrips their potential for economic development. However it should be remembered that a closer analysis of migratory processes reveals that they are not exclusively one-way. The crude statistics of rural–urban migration may disguise not only the frequency of return migration but also the existence of persons and families who regularly alternate their residence between rural community and town.

We may approach the anthropological study of migration either in terms of the impact of migration rates and processes on the rural community: in terms of its family structure, its economic organization and its cultural or ethnic identity. Or we may approach migration from the urban perspec-

tive (*see* CITY, ANTHROPOLOGY OF THE), studying how the migrants are incorporated into the urban environment, how migrant communities respond and change as a result of urban life, and how the communities they form (often SHANTY TOWNS in Third World cities) in turn change the nature and characteristics of the city itself.

Because of the the nature of the migratory phenomenon, most analyses automatically take as their starting point the economic and ecological aspects of migrant motivation and social organization. From these it is evident that rural–urban migration is basically a response to the lack of economic opportunities in rural areas, plus the lack of support for the small-scale producer or peasant, often allied to other factors such as the concentration of land or other resources in the hands of a wealthy elite at the expense of the poorer sectors of the population. At the same time we should not forget that a degree of social and cultural dominance over the rural area by the city also contributes to migratory processes, since the city is perceived as the locus not only of politico-economic and social power but also of dominant cultural values. The rural–urban migrant, permanent or semi-permanent, meets with the perpetuation of this pattern of dominance within the city itself, since he or she is generally incorporated into marginal or 'spontaneous' population settlements characterized by lack of employment opportunities and by a concentration of urban POVERTY factors.

Migration studies generally pay particular attention to demographic factors (sex, age, and family characteristics) of migrants, relating these factors to socio-economic and cultural aspects of the migratory process. The sexual differentiation of migrants is dependent not only on the type of economic opportunities available in the city (domestic work is available mainly to women, industrial labour may be available preferentially to men, etc.), but to cultural, economic and social structural features of the home community, which influence the decision as to who will move. In South Africa labour migration to the white-controlled cities is restricted to men, who may migrate to the city if they possess a work permit, but whose wives and families must remain in the African 'homelands' which have been created in order to keep the majority of the black population at bay (*see* APARTHEID; RACISM). This is an extreme example of how racist ideologies act to support and maintain systems of economic exploitation of migrant labour, but similar if less extreme phenomena may be observed in most modern nations and cities, where the fact of being a migrant of subordinate ethnic group status is sufficient to deprive the individual of what are otherwise regarded as inalienable civil or human rights.

Specific studies within urban anthropology may focus on the particular economic conditions and opportunities in given urban settings, and the processes whereby migrants may either progressively improve their situation or alternatively become 'entrenched' in marginal squatter settlements and urban poverty. A separate but related phenomenon is that of the changing ETHNIC identity of migrants. However we should not assume that 'successful' migrants necessarily lose their ethnic identity or cease to value the culture of their region or country of origin, just as it is not necessarily true to say that 'unsuccessful' or poor migrants are more likely to retain their ethnic identity. Rather, the interrelationships between migration and ethnicity must be studied in each case in terms of the development of ethnic politics in the nation or region concerned.

But this type of migration, which is a relatively permanent move from the rural areas to the city, is only one form among many. Migration in its more general sense however includes a wide range of population movements, including NOMADISM among certain HUNTING AND GATHERING and PASTORAL peoples, and involuntary (*see* REFUGEES) and planned migration, all of which have distinctive characteristics. Planned migration, as opposed to spontaneous migration, is often created by government policy either in order to build up new cities or towns with planned economic or industrial development, or to populate or colonize supposedly underexploited regions. The problems of planned migration or colonization are part of the field of DEVELOPMENT and planning studies. It should be noted that planned colonization in the Third World may be to the detriment of existing native populations in the designated areas, and often obeys the dictate of political rhetoric

rather than that of ecological or economic rationality, as in the so-called 'conquest of the Amazon'.

Return migration is a special phenomenon which may relate either to the sense of a change in comparative economic opportunities in rural and urban areas, or to a particular stage in the developmental cycle of the domestic group and the individual ageing process. In addition, factors which influence return migration include the revival of interest in the cultural or ethnic patterns and values of the community of origin.

migrationism. A CULTURE HISTORICAL theory associated with the British anthropologists Smith, Perry and Rivers, who explained cultural variation and development in terms of processes of migration and DIFFUSION. Interest in migration and diffusion declined in the 1930s due to the rise of FUNCTIONALIST and STRUCTURAL FUNCTIONALIST theory.

millenarianism. Millenarian or millenial movements are types of religious, in many cases politico-religious movements, characterized by a doctrine in which the central tenet is a belief in radical changes in the order of things. These changes are often characterized as the overthrow of dominant powers and the revindication of the rights of native populations. The term 'millenium' meaning 1000 years, is derived from the Christian tradition, but has been extended to other types of religious movement which predict a 'paradise on earth' or the overthrow of the established order by supernatural means. The coming of the millenium may be regarded by believers as imminent, or it may be put off as an indefinite expectation, especially in those millenarian cults which have become relatively established. Millenarian movements exist both within the Christian religion and also in other religious traditions as a result of their contact and interchange with Christianity.

In his classic study of millenarianism in Europe during the Middle Ages, Norman Cohn (1957) relates these movements to socioeconomic and political factors, including the dislocation of large proportions of the rural population who lost their lands to large landowners under a process of increasing concentration of landed property in the hands of the ruling class. This dislocated peasantry, he argues, formed the mass of membership of millenarian movements which were in part a response to social and politico-economic injustice and marginalization. This association of millenarianism with dispossessed peoples has continued throughout history, and has recurred consistently in conjunction with processes of colonization. Thus millenarian movements have been reported for a wide range of ethnographic areas, some of the better known examples being from Melanesia (*see* CARGO CULT) and from North America where cults such as the Ghost Dance of the Plains Indians have been extensively documented by historians and anthropologists.

The dispossession associated with millenarianism is not only economic but cultural: in millenarian movements there is an evident element of cultural dispossession or alienation. Features of traditional culture often come to serve as symbols of an idealized past, and indeed some movements characterize the millenium as a return to the precolonial past, rejecting all that is associated with the new order of things. But in contrast there is also often an ambivalent relationship with the new order and with the symbols of power associated with colonial dominance, and in some cases these symbols may be embraced to the point of a rejection of all that is associated with the past. Though millenarian movements vary in the symbolic significance they attach to traditional and new cultural elements, all are characterized by a degree of alienation from traditional culture to the point where this becomes an external symbolic value either to be praised or rejected. Millenarian movements have also been interpreted in psychological and symbolic terms, by writers who stress congruences and incongruences between traditional doctrines, beliefs and psychological orientations and the new ones imposed by conditions of social CHANGE. However interpretations of millenarianism in terms of psychological and symbolic or religious factors alone are not sufficient, since they fail to take into account the global social and politico-economic context within which these movements occur. It is therefore important to remember that millenarian movements do not occur in isolation from each other or from the regional, national and international systems. Instead they appear to be historically and geographically interrelated in such a way that we must interpret them not in terms of local psychological or cultural peculiarities, but rather in terms of the historical development and spread of CAPITALISM and colonialism.

As responses to colonial exploitation and its accompanying RACIST ideologies, millenarian movements in the Third World may be interpreted as incipient political movements. To the extent that they actually operate as movements for ethnic revival and political organization in this world rather than the next, millenarian movements may be analysed as political strategies whose symbolic and magical dimensions should not be allowed to obscure their actual function in the manipulation of political relations and the organization of resistance to colonial or neo-colonial power structures. The fact that there is a causal connection between millenarianism and more direct political action is demonstrated by the fact that in those areas where millenarian movements were most frequently reported in the past they have been largely superseded in modern times by political organizations demanding the revindication of the rights of indigenous populations. As Keesing points out (1978), the anthropologists' focus on the religious and psychological aspects of millenarianism as a mixture of fantasy and magic has led them to subscribe to the dominant colonial ideology which, by defining millenarianism as an irrational and deviant phenomenon, permitted the colonial elite to continue to ignore the legitimate political claims which these movements in fact represented.

minority. In the most general sense, a subordinate or marginal group, which may be defined in racial or ETHNIC terms or in terms of some special characteristic or STIGMA. Minority groups in this sense are not necessarily numerical minorities: since the criterion of minority is determined by subordinate or marginal status rather than by numbers, they may be more numerous than the 'majority'. This usage may however lead to confusion where subordinate groups constitute the numerical majority.

misrepresentation. *See* IDEOLOGY; FALSE CONSCIOUSNESS.

missionaries. Those who attempt to promulgate religious beliefs and adherence to specific churches or sects among the unconverted. Missionaries work both in their own countries and abroad, but for the purposes of anthropology overseas missionaries, particularly those who operate in the Third World, have attracted the most attention. The traditional opposition betwen anthropologists and missionaries has led to a vast oversimplification within the folklore of the anthropological profession of the role and characteristics of the missionary, and of the historical importance of missionary scholarship and missionary action within colonial and neo-colonial settings. However, recent works – most of them not surprisingly by missionaries and some by missionary–anthropologists – have encouraged a closer scrutiny of the historical and contemporary functions of missionaries. It is certainly an oversimplification, for instance, to regard the work of all missionaries as practically identical: we have only to compare the missionary style and work of the Summer Institute of Linguistics with that of missionaries working within the boundaries of LIBERATION theology for this to become immediately apparent.

Historically it is evident that missionaries' overwhelming importance in COLONIALISM has been as part of the apparatus of ideological 'conquest', often as direct agents of the political and economic domination of colonial peoples. Christianity was introduced into the Americas, for example, as an essential part of the apparatus of military conquest and as an ideological justification of RACIST and exploitative policies. The native population of Latin America was thus placed under the direct control of the Church, which under the pretext of missionary zeal performed the task of subjugating them to an alien order. In modern times, too, missionary contact has often served as the bridge which has effected the eventual subordination of indigenous peoples, making them receptive to the new culture in general and eroding their own cultural values. In economic terms missionaries often act as intermediaries who create new demands and necessities in the indigenous population, demands which traders and patrons may then step in to meet.

The missionaries' reply to these accusations, which are frequently levelled at them by anthropologists, is not only to point out those among their ranks who have performed great services both to scholarship and to the defence of the rights and humanity of indigenous peoples, but also to question the anthropologist's own self-righteousness. We should remember that if missionary work in general may be criticized as a product and servant of IMPERIALISM, so too may anthropological work. It is true to say that there are many anthropologists who are just as or more insensitive to the practical plight of indigenous minorities as missionaries are: and indeed missionaries dedicate a large part or all of their lives to coexistence with and struggle on behalf of these minority groups far more frequently than anthropologists do. Furthermore we should remember that the missionary, with his belief in the Christian religion, may be better understood by an indigenous group which also believes in its own traditional religion than an anthropologist, who is usually awkwardly atheistic and whose presence serves no apparent purpose.

This is not to say that the evangelistic aspect of even the most enlightened missionary work is not problematic in the extreme from the anthropological viewpoint, and enlightened missionary work is regarded by some as even more insidious and dangerous than crude 'bible-thumping' evangelization. A complete treatment of this topic would include a historical study of the political role of the Catholic Church and other churches and sects, and would perhaps be unable to reach unequivocal conclusions, since within the Christian religion itself there are different and contradictory political trends and allegiances. However it is as well for the anthropologist to remember that his or her own profession is subject to the same critiques, and that in practice the anthropologist is as far or further from the reality of the ethnic groups he or she studies as is the missionary.

mobility. In systems of social STRATIFICATION individuals and groups are located in a given position in the hierarchy and also have a potential to change that position. The potential for change in position may be great, as in 'open' systems, or very reduced, as in 'closed' ones. Conventionally it has been stated that traditional agrarian-based societies are closed in this sense, and modern industrial ones more open (*see* ACHIEVEMENT AND ASCRIPTION). However this received wisdom has been increasingly challenged in recent years. For example, studies in Africa have shown that modernization, in particular change in the educational system, has produced a more closed pattern than the traditional agrarian society. Similarly, sociological studies comparing mobility rates in different types of society have failed to show systematic differences. The concept of social mobility has received little attention in anthropological studies of communities with little internal status differentiation.

modal personality. A concept developed within the CULTURE AND PERSONALITY school, which represented the attempt to develop a more objective measure of personality traits in society using statistical methods. The modal personality is the pattern of personality traits, manifested in patterned observable behaviour, which occurs with most statistical frequency in a given population. The term was first employed by DuBois.

model. A device employed in order to aid the interpretation of reality and the building of THEORY. The exact significance of the concept of a model and its relationship to theory and to empirical evidence is not always clearly defined in the social sciences, though it is generally agreed that a model occupies an intermediate status between the levels of empirical observation of specific cases and abstract or general theory. A model seeks to account for the relationships between a specified set of phenomena or variables by representing them in simplified form, but the use of the term is extended to various kinds of generalization or representation, ranging from analogies which are intended to aid understanding to IDEAL TYPES or to 'models' which approximate to theories in their explanatory aims. There have been considerable disagreements in the social sciences and anthropology about the theoretical significance and status of models. These differences have been discussed as one aspect of the opposition between STRUCTURAL and empiricist anthropology. Empiricists, according to Levi-Strauss and others within the structuralist school, have fundamentally misunderstood the notion of structure, mistaking it for a superficial phenomenon which may be abstracted from empirical observation. Levi-Strauss argues that structure is not directly observable, nor is it a simplified model of empirical reality. Rather it is a set of governing principles which underlie empirical reality and the operation of which can be detected by its empirical manifestations. Its nature is, however, fundamentally different from these aspects, since it operates upon a different and unconscious level.

Apart from the debate between empiricist and structuralist anthropology, there is in anthropological theory and writing generally a considerable degree of variation in the way in which models are seen. They may be taken to be actual representations of reality which truly correspond to the phenomena they represent, or merely selective heuristic devices which are more or less arbitrary in their relationship to empirical reality and whose only test of validity is the extent to which they aid us to advance in our comprehension of the phenomena under study. The failure to clarify the level at which a model is intended to be interpreted leads to much sterile debate in anthropology.

mode of production. A central conception within Marxist and neo-Marxist social and historical theory. Its development and interpretations of it are far from uniform, since varying theories and schemes exist of the relationship between modes of production and SOCIAL FORMATIONS and of the historical transformation from one mode of production to another. Essentially the mode of production is constituted by the relationship which exists between the MEANS OF PRODUCTION and the RELATIONS OF PRODUCTION. Thus Marx affirmed that in producing goods for the economy humans also produce specific sets of social relations, which include the OWNERSHIP of the means of production and the social relationships entailed by the productive process.

According to Marx, the real economic foundation of society is given by the material forces of production, which he also asserts manifest a universal historical tendency to develop and evolve. The forces of production at any given stage of social evolution give rise to a specific set of social relations of production, by which we may characterize the mode of production in the society under study. The social relations of production which at a given moment are appropriate for a certain level of development of the productive forces will however inevitably become anachronistic due to the ever present tendency of the productive forces to develop and thus outgrow the productive relations within which they are bound. Thus social systems which are at one point of evolution progressive become retrograde at a later date, and the contradiction between productive forces and productive relations eventually culminates in REVOLUTION, which is the transition from one mode of production to another. Such revolutionary changes in pre-class society may be identified primarily by technological change (*see* NEOLITHIC REVOLUTION) and in class-based societies are characterized by the overthrow of one dominant class and its replacement by another as owners or controllers of the means of production.

The concept of mode of production and the theory of the determining role played by the evolving forces of production in social evolution have given rise to some theories which equate Marxism with crude economic or material determinism, though these theories have not found favour in Western social science in general. There exist also a number of more sophisticated interpretations of economic determinism, and within MARXIST ANTHROPOLOGY the concept of mode of production has been found to be of central explanatory value. However some Marxist theorists have criticized interpretations of the concepts of mode of production and social formation by writers such as ALTHUSSER (1966). They believe that the attempt to make these concepts more sensitive to the particular and complex interrelations of economic, ideological and political domains within given historical contexts has allowed such writers to lose sight of the primary aim of Marx's own work, which was to provide an explanation of the transition from one mode of production to another in materialist terms. However, the proper use of the concept of mode of production,

combined with historical and anthropological research methods which elucidate the special properties of any given social system, should allow us to resolve this problem. The two perspectives are not in fact contradictory but complementary, as they refer to different levels of analysis much in the same way as micro- and macro-evolutionary theories. In this respect the theories of Godelier (1978) are important, since he clarifies the issue of economic determinism in anthropological contexts where as it has been frequently observed it is not economic relations *per se* but other relations, such as those governed by kinship or religion, which are the dominant factors in social organization. Godelier points out that in such cases we should examine individually why it is kinship relations, or religious systems or legal systems which are dominant. The answer, he asserts, lies in the centrality of these domains to the organization of the relations of production. Thus in kinship-based societies it is the kinship system which organizes the social relations of production, in societies dominated by religion it is the religious system which performs this function (*see* CASTE; JAJMANI) and so on.

An additional confusion in the anthropological use of the concept of the mode of production has been derived from discrepancies with Marx's original scheme, itself not entirely consistent throughout his writings. Since Marx was less concerned with the description of pre-capitalist modes of production than with the analysis of capitalism itself, his theories of pre-capitalist modes have been found wanting by many anthropologists whose special interest in pre-capitalist society combined with the availability of modern ethnographic data have led to the formulation of new 'modes of production' not contemplated by Marx (for example the DOMESTIC MODE OF PRODUCTION, lineage mode of production, peasant mode of production, and colonial mode of production). However there is no general agreement as to the adoption of these new terms, and there is disagreement also over the acceptance of some of Marx's own categories: the SLAVE mode of production, the ASIATIC MODE OF PRODUCTION, and so on. Even the more generally accepted categories like FEUDALISM and CAPITALISM have been subject to extensive debate and attempts at subclassification and differentiation in order to accommodate the historical and regional variability of socioeconomic forms. Marx held that the original or most primitive mode of production was PRIMITIVE COMMUNISM, though anthropologists have naturally found it necessary to refine and internally differentiate this category in order to do justice to the variability of social and economic forms found in pre-class societies. The emergence of AGRICULTURE and the increased DIVISION OF LABOUR to which this eventually gave rise, together with the possibility of larger settlements and considerable sectors of the population able to subsist upon the surplus produced by the agricultural sector, led to the development of private property and social classes, giving rise to what Marx called the 'ancient' or in some of his writings the 'slave' mode of production. Anthropologists have however questioned whether all societies underwent this stage, and whether slavery can be said to characterize ancient modes of production, since slavery has formed a part of a variety of different productive systems (including capitalism) in modern times. According to Marx, the ancient or slave mode gave way to the feudal mode, characterized by the dominance of the landholding nobility and the extraction of surplus production from the agricultural producers. These were maintained in a condition of SERFDOM or bound labour. The considerable debate among historians and other social scientists about the essential characteristics and historical role of feudalism have been supplemented by the anthropological debate about the applicability of this concept outside its original historical and geographical reference.

Feudalism gave way in modern times to capitalism, which is the mode of production most extensively studied by Marx himself. In capitalism the control over the means of production passes from the landed aristocracy to the BOURGEOISIE, and the dominant historical oposition becomes that between the bourgeoisie and the PROLETARIAT. The eventual overthrow of the former by the latter constitutes the revolutionary transition to SOCIALISM or COMMUNISM and is in accordance with the underlying development or evolution of the productive forces which establishes a productive system that is essentially collective or socialized in form and is thus in contradiction with the private ownership of the means of production.

One of the most interesting aspects of modes of production from the anthropological viewpoint is the fact that different modes of production may coexist within a given context, as when the capitalist mode of production comes into contact with pre-capitalist modes in colonial settings. The study of the resulting ARTICULATION OF MODES OF PRODUCTION is one of the most challenging and promising areas of Marxist anthropology.

modernization. *See* DEVELOPMENT; INDUSTRIALIZATION.

moiety. From the French *moitié*, meaning 'half', this refers to the division of a group or society into halves. The division into moieties is usually considered to be based on DESCENT, giving rise to the division of the group into two 'patrimoieties' (patriclans) or two 'matrimoieties' (matriclans). However, moieties may also be based on marriage rules, residence or ceremonial relations, or any combination of these with or without the operation of a descent rule. (*See* DUAL ORGANIZATION.)

monarchy. A term used in two separate senses. As a form of government, it refers to the concentration of power in the hands of a hereditary ruling family. As an institution, it refers to the existence of such a hereditary ruling family, whether or not the overall type of government in the society concerned is monarchical. Monarchies may thus exist within types of political system where power is not exclusively concentrated in the hands of the monarchy itself, and where other mechanisms of decision-making and government are dominant. Speculations as to the origins of monarchies have often pointed to the connection between spiritual and religious power and political office. Monarchs in traditional African states, in Polynesia, in the Americas and other ethnographic areas were invested with special supernatural powers and divine or sacred status. Lowie (1920) suggests that the combination of chiefly and SHAMANIC or priestly powers in a single office is what permitted the development of monarchies out of the egalitarian political systems of the aboriginal population of the Americas. Historical and ethnographic accounts of traditional monarchies show wide variation both in the degree and type of power concentrated in the hands of the sovereign and in the relationship between the monarchy and the overall system of hereditary or achieved rank in society. Studies of traditional African kingships have shown that the sacred or divine attributes of the monarch do not necessarily imply that he is all-powerful in the political domain: indeed these very attributes and the ritual precautions and observances surrounding him may effectively isolate him from actual decision-making and government, which devolves in practice on counsellors or other political institutions. Evans-Pritchard stated that the Shilluk king 'reigns but does not rule', since his attributes are almost exclusively ritual rather than governmental (1948).

Peter Lloyd, reviewing the literature which attempts to classify African kingdoms (1965), mentions the classification suggested by MURDOCK of 'African despotism'. Among the common features which Murdock proposed for such despotism are divine kingship where the ruler is considered owner of his subjects and their land, and the existence of a corps of advisory and/or administrative officials. SUCCESSION is generally not by primogeniture, and after the death of the monarch rival princes compete for the throne and for the support of the officials who must elect the new monarch. Vansina, on the other hand, defines a kingdom as a sovereign political group divided into territorial units which are under the authority delegated by the ruler to his local representatives, and bases his classification of African kingdoms on their degree of centralization – that is to say, the degree to which provincial rulers have independent power or authority. Lloyd points out that many writers have emphasized the incompatibility of LINEAGE and STATE as forms of sociopolitical organization, and following Fortes and Evans-Pritchard (1940) have divided African societies into the 'segmentary lineage' and 'centralized state' dichotomy. As Lloyd points out, however, the empirical evidence does not bear out a sharp distinction between 'lineage-based' societies and states, since we may observe both that in the 'lineage' societies other principles of

political organization and decision-making (age grades, titles, associations) are important, while lineage organization may also be of great significance in decision making and political organization in the states. While Mair (1962) defines the state as a polity where the territorial agents responsible for local administration are appointed by the ruler, such a definition would exclude many African kingdoms where lineage or other principles of sociopolitical organization rather than appointed administrative officials are responsible for local decision-making. Many attempts to classify African kingdoms have focused on the one hand on the role played within them by lineage organization, age grades, title associations or by appointed officials, and on the other on the degree of centralization or local independence within the different territorial units which compose the kingdom.

Lloyd's own classificatory model of African kingdoms is based on types of recruitment to the political elite, and draws on the criticisms of earlier classifications made by D. Easton (1959) and by M.G. Smith (1960). Taking into account the four principal variables, which are the political power of the royal lineage, the rights over land, the control of physical force and the preservation of individual rights, Lloyd discusses three variants which he terms the 'open, representative', the 'open, by political association' and the 'closed' types of government. In the first type, recruitment to political elites is open in the sense that each descent group is represented as a fixed constituency. In the second type recruitment to political elites is via political associations, through which any individual may rise to a high office. In the third or closed type however, political office is reserved for members of a ruling class which may be defined as an ETHNIC group, by the ranking of descent groups (a royal lineage) or as a hereditary ARISTOCRACY.

Many authors writing on African traditional monarchies have stressed the different systems of checks and balances which operate to limit and control the power of the monarch, and which include ritual, ceremonial and political elements. Thus Beattie in a review of four traditional African monarchies (1967) lists 17 different types of norms ranging from ceremonial admonition and the existence of advisory and consultative relations or councils to the rights of subjects to revolt or move out of the area of authority of the monarch.

Checks and balances on a ruler's authority should be considered not only in the context of the relationship of monarch to commoners but also in view of that between different elements within the aristocracy or hereditary nobility. Status rivalry within the nobility is an extremely important factor in the historical evolution of monarchies, which display varying degrees of centralization or of success in controlling the political ambitions and governing power of the lesser nobles or chiefs within the state. This topic has been examined at length within the study of FEUDALISM, where a constantly recurring theme is the opposition between the central authority represented by the monarchy and local authority and networks of personal allegiance. The same theme characterizes anthropological studies of traditional monarchies in different ethnographic areas, where problems of succession to the monarchy as well as problems of rivalry between the monarchy and lesser chiefs and nobles constitute an important element. Were we to possess more detailed historical information about many of these traditional monarchies before European contact we should almost certainly discover a considerable degree of historical instability and change as a result of the changing balance of power between different components of the sociopolitical hierarchy. Thus the traditional history of Tonga demonstrates that the original office of priest-king or *Tui Tonga* was subject to continual attack, as monarchs were assassinated by ambitious lesser chiefs. As a result, traditional accounts relate that in the 15th century a Tonga ruler created a special secular office for his son, with responsibility for the supervision of land, in order to create a buffer between the monarchy and the chiefs. This secular inherited office in turn led to the gradual usurpation of governmental power from the *Tui Tonga* to the *Tui Kanakupolu*, as the new office came to be called. Later continued wars over succession, according to Goldman in his account of Polynesian political evolution (1967), led to the 'feudalization' of Tonga society as the Tongan islands became divided into small fortified garrisons.

It is evident that another important element in the nature and development of traditional monarchies is the degree and type of military power which is under their control. The organization of such power and the constitution of armies, whether under the direct control of the monarch or under the control of lesser chiefs or nobles, is of vital historical importance. The development of military power directed towards conquest of other regions (*see* IMPERIALISM) is correlated with the increase of social stratification and centralization of power at home: the traditional Aztec and Inca empires, for example, combined their expansive strategy of imperial conquest with the increasing concentration of power and political decision-making in the hands of the sovereign.

The evolution of monarchies and the functions performed within the political system by the monarch should thus be considered in the light of the overall political evolution of the society concerned. Attention should at the same time be paid to its regional context, taking into account both ecological and economic factors as well as the historical development of social stratification and status rivalry within strata. Similarly, the study of the ritual attributes of the monarch and the ceremonial or religious practices connected with the monarchy should be studied within the context of the ideological functions of religion and the separation or conjunction of religious and political power within the society as a whole.

money. A generalized medium of exchange, that is to say, one by means of which a relatively large number of commodities may be measured and transferred. However even in money-dominated economies there are always certain things which cannot be directly measured or exchanged by this standard, and other areas where money exchange is regarded as immoral or inappropriate. In pre-capitalist economies money may be either absent or very restricted in its use, and we may observe the existence of 'special purpose money' whose use is limited to a fixed and restricted set of transactions for specific types of commodity, as opposed to modern 'general purpose money'. Non-monetary economies have been analysed anthropologically in terms of the existence of discrete SPHERES OF EX-CHANGE or scales of value which establish equivalences between commodities within different domains of economic activity. In money economies however the existence of a general purpose medium of exchange permits the establishment of equivalences between any given set of commodities, thus breaking down the barriers between geographically and socially separate producers and consumers and performing an essential function in ensuring the agility and flexibility of a market economy.

Money should not be confused with currency or physically circulating cash. In modern industrial economies currency itself is too cumbersome for many exchange operations, and the symbolization of exchange value has reached a further stage in such economies whereby physical currency is bypassed and transactions are carried out at the level of abstract accounting procedure. (See ECONOMIC ANTHROPOLOGY; RECIPROCITY.)

monogamy. A rule by which persons of either sex are permitted only one spouse. In some cases this rule extends to the prohibition of remarriage after the death of the original spouse and/or the prohibition of divorce and remarriage. Where remarriage is permitted, and especially where it is common for persons to pass through a series of marriages in succession, the term 'serial monogamy' or 'serial polygamy' may be employed. (See DOMESTIC GROUP; FAMILY; MARRIAGE; POLYGAMY.)

monotheism. The origin and cause of monotheistic RELIGIONS attracted considerable attention in 19th-century anthropology, especially from theorists such as TYLOR concerned with the general or universal evolution of religious forms. Tylor thought that religion in human society had evolved from an original stage of ANIMISM, through ANCESTOR worship to POLYTHEISM and finally monotheism. He viewed the development of a belief that a single supreme being was the primary and final cause of events as the result of a philosophical advance in human thinking, in which the separate deities of polytheism were fused into a single explanatory principle.

There is some debate in anthropology as to whether monotheistic religions occur in traditional or small-scale societies. When broadly defined as those religions which postulate a supreme deity upon which all lesser spiritual beings depend, we may identify monotheistic religions in a wide variety of ethnographic areas. However some authors would limit the definition of monotheism to a few religions such as Christianity, Islam and Judaism where the belief in a high god is linked to concepts of morality and salvation (the 'ethical' religions). Swanson (1960) in a cross-cultural study of the occurrence of beliefs in a high god found them to be related to the degree of social complexity and hierarchy.

Montesquieu, Charles-Louis de Secondat, Baron de la Brède et de Montesquieu (1689–1755). French philosopher and social theorist whose influence on the development of the social sciences has been profound. Montesquieu was one of the first social theorists to advocate a form of CULTURAL RELATIVISM, asserting that each society should be judged in terms of the peculiar conditions which influence and shape it, and also employing this principle to turn a satirical gaze onto French society itself as seen through the eyes of imaginary foreigners to whom French customs appear strange and absurd. His best known work is *L'Esprit des lois* (1748), a collection of books in which he developed many of the ideas later to be taken up by the founding theorists of anthropology and other social sciences. Apart from discussing at length the origin and nature of different types of legal system and different forms of government, Montesquieu paid particular attention to the influence of climate and material factors in shaping social systems, and was the first to propose the classification of societies into the evolutionary stages of SAVAGERY, BARBARISM and CIVILIZATION.

morality. The domain of NORMS which relate to the behaviour of persons and which are characterized in that they are justified not in terms of their practical consequences but rather in terms of their intrinsic 'goodness' or 'badness'. Moral values or attitudes are thus those connected with the control which is exercised by social groups over the behaviour of their members, a control internalized by the individual and a part of his or her own set of values, to which emotional importance is attached. Anthropology is generally characterized by a high degree of moral relativism, and the bulk of ethnographic and anthropological discourse tends towards the accumulation and presentation of evidence which supports the notion that moral values are highly variable and relative both between cultures and from one historical period to another. Since DURKHEIM (1961), anthropology has also explored the manner in which morality functions as part of systems of SOCIAL CONTROL and SOLIDARITY, demonstrating that moral values, attitudes and 'issues' are part of a process of definition and demarcation of social roles and social groups (*see* ETHNOMETHODOLOGY; LAW, ANTHROPOLOGY OF; SYMBOLIC ANTHROPOLOGY; RELIGION, ANTHROPOLOGY OF).

In spite of the centrality of concepts relating to morality within anthropological theory there has not so far been a systematic anthropology of morality, and anthropologists seem to have shied away in particular from a closer inspection of the real implications of moral relativism. The examples which are cited of exceptions to 'universal' moral rules such as the permissibility of killing under such diverse circumstances as war, revenge, euthanasia, capital punishment, and so on, need closer investigation, since they are in fact probably also 'exceptional' cases in the societies where they occur. Moral relativism may consequently be reduced to the level of asserting that there are are no universal moral rules which apply under all circumstances in every society, but this is not to say that there are not universal moral problems which are perceived as such in all societies. Anthropologists would have to demonstrate the existence of a society in which killing was generally regarded with moral indifference in order to substantiate a theory of total moral relativism. In fact it is probable that acts such as killing present a moral problem in all societies – a problem which of course receives different treatment in each sociocultural context, with the result that it may be permitted under a wide range of circumstances in some societies while being forbidden under nearly all circumstances in others. Another example of a domain which is universally problematic in moral terms while at the same time offering a vast array of different moral values and attitudes across space and time is the domain of family and sexual/marital relations. Moral relativism should thus be complemented by a study of the universal moral problems which confront all human groups, recognizing at the same time that the complex nature of moral norms and values means that there are infinite possibilities for cross-cultural and historical variation in the actual expression of such problems.

In addition, a certain degree of common perception of moral problems is probably a prerequisite for the mutual comprehension of different cultures, since it can be seen that the differences in specific moral codes are responsible for many of the more emotively charged failures in intercultural communication and comprehension. The moral rejection of another culture, which we term ETHNOCENTRISM, occurs precisely because what is perceived in both cultures as a moral problem is subject to a different resolution in each, with the result that each solution offends the other's moral values. Were the moral problems in each society perceived as entirely different, the reaction to an alien morality would be indifference rather than outrage.

The theories of moral development advanced by Piaget (1960) and other developmental psychologists offer an important contribution which might be employed by a moral anthropology in order to clarify the relationship between COGNITIVE and moral domains, and to suggest universal elements or stages of moral reasoning which could be tested cross-culturally. Similarly, the field of moral anthropology would need to develop and test hypotheses relating different types of moral code to different levels of technological, economic and social development or complexity. The theory of morality in this latter aspect is closely linked to the theory of IDEOLOGY, since the moral pressure supporting dominant ideologies is a vital element in their successful imposition upon subordinate groups.

mores. The moral norms of a human group or society. (*See* MORALITY.)

Morgan, Lewis Henry (1818–81). A lawyer whose interest in Iroquois Indian affairs led him to study their customs and social system, giving rise to what is often cited as the first modern ethnographic study of a native people, the *League of the Iroquois* (1851). In this work he considered ceremonial, religious and political aspects and also initiated his study of KINSHIP and MARRIAGE which he was later to develop into a comparative theory in his *Systems of Consanguinity and Affinity* (1871). This latter work is also a milestone in the development of anthropology, establishing kinship and marriage as central areas of anthropological enquiry and beginning an enduring preoccupation with KINSHIP TERMINOLOGIES as the key to the interpretation of kinship systems. His *Ancient Society* is the most influential statement of the 19th-century cultural EVOLUTIONARY position, which was later to be developed by later evolutionists and by MARX and ENGELS in their theory of social evolution. Employing MONTESQUIEU's categories of SAVAGERY, BARBARISM and CIVILIZATION Morgan subdivided the first two categories into three stages (lower, middle and upper) and gave contemporary ethnographic examples of each stage. Each stage was characterized by a technological advance and was correlated with advances in subsistence patterns, family and marriage and political organization.

mortuary rites. The study of mortuary rites has always been of great importance in anthropology. Some archeologists see evidence of mortuary rites as one of the earliest signs of human culture. Theories about mortuary rites, especially insofar as they are connected with ideas of fertility and of the immortality of the SOUL dominate the work of such early anthropologists as BACHOFEN, TYLOR, FRAZER and Hocart. Perhaps the first attempt to relate the type of rites to the type of social organization goes back to the essay by the French anthropologist R. Hertz, which has been published together with another essay in English under the title *Death and the Right Hand* (1960). Hertz was particularly interested in a theme later stressed by such other writers as VAN GENNEP (1909) and RADCLIFFE-BROWN (1952): how society coped with the disruption caused by the disorganizing effect of the death of one

of its members. He paid special attention to what have been called 'double obsequies' which occur in their most well-known form in Southeast Asia and Madagascar, but which in somewhat different forms are found in a great number of countries including China, Japan, Greece and Melanesia. What struck Hertz was how the division of the funeral into two parts, sometimes separated by a number of years, enabled people to mourn the disruption of society, but later to re-establish its order, often at the same time as establishing the dead as an immortal ANCESTOR. In this way he was able to point out striking similarities between mortuary rites and INITIATION rites. This is a theme which has been echoed ever since in both the theoretical and the ethnographic literature on many areas of the world.

Double obsequies are often linked to beliefs that the body is made up of two elements: one 'this earthly', and the other transcendental. These elements may be in some cases identified with the bones as opposed to the flesh, the 'dry' or transcendental elements of the skeleton as opposed to the 'wet' or temporal elements of the flesh.

One word must be said about the sadness of death which is often manifested by weeping. Although often genuine, it is always orchestrated and organized and very commonly the women of the community have the task of acting out sorrow. This is significant, as mourning often implies guilt in some direct or indirect way.

Finally, a very important aspect of some mortuary rites is that they are occasions for disposing of the possessions of the deceased. These may be destroyed, but when significant property is involved it must be transmitted. This often involves complex rituals in itself.

mother right. *See* MATRIARCHY.

multi-ethnic system. *See* ETHNICITY.

multilineal evolution. *See* EVOLUTION.

multilingualism. The ability to use or understand more than one language. The term does not necessarily imply that the subject is perfectly or equally fluent in all of the languages referred to. The term also refers to the use of several languages within a given community or population unit. Multilingualism is generally considered together with BILINGUALISM, although strictly speaking 'bilingualism' implies only two languages and 'multilingualism' should therefore be the more inclusive or general term. However the term 'bilingual' in its modern usage includes a wide range of situations of linguistic pluralism both at the level of individual speakers and that of entire communities or population units.

multinational and transnational corporations. Multinational corporations are those based in one industrial centre, possessing subsidiaries or branches in other countries. Transnational corporations are those whose operations transcend national barriers and are thus not linked to any one home base. J. Nash (1979) points out that anthropologists have studied the effects of these corporations throughout the world to some extent, but have not devoted sufficient attention to the organization of production, distribution and exchange on a global level (*see* WORLD SYSTEMS). The study of the implications of the supranational integration of industry has been pioneered by Wolfe, who points out that this has resulted in the disintegration both of national polities and of labour organization. Transnationals shift productive activities to those countries where raw materials and labour are cheap and where government and unions do not obstruct them. Nash points to some areas for future anthropological investigation, including the effects of transnationals and their employment practices on social organization, on family and household, and on class consciousness, and the investigation of what she terms the 'logico-meaningful integration' of the new economic and ideological system which transnationals bring about. (*See* DEVELOPMENT; INDUSTRIAL ANTHROPOLOGY; LABOUR ARISTOCRACY.)

murder. The unlawful killing of a person. The definition of murder consequently varies in each society according to its legal system and to its customary norms relating to the circumstances under which killing is regarded as justifiable. Contexts within which killing occurs and which are subject to differing interpretations cross-culturally as

well as between different sectors or persons within a single culture include INFANTICIDE, WAR, revenge killing, euthanasia, capital punishment and ritual killing or SACRIFICE. (*See* LAW, ANTHROPOLOGY OF; MORALITY.)

Murdock, George Peter (1897–1985). Murdock studied at Yale University and worked largely independently from the dominant BOASIAN tradition of his day. He was concerned with establishing a methodology which would apply to sociology and anthropology alike, and whose subject matter would be cultural (non-biological) behaviour. In order to make CROSS-CULTURAL COMPARISON and generalization possible he initiated the cross-cultural survey, now known as the Human Relations Area Files at Yale, later to attract the participation of many other institutions. His best known work is *Social Structure* (1949) in which he focused on family and kinship organization, seeking sets of functionally interrelated traits in a wide range of societies.

museums and anthropology. As well as acting as centres for scholarly research, museums are of great interest in themselves as objects of anthropological study, since they represent the interaction between trends in educational and academic theory and the pressures from government and bureaucratic sectors towards the display or encouragement of an 'official' version of science, history, or other disciplines. Museums are often impressive examples of the ARCHITECTURE of their day and in this sense too reflect the prevailing definitions of a 'public' building and the expected behaviour of the persons who enter it.

Museums cover an increasingly wide range of areas of human culture and scientific enquiry, from science and natural history to archeology, ethnology and diverse aspects of local history, to mention but a few. More narrowly, museums devoted to archeology, to ethnology or anthropology are of especial interest both to the student and scholar in anthropology and as a means through which anthropological knowledge may be disseminated to a wider public. Students and scholars employ museum materials in order to study the relationships between collections of material artifacts from different cultures or CULTURE AREAS. As an educational tool for the dissemination of anthropological knowledge or awareness the 'traditional' museum has been much criticized by anthropologists both for its bias towards the display of objects of traditional material culture divorced from their sociocultural context and its failure to take into account the modern conditions under which ethnographically studied peoples live. Modern museums attempt to overcome these limitations both by extending their educational activities to include talks, performances, ethnographic film, and so on, and by attempting to integrate into their displays information about the total social and cultural context within which material objects occur.

music. *See* ETHNOMUSICOLOGY.

mutilation. The mutilation and deformation of parts of the human body are commonly employed both for decorative and ritual purposes (*see* BODY, ANTHROPOLOGY OF). Bodily mutilations, which take a wide variety of forms ranging from genital mutilations (CIRCUMCISION, CLITORECTOMY etc.) to tattooing, scarification, and deformation of the shape of parts of the body (the head, foot, or neck, for example) are sometimes part of RITES OF PASSAGE. In these cases, the bodily change serves as a visible mark of a change of social status. In other cases bodily mutilations and deformations are regarded as more purely decorative, though even in these cases they lend themselves to the marking of different levels of status or categories of person. Such manipulations of the human body for expressive and decorative purposes have been subject to a range of psychoanalytical explanations, as well as to other types of explanation which emphasize their social rather than personal symbolic significance.

Mutterrecht. This term was employed by BACHOFEN and is translated as 'mother right'. (*See* MATRIARCHY.)

Myrdal, Gunnar K. (1898–). Swedish economist and theorist of DEVELOPMENT who has studied RACE in the USA and economic development in Asia and other regions. Myrdal stresses the importance of institutional factors in influencing underde-velopment, and has put forward the theory that international aid is in fact an obstacle which impedes the progress of Third World nations. Major works include *Economic Theory and Underdeveloped Regions* (1958) and *The Asian Drama* (1968).

mystical attack. *See* WITCHCRAFT; SORCERY.

myth. The term 'myth' is generally reserved for tales which are sacred or religious in nature, are social rather than individual or anecdotal in their subject matter, and are concerned with the origin or creation of some phenomenon which may be natural, supernatural or sociocultural. However the definition of myth and the distinction between this and other types of ORAL LITERATURE such as the folktale, or LEGEND is not rigid, and attempts to isolate the study of myth from the study of other forms of the oral tradition have not been particularly fruitful (*see* FOLKLORE). The term 'mythology' has two distinct meanings: on the one hand it refers to a body of myths found in a given region or human group, and on the other it refers to the study of myth. We should also distinguish the anthropological sense of 'myth' from the popular use of the term to refer to a false belief.

Anthropologists have observed over many years the connection between myth and RITUAL. This connection, which manifests itself in the ritual 'acting out' of myth and in the SYMBOLIC elements common to both myth and ritual, has led to extensive anthropological debate and discussion about the relationship between these two areas. There was for some years a debate about whether myth or ritual is primary. Some anthropologists have proposed that the myth is the primary factor and the ritual acts it out, others that the ritual is primary and the myth is to be regarded as a commentary on it. The debate has however been largely superseded in modern anthropology. It is generally recognized today that myth and ritual are mutually interrelated, and indeed each may be a commentary upon the other. Rather than attempting to ascribe primacy to what are evidently two different and complementary aspects of a society's creative and religious expression, anthropologists have devoted their attention to tracing the relations which exist between myth, ritual and social organization.

We may distinguish several different approaches to the anthropological study of myth. One approach is to trace the historical relationships between myths or bodies of myths, using mythological data as evidence of historical and geographical relationships between cultures and culture areas. This approach was criticized by MALINOWSKI (1948), as were other types of speculative or psychological interpretation of myth. Malinowski proposed that myth should be interpreted instead as a kind of 'social charter': that is to say, as a rationalization of the customs and behaviour of the group. At the same time, he insisted that myths were to be understood in their present-day social context, not as evidence of evolutionary or diffusionist hypotheses nor as abstract texts for psychological or psychoanalytic interpretation. The sociological approach to the study of myth became general in British social anthropology during the period 1930–60, while in the USA students of BOAS during this period generally studied myth as a repository of information about culture and culture traits and also as a guide to the regional historico-geographical relationships between different tribes or population units. The social charter approach pioneered by Malinowski came under criticism in its turn by later anthropologists, since it failed to do justice both to the symbolic complexity of myth and to the often ambiguous relationship between the content of mythic narratives and the features of social structure or social organization which it supposedly justifies.

Another approach to myth which has been consistently maintained by a sector of the anthropological community is the psychoanalytic one. FREUD himself employed mythical data as part of his theory of human history and of the basic characteristics of the human personality, and following Freud many psychoanalytically-oriented psychologists and social scientists have attempted to trace in myth the expression of themes of psychic conflict (the Oedipus complex, male-female envy or tension, and so on) in myth and in other areas of symbolism such as ritual and art. The degree of flexibility in the application of orthodox Freudian theory (or other variants of the psychoanalytic ap-

proach such as Jung's theory) to the context of non-Western cultures varies considerably among these scholars, because some seek to establish the universal validity of quite specific symbolic contents and psychological conflicts while others are more open to the span of variation in the symbolic and psychological expressions of different cultures. Freudian theories have however been profoundly influential in the study of myth and symbolism, and even those authors who reject or modify Freud's own scheme of psychological and social development and structure often owe much to his pioneering technique of symbol analysis.

An important and influential approach to myth has been that of the French structuralist anthropologist LEVI-STRAUSS, whose early interest in this theme culminated in his massive *Mythologiques* (1964–72). Levi-Strauss was concerned with myth as a type of thought, and also as an example of the working out of the universal structural principles which underlie all human cultural and social systems. He analysed myth as an intellectual tool which is used to reflect upon (and at a symbolic level to mediate or resolve) both universal and culturally specific contradictions. The universal contradictions or oppositions such as the problem of death, of creation (creation from a single first ancestor or from a pair), the opposition of nature and culture and of maternal and paternal relations are expressed and worked upon in mythology, which endlessly combines and recombines the different symbolic elements. An important feature of Levi-Strauss' approach is that it regards the myth not as an original version with a series of derivations or distortions but rather as all the existing and potential versions. He thus moves away from the search for an original or 'authentic' version of myth and towards a vision of the constant creation and modification of mythical knowledge and thought.

In his analysis of the story of Asdiwal Levi-Strauss echoes Malinowski's social charter theory at a more sophisticated level by suggesting that the ultimate function of the myth is to prove that of all possible arrangements only the one actually adopted by the group is feasible. The myth is thus regarded as an elaborate discourse on the possible combinations of social relations, leading to the conclusion that none is viable except the one practised by the group. This interest in the linkage of myth to social organization, and the interpretation of individual myths in relation to their social context, gives way in *Mythologiques* to the tracing of relationships between a vast array of myths from a wide range of ethnographic areas, stressing the manner in which mythology oversteps sociological boundaries and forms an ever-widening web of symbolic transformations, inversions and combinations. The interpretation of myth in *Mythologiques* is in terms of universal features of human thought and symbolic patterning, largely bypassing the level of specific types of social organization or social institution and their relationship to mythic themes and mythic forms.

The different approaches to myth briefly outlined above should not be regarded as mutually incompatible. Indeed they are all to some extent complementary, and each may reveal different aspects of the relationship between myth, symbolic-cognitive domains and social organization. Thus the social charter theory may be enriched both by Levi-Straussian techniques of myth analysis which help to elucidate the underlying symbolic structure, and also for example by Marxist theory of ideology which enables us to develop a more sophisticated view of how tales of the past and of the creation of things may serve as justifications and mystifications of the present state of affairs, making this seem eternal and sacred or natural. Similarly this does not rule out the judicious use of mythical data in order to aid in the reconstruction of historical relationships between population units and culture areas.

N

naturalization. The presentation by a given IDEOLOGY of socially specific situations, conditions or norms as if they were natural and inevitable phenomena. This process of ideological naturalization of the social order is linked to the process of MYSTIFICATION or ideological disguising of the true origin and nature of social relations.

nature/culture. One of the principal BINARY OPPOSITIONS which LEVI-STRAUSS considers fundamental to patterns of human thought, and which is elucidated by STRUCTURAL analysis of MYTH, RITUAL and other domains of SYMBOLISM.

nature/nurture. The controversy over the respective contributions of nature and nurture, of heredity and environment, and of 'instinct' and learning, is one which consistently recurs in the social sciences and has complex and deep-set historical, ideological and philosophical roots. The recent upsurge of interest in and debate over SOCIOBIO-LOGY, for example, is a modern expression of this controversy. Other fields of continuing debate include the field of GENDER studies, that of RACE, and the debate within educational theory and policy over the inheritance and development of intelligence. Such debates are often characterized by the confrontation of extreme positions: on the one hand the 'biological determinists' attempt to reduce all human phenomena to the expression of biological or biopsychological programming, while on the other the sociological or cultural determinists, often taking refuge in the dictum that social or cultural systems are *sui generis* and are not to be reduced to other levels of explanation, maintain that biology is irrelevant to the social sciences.

Modern developments in fields such as ETHOLOGY, in sociobiology itself, in PSY-CHOLOGICAL ANTHROPOLOGY and others would suggest that it is necessary to view biological and sociocultural systems as mutually interrelated. Both the biological determinist and sociological determinist positions are inadequate, in that they fail to take into account the fact that it is humans' biological nature to be cultural and social beings. That is to say, our behavioural and psychological 'programming' includes abilities like LANGUAGE, and other complex symbolizing capabilities, and the predisposition towards social and cultural organization. These capabilities and predispositions are however 'empty' in the sense that they do not carry any predetermined content (all normal humans are born with the inbuilt capability to learn and employ language, for example, but the particular language to be learned is given by each specific context within which the individual develops.) We may agree in the same way that there is a common universal repertory of human emotions, while recognizing nonetheless that different cultures and social systems may permit and encourage the expression of these universal emotions in differing degrees, combinations and forms. To recognize the importance of biological predispositions and conditions in shaping human sociocultural systems, however, should not be confused with the political or ideological process of proposing a carefully selected model of biological determinism in order to justify the subordination of given racial, ethnic or social groups and categories. This is to say no more than that investigations of the biological aspects of behaviour and sociocultural systems should be submitted to the same process of critical analysis to which we should submit all theories in the social sciences, an analysis which examines the actual and potential ideological implications (intended or unintended) of the theory concerned.

necronym. A name given to Ego by virtue of his or her relationship to a deceased person.

needs. The concept of needs and the relationship between these and sociocultural systems is one which has been particularly important in FUNCTIONAL social theory. Unfortunately many discussions of needs introduce a confusion between individual physical and psychological needs and social ones. In order to avoid this confusion, some functionalist theories refer to the social set as 'necessary conditions', 'functional imperatives', 'functional prerequisites', and so on. The concept of needs has not been applied with any great analytical precision, and its application is indeed problematic since we do not possess the means of distinguishing analytically or empirically between for example 'wants' or 'desires' and needs, or on the other hand between needs and limiting conditions beyond which survival is impossible. Thus on the one hand needs may be conceived of as those conditions which must be maintained in order for the human being or the social group to continue to exist (objective needs), while on the other they may be defined in terms of people's consciousness of the conditions they require (felt needs). In addition, different needs and different kinds of need (objective and subjective, individual and social) do not coincide perfectly and the simultaneous pursuit of these different needs may in itself lead not to a harmonious functioning whole but to CONFLICT and CONTRADICTION.

negotiation. A term with two distinct though related senses. In one sense it refers specifically to a type of process of DISPUTE SETTLEMENT in which the parties to the dispute directly attempt to find a solution acceptable to both or all. The term is also applied to a wide range of social contexts including those where there is no overt conflict or dispute involved, but in which two or more parties attempt to reach an agreement from initial positions which differ in some way. Negotiations in this second sense may thus occur, among other contexts, within the context of dispute settlement by other modes such as ADJUDICATION, ARBITRATION, and MEDIATION. All modes of dispute settlement may involve elements of negotiation inasmuch as

the parties involved in the conflict, their representatives, lawyers, judges and mediators, agree to discuss and bargain over the outcome of the legal process. Negotiation also occurs in a wide range of other contexts: for example, whenever two or more persons enter into a social relationship or are united by a common activity or by their participation in a social institution, negotiations will occur as the persons involved distribute power and leadership roles among the group and their opinions converge (or fail to) upon common definitions of each others' roles or positions.

The negotiating process implies that the parties are of more or less equal STATUS, or at least that for the purposes of the negotiation they agree to put aside differences of POWER or status and enter into the process as if they were equals. This equality may be more or less real, however, since behind the apparently democratic negotiation process there may be differences of power which condition the terms and outcome of the negotiation. We may thus distinguish negotiation between status equals from negotiation between persons of differential status or power. Minimally, however, each party must have something to bargain with, and this gives the negotiation process at least a temporary illusion of equality. The study of processes of interpersonal negotiation is important in the fields of ACTION THEORY and ETHNOMETHODOLOGY among others.

negro. *See* BLACK; ETHNICITY; RACE.

neo-colonialism. A term employed by some authors to denote the mechanisms by which an ex-colonial power retains control and politico-economic dominance over its former colony even after the granting of formal independence. Neo-colonialism in this sense depends upon the creation of an elite within the colonized nation which will perpetuate relationships of DEPENDENCY with the former colonial power, as well as the maintenance and continued control of international markets and economic conditions in such a way as to limit the opportunities and strategies of the former colony for independent economic or industrial development. The term is also often applied with the broader sense of strategies or policies within the industrialized nations which are designed to maintain or establish colonial-type or dependent relationships among Third World nations, independently from previous colonial relations. Through this second usage, neo-colonialism is defined as a strategy of the industrialized nations which, faced with the impossibility of creating and maintaining new colonies under direct administrative control, nevertheless attempt to perpetuate HEGEMONY and to create new relations of international dependence. (*See* COLONIALISM.)

neo-imperialism. Like NEO-COLONIALISM, this term is employed to refer to the new strategies of industrialized nations which seek to preserve their politico-economic hegemony over Third World nations under the new historical conditions which make the pursuit of traditional imperialist strategies impracticable. (*See* IMPERIALISM.)

neolithic. A stage of technological and sociocultural evolution characterized by the use of ground and polished stone tools (hence the name 'neolithic' meaning 'New Stone Age') and by the advent of AGRICULTURE and the domestication of animals. Archaeologists and anthropologists following CHILDE have classed the neolithic as the first great REVOLUTION in human development, representing as it does the overthrow of a pre-agricultural by an agricultural economy, with the concomitant social and cultural changes.

neolocal. The pattern of post-matrimonial RESIDENCE whereby the married couple reside in a new household or locality, independently of the parents of either. Neo-locality as well as bilocality (where the couple may choose whether to reside with husband's or wife's kin) or ambilocality may be associated with fluid local group composition, with independent domestic groups based on a nuclear family, with bilateral kinship systems, or with societies where factors other than kinship are the principal determinants of residence.

neo-Tylorianism. A school of thought in the anthropological study of RELIGION, led by Robin Horton (1967), which attempts to revive TYLOR's intellectualist approach to religion, and opposes neo-Durkheimian or functional-sociological explanations of religious phenomena.

network. In the social sciences the study of networks is that of interpersonal relationships and the manner in which these are arranged to form a pattern which we may term a social network. Whitten and Wolfe (1974) define a social network as a 'relevant series of linkages existing between individuals which may form a basis for the mobilization of people for specific purposes, under specific conditions'. According to this definition networks may coincide with, cross-cut or exist apart from specific social INSTITUTIONS, and the study of network formation and the mobilization of networks may thus be carried out in different contexts and at different levels: within a formal organization, within a community, within a dispersed set of persons linked by some common interest. Network study, with its emphasis on personal behaviour and choice or strategy, is closely linked to ACTION THEORY in anthropology.

New Archaeology. An approach in ARCHAEOLOGY pioneered by Lewis Binford (1972) which emphasizes on the one hand the rigorous processing and ordering of archaeological data and on the other the use of this data in order to construct and test hypotheses on human sociocultural development. The new archaeology thus draws closer to the concerns of anthropology and is linked to anthropological theories of human sociocultural evolution.

New Ethnography. *See* COGNITIVE ANTHROPOLOGY.

nicknames. Names given to persons apart from their proper personal name. Nicknames may be invented for each person or may come from a standard set. They may serve as means of indicating or addressing persons in those societies where the use of personal names is forbidden, or may function in order to express on the one hand friendliness or familiarity or on the other disapproval or social distance. (*See* INSULTS; JOKING RELATIONSHIP.)

nobility. A social CLASS identified by its possession of hereditary rights to land and other property as well as to honorific titles which are accompanied by some degree of privilege or political power. Also termed ARISTOCRACY, though strictly speaking this latter refers to a type of government rather than the class in itself. (*See* FEUDALISM.)

nodal kindred. A type of corporate KINDRED organization described by Goodenough (1970) and found for example among the Lapps and Lakalai. Kin ties are centred around a dominant core sibling set, to which other 'peripheral' sibling sets are attached, often by marriage.

nomads. Derived from the Greek *nemo* (to pasture), the term is used in anthropology to refer to the lifestyle not only of PASTORAL NOMADS but also of other social types characterized by the lack of a permanent residence or settlement. HUNTERS AND GATHERERS are also referred to as nomadic. Groups who alternate periods of nomadism and population dispersal with periods of population concentration and more extended residence in a single location are called semi-nomadic. This alternation relates to ecological and seasonal factors but also to symbolic and sociopolitical ones. Shifting agriculturalists are also sometimes called semi-nomadic because their residence in a single location is for a limited period of time, after which they abandon the site and move on. In the Amazon region shifting agriculture may be practised seasonally, and alternated with periods of nomadic hunting and gathering, thus combining the two types of semi-nomadic existence.

Populations who move around seasonally according to the pasturing needs of their animals are said to be TRANSHUMANT.

nomads, pastoral. *See* PASTORAL NOMADS.

non-unilineal descent. This term has been used by anthropologists to refer to DESCENT systems which do not operate exclusively according to UNILINEAL principles: that is to say, are not MATRILINEAL, PATRILINEAL or DOUBLE UNILINEAL. Keesing (1975) has suggested that for greater precision we should use the term COGNATIC descent to refer to those systems which trace descent through male and female links indiscrimi-

nately. Other authors have employed the terms ambilineal, BILINEAL or BILATERAL for this type of system, though the reader should carefully clarify the author's precise meaning in each case, as these terms have been defined quite differently by different writers. In traditional anthropological LINEAGE THEORY it was frequently asserted that bilateral, or cognatic, kinship could not provide the basis for the formation of viable descent CORPORATIONS, because cognatic kinship reckoning does not produce discrete groups but a series of overlapping affiliations. Modern kinship theory has shown however that cognatic descent reckoning is compatible with discrete kinship groups or corporations, and that in practice the problem of overlapping allegiances is resolved by the application of other mechanisms or principles which narrow down individual membership to a single corporation. These principles or mechanisms may include residence patterns, marriage rules and the emphasis on either matrilateral or patrilateral relations within the cognatic descent system. (*See* KINDRED.)

norm. Two categories may be distinguished, the 'statistical norm' and the 'ideal norm'. In the statistical sense, the norm is the average or modal phenomenon. In the ideal sense, it is the prescribed or expected pattern or standard of behaviour in a given social group or social context. However there is often some confusion between these two senses of the term: when we refer to a norm as 'expected behaviour', we often introduce a confusion between behaviour which is considered morally recommendable and that which is in fact likely to occur. Thus under certain circumstances it may be 'normal' (in the sense of statistically probable, and also in the sense of behaviour which is expected and encouraged) to transgress 'norms' of an ideal legal or moral nature. For example, a person may experience peer group pressure to transgress norms which at another level he or she upholds. Thus theories which stress the moral commitment to norms in society are problematic in their application, as pragmatic considerations are as important or more important than moral ones in determining the pattern of standards or expected behaviour. (*See* ATTITUDES; CONSENSUS; VALUE.)

nuclear family. *See* FAMILY.

numbers. Systems of numbering in different societies vary widely in their complexity and scope. While some languages possess only the words for a very few numbers (one and two, or one, two and three, for example) others possess very many distinct number words. Numbers should be considered in relation to systems of counting and arithmetic, and to their applications, which are both practical or economic and ritual. In general less attention has been paid to numbers and numeracy than to LITERACY, though like literacy numeracy and the form it takes in a given culture is an important element in shaping and facilitating the development of more complex social, economic, political and administrative structures. The anthropological study of numbers has focused to as great extent on number names and the ritual significance of numbers, to the exclusion of the study of mathematical and arithmetic systems. LEVY-BRUHL (1923) argued that the mystical qualities of numbers in primitive societies made them unsuitable for arithmetic operations. Barnes in his study of the Kedang (1982) shows that they have both a symbolic use of numbers, involving the symbolic opposition odd/even and its relationship to other cultural categories, and a mathematical use.

O

oblique discontinuous exchange. The hypothetical model of the exchange pattern created by a norm of marriage with Ego's sister's daughter or an equivalent category. The marriage exchange is 'oblique' in the sense that it is between persons of different generational status and 'discontinuous' in the sense that the reciprocation of a woman is not direct but delayed. Thus if a group A gives a woman to a group B, the alliance will be reciprocated in the succeeding generation when the daughter of this marriage is returned to her mother's brother in group A.

office. In POLITICAL ANTHROPOLOGY, an office is a formally constituted position within a political or administrative system. Offices may or may not be accompanied by honorific or ceremonial and ritual attributes. The office differs from position in that it has an independent existence which transcends that of the person who occupies it. In certain political systems the concept of office is inapplicable since there are no political positions which have an independent existence apart from their occupants (*see* BIG MAN; HUNTING AND GATHERING; LEADERSHIP.)

The rules of succession or election to office are an important element in the study of political systems, as is the examination of the manner in which LEGITIMACY is conferred upon office holders within different systems of political AUTHORITY. Office implies both a ROLE and a STATUS occupied by a specific individual for a certain time through a 'mandate from society', as Balandier has expressed it (1970). Ceremonials or rituals of investiture or of accession to office highlight this distinction between the person and the office. An office has both technical and rational-legal aspects as well as moral/religious ones. The former predominate in BUREAUCRATIC systems, while the latter may be as or more important in traditional societies where office is linked to kinship and/or religious systems. STRUCTURAL FUNCTIONALIST social anthropology emphasized the moral and religious components of office as expressions of the moral unity upon which the social structure depends, while Marxist anthropologists on the other hand have emphasized the IDEOLOGICAL functions of the ritual and religious attributes of office holders in maintaining and justifying the dominant position of a ruling group or CLASS. (*See* MONARCHY; STRATIFICATION.)

oligarchy. From the Greek, meaning 'rule by the few'.

Omaha. A type of KINSHIP TERMINOLOGY which is the mirror image of the CROW system. In the Omaha terminology the terms for matrilateral and patrilateral cross-cousins are distinct, and the cross-cousin terms are subject to generational 'skewing' such that MBS=MB and FZS=ZS. The Crow and Omaha terminologies have often been interpreted in terms of matrilineal and patrilineal descent systems respectively. However the empirical coincidence of terminological and descent systems is not perfect. ALLIANCE theorists have similarly linked these terminologies to the practice of matrilateral and patrilateral cross-cousin marriage respectively, though once again the correspondence is questionable, as these types of terminology may occur in conjunction with different types and combinations of marriage and descent rule.

ontology. The study or theory of being or existence. In philosophy and metaphysics ontology is the study of assumptions about reality and the nature of existence.

Opler, Marvin Kaufmann (1914–81). Cultural anthropologist who has worked in the field of PSYCHOLOGICAL ANTHROPOLOGY and the ethnography of North American Indians.

Opler, Morris E. (1907–). Cultural anthropologist who advocated the 'thematic' approach (*see* CULTURE AND PERSONALITY) and who has carried out field research among North American Indians and in South Asia (e.g. 1968).

oppression. Oppression may be social or economic, political or ideological, cultural or any combination of these. It refers to the subjection or domination of one people or group by another, and the use of the term implies that there is a subjective perception of domination as well as its existence in objective conditions.

oral literature. Part of the ORAL TRADITION, oral literature has been defined by W.P. Murphy (1979) as 'a form of communication which uses words in speech in a highly stylized, artistic way'. It is thus the more expressive end of a continuum ranging from referential to stylistic communication, and would include such forms as MYTH, folktale, legend, proverb and poetry. In the study of FOLKLORE, oral literature has had a central place. The historical-geographical method initiated by Grimm was long dominant in this field, and this concentrated on reconstructing the origin and diffusion of a folktale or other element by studying its distribution and variations. Another very influential approach has been psychoanalytic, whether the Jungian view which defines symbols in oral literature as manifestations of archetypal images from the 'collective unconscious', or the Freudian model of oral literature as a reflection of unconscious personal drama. Thus Dundes (1965), following the latter model, sees oral literature as a form of 'therapy' meeting the unconscious needs of individuals. LEVI-STRAUSS attempts to uncover unconscious meanings in a different way: he deals with a deep structure of cultural categories built up from oppositions and their mediation, and the analysis of myth and oral literature in STRUCTURAL ANTHROPOLOGY has carried on this concern with the underlying structures governing form and meaning.

Recent studies of oral literature have been influenced by developments in sociolinguis-

tics and COGNITIVE ANTHROPOLOGY to shift their emphasis from the text in itself to the study of the relationship between the text and its linguistic and social context. Thus for example, in an essay on legend, Degh and Vazsonyi show how an audience's shared knowledge of the beliefs underlying legend affects the nature of the genre, favouring the development of a brief and fragmented style. Similarly Abrahams classifies types of folklore in terms of different kinds of performer/audience involvement: compare the riddle, characterized by a high degree of interpersonal involvement, with the epic, where it is low. Other analysts relate oral literature to the RITUAL context in which it is employed, as in Herzfeld's study of the variations in Greek songs.

The contextual approach to oral literature, which concentrates on different kinds of meaning and the importance of speaker's intentions and interpretations, has links with the anthropological study of myth and of ORATORY as well as of ritual. The term 'oral literature' itself is however normally associated with the study of folk traditions and with European ETHNOLOGY.

oral tradition. The concept of the oral tradition is linked to that of the FOLK society and FOLKLORE. The oral tradition is that part of a society's cultural knowledge or 'traditional culture' which is passed on orally rather than in written form, and thus stands in implied opposition to the 'literate tradition' (*see* GREAT AND LITTLE TRADITION). Oral traditions are a source of information not only about contemporary cultural and social systems but also about the history of the group (*see* ETHNOHISTORY; HISTORY AND ANTHROPOLOGY.)

oratory. Oratory, the art of public speaking, is of great interest to anthropologists because of the central importance it has for many preliterate people. This importance is twofold: aesthetic and political.

In many parts of the world, such as among the Maori and other Oceanic peoples and among the native Americans of North America, the art of public speaking is highly valued for itself. This involves the ability to use well-illustrated language which refers to such communal sources as traditional history and proverbs. Also of value are the form of delivery, the wit of the speaker, his tone of voice, his posture, and so on.

The aesthetic aspect is however never totally divorced from the political. It is never enough to be skilled in oratory – one must also be the right kind of person from which such behaviour is acceptable. The oratory of political leaders can take one of two forms. The first is the oratory of a person whose rule is seen to embody all the moral values of the society. Such people are typified by the rulers of South East Asian and African states. Their oratory tends to follow precedent, they repeat well-accepted ideas using well-known examples. In their oratory, such rulers dissolve into the persona of their ANCESTORS and predecessors and so it is not surprising that it is sometimes difficult to draw the line between such oratory and spirit POSSESSION.

The other form of political oratory is characteristic of political leaders whose position is represented as the fruit of a successful struggle with other contenders. Such is the oratory of the New Guinea BIG MAN. Their oratory is highly assertive and therefore much more original, their speeches do not express the moral values of their communities, often the very opposite. Such oratory is often seen, as it is in New Guinea, as an essential tool of a successful warrior.

In some parts of the world it is not the political leader himself who speaks; he has a specialist orator speak for him. Such a situation is linked with those systems where the political and ritual aspects of leaders are separated or in cases where the speech maker runs the risk of humiliation.

ordeal. A part of mechanisms of DISPUTE SETTLEMENT or LEGAL process in certain societies. It is a test of physical endurance or a painful experience which the accused person undergoes, and the results of which are interpreted in order to establish his or her guilt or innocence. Physical ordeals also form a part of some INITIATION rites or other RITES OF PASSAGE including SHAMANIC initiation and other forms of religious training. In these cases, the physical ordeal may be intended not only to test the initiate but also to induce ALTERED STATES OF CONSCIOUSNESS which permit contact with the spiritual world.

organic analogy. See FUNCTIONALISM.

organic solidarity. See MECHANICAL/ORGANIC SOLIDARITY.

organization. This term has two distinct senses, that of SOCIAL ORGANIZATION in general and the more limited sense in which we refer to an organization or a formal organization as a purposive device for the achievement of specific goals or the carrying out of given functions in society. Organizations in this second sense may be BUREAUCRATIC or not, and occur in a wide variety of forms ranging from commercial organizations to voluntary ASSOCIATIONS and other kinds of formal grouping. The study of formal organizations is not well-developed in anthropology, though in recent years a minority of anthropologists have increasingly turned their attention to the analysis of complex INDUSTRIAL societies and the organizations which exist within them.

Oriental despotism. A term used by Wittfogel (1957) in order to describe the political structure or political type of Asiatic societies characterized by the centralized BUREAUCRATIC control of water supply and extensive irrigation works (irrigation civilizations or hydraulic civilizations). According to Wittfogel, the hydraulic or irrigation system prevalent in these societies led to the development of despotic political systems. The concept relates to that of the ASIATIC MODE OF PRODUCTION proposed by Marx. The features which Wittfogel considers as essential to oriental despotism as a type include the control over key elements of the MEANS OF PRODUCTION (in this case, the irrigation system) by the ruling class, and the existence of a state bureaucratic apparatus with extensive control over all areas of social life, as well as the state monopoly of military power. Wittfogel argued that the state comes to be more powerful in these systems, and more organized than local PEASANT communities which are reduced to atomistic and disorganized masses. Wittfogel's work regarding this social type has been widely criticized, and there is continuing controversy regarding both the nature of 'hydraulic' civilizations in Asia and the applicability of the concept to other regions of the world where extensive irrigation systems are found as the basis for agricultural production.

ostracism. A mechanism of punishment or SOCIAL CONTROL which is found in many societies, and which consists in isolating a person from social interaction or conversation. In its extreme form ostracism may involve treating the person as if he or she were 'dead', and may indeed lead to the death of the person.

P

palaeontology. The study of fossil remains. Human palaeontology is a branch of PHYSICAL ANTHROPOLOGY concerned with the study, dating and evaluation of the fossil remains of human and hominid species.

paradigm. A pattern or model. The term was employed by T.S. Kuhn in his theory of 'scientific revolutions' (1962) to designate the prevailing 'model problems and solutions' which dominate scientific activity at any moment in time. According to Kuhn, as the weight of evidence against a given paradigm accumulates over time, it is held in suspense until such time as it becomes overwhelming and results in the overthrow of the current paradigm and its replacement by another.

parallel cousin. The parallel cousins are those linked to Ego by same sex links in the first ascending generation (father's brother's and mother's sister's children).

parallel cousin marriage. This type of ALLIANCE is comparatively rare in the ethnographic record, the most common type of cousin marriage being with the cross-cousin or an equivalent category. Parallel cousin (FBD) marriage occurs in the Middle East and North African region and has been the subject of differing anthropological interpretations linking it to property transmission and LINEAGE ideology. ROBERTSON-SMITH (1885) interpreted this type of marriage as a form of inheritance by close male kin of the right to marry the wife or daughter of deceased Ego. Later interpretations have pointed to the possible ecological advantages of FBD marriage in the sense that it permits agnatic segmentation to extend to nuclear family level and is thus functionally flexible in situations of frequent feuding and fission. Other authors have emphasized the symbolic and ideological aspcts of FBD

marriage, while still others have pointed out that empirically this form is not as common as was once believed, and often coexists with other exogamous marriage norms. Thus the emphasis in recent studies has shifted from marriage structures in themselves towards the study of marriage choices within a broader socioeconomic and political framework.

parallel descent. A form of DESCENT in which there exist single sex descent groups where membership is passed from M to D and from F to S.

parricide. Parricide or patricide refers to the murder of the father. According to the PSYCHOANALYTIC theory of FREUD, the origin of the INCEST TABOO lay in the guilt experienced by primitive men at the crime of parricide committed to eliminate the father and enjoy sexual access to the mother. (*See* PATRIARCHY.)

Parsons, Elsie Clews (1875–1941). US anthropologist whose ethnographic studies of the Pueblo Indians, among others her *Pueblo Indian Religion* (1939), are well-known for their scope and detail.

Parsons, Talcott (1902–79). US sociologist who was a major contributor to FUNCTIONALIST sociological theory. Parsons was influenced by, and himself influenced, anthropological functionalism. Major works include *The Structure of Social Action* (1937), *Toward a General Theory of Action* (1951), and *The Social System* (1951).

participant observation. A technique of anthropological research associated with MALINOWSKI (1922), which has been incorporated into modern cultural and social anthropological FIELDWORK as a fundamental element. Indeed participant observation has come to be almost synonymous for many with ETHNOGRAPHY or anthropological field research as a whole. Malinowski advocated extended periods of fieldwork in which the anthropologist should attempt to immerse him or herself in the daily life of the people studied, thus minimizing the interfering effect of his or her presence and permitting a full appreciation of the cultural meanings and the social structure of the group with all its FUNCTIONAL interrelations between customs and beliefs, which at first sight appear inexplicable and incoherent. Participant observation is a technique which is necessarily directed towards the study of small and relatively stable human communities, which have hitherto been the favoured province of anthropologists.

Participant observation continues to be a basic element in modern anthropological research, and the type and depth of insight and interpretative material which it yields are difficult or impossible to gather using other research methods. However in recent years there has been in some quarters an increasing interest in supplementing, orienting and refining participant observation by introducing increasingly sophisticated methodology, and in others an increasing tendency to appraise critically the underlying premises of traditional anthropological fieldwork, including the implicit assumption of the 'neutrality' of the participant observer. Those who thought that the method of participant observation lacked vigour and objectivity have begun to look beyond it and have employed methodological approaches derived from, or influenced by other social sciences. While few would reject participant observation completely, the need to make the theoretical and methodological guidelines and the participant observer's assumptions or hypotheses more explicit and more rigorous has been pointed out as has the need to link the data gathered by means of participant observation to some more objective means of testing, whether in quantitative terms (*see* COMPUTERS IN SOCIOCULTURAL ANTHROPOLOGY; MATHEMATICAL MODELS IN SOCIOCULTURAL ANTHROPOLOGY; STATISTICS IN SOCIOCULTURAL ANTHROPOLOGY) or in terms of theoretical schemes. CRITICAL ANTHROPOLOGY on the other hand has pointed to the need to subject traditional assumptions of partici-

pant observation and of ETHNOGRAPHIC WRITING to critical scrutiny, arguing that the traditional stance of the anthropologist is both philosophically and politically naïve.

Modern anthropology has also rejected the stereotype of a discipline devoted to the study of small-scale societies, and in the anthropological study of complex INDUSTRIAL societies the participant observation method is more limited in its scope and possibilities. In modern anthropology it is impossible to maintain in consequence that participant observation is synonymous with ethnography or anthropological research in general, since it is evidently only one of a set of research techniques which may be employed by the cultural and social anthropologist.

pastoral nomads. Pastoral nomads constitute a social type which according to R. and N. Dyson-Hudson in their review of this topic (1980) may be defined by the coexistence of dependence on livestock with spatial mobility or nomadism. Such societies have been and are found in many parts of the world, including Africa, Asia, southern Europe and South America, where they have been the subject of anthropological study. However the principal geographical focus of the study of this social type has been on East Africa and the Middle East.

'Pure' pastoralists, or those who are totally dependent on their herds with no agricultural activity, are comparatively rare, and a combination of pastoral and agricultural activities is more common. There is considerable variation in social, economic and demographic patterns among societies broadly labelled 'pastoralist'. The category embraces a number of different groups whose population movements and social organization are subject to the influence of widely varying ecological, political, economic and cultural or cognitive factors. Nevertheless there have been many attempts to formulate a general theory or model of this type of society.

Before 1970 the predominant interest in pastoralists was as paradigmatic cases of the SEGMENTARY LINEAGE society within British STRUCTURAL FUNCTIONALISM. During the 1970s however there was an upsurge of different and competing views, many centred on ecological and/or economic interpretations of pastoral social organization. Barth (1961) proposed as a general characteristic of pastoral social systems their greater potential dynamism compared to agricultural ones, since animals as capital reproduce and increase whereas land does not. Spooner (1973) suggests that there is a consistent relationship between pastoralism as an ecological adaptation and certain specific cultural-ideological features such as egalitarianism and independence. Schneider (1984) argues that lineage-based organization in pastoral societies is linked to the existence of pressure on resources, while the lack of such pressure leads to the development of age-based systems. There has thus been a continuing interest in the themes established by EVANS-PRITCHARD's classic study of the Nuer (1940): the relationship between ecology, social forms and values or cultural pattern. However the hypotheses proposed, as R. and N. Dyson-Hudson point out, have not been adequately tested. It is clear that pastoralists are not a unitary social type, yet some authors consider the notion of a pastoral MODE OF PRODUCTION valid while others would dispute the creation of a special category for pastoral societies. On the other hand, in modern anthropological studies of pastoralists it has also been recognized that these groups cannot be studied in isolation from the national and regional context of inter-ethnic relations and their relationship to a dominant state system and/or to neighbouring agricultural peoples. Another important theme which has only recently been taken up by such anthropologists as M. Llewelyn-Davis (1981) is the study of the role of women, long-neglected by ethnographies, which have shown a clear PATRIARCHAL bias.

pater/genitor. This distinction, following Roman law, separates the physiological father of a child from the social father. According to Roman law the *pater* was the mother's legal husband, irrespective of who may have been the *genitor* or actual physical father. This distinction is sometimes employed in anthropology, and a parallel distinction between *mater* and *genetrix* has been suggested, although this latter has little practical applicability since the physiological and social mother are generally (though not always) identical. (*See* CONCEPTION; KINSHIP.)

paternity. *See* SOCIOLOGICAL PATERNITY.

patriarchy. In its original and more restricted sense, this term refers to a type of social system dominated by the principle of 'father-right' or the sole control of domestic and public-political authority by senior males within the group. 19th-century anthropological theory of kinship and social evolution was dominated by the controversy between those who advocated MATRIARCHY as the original form of society, followed later by patriarchy (BACHOFEN (1867) and MORGAN (1977) among others) and those such as MAINE (1861) and WESTERMARCK (1861), who held the opposing view that the original form of society was patriarchal. Outside anthropology, ENGELS (1884) and FREUD (1913) are the most celebrated champions of the matriarchal and patriarchal theories respectively. Freud argued that human society commenced with the patriarchal horde where the senior male or father dominated and thought that the patriarchal regime was overthrown by the primordial crime of PARRICIDE committed by the sons in order to gain sexual access to the mother (*see* INCEST.)

There is no generally accepted or rigorous definition of patriarchy, however, and in particular there is some confusion as to the domestic and the public or political aspects of male dominance which are necessarily present in order for a type of society to be called 'patriarchal'. Thus 'father-right' may be viewed as the absolute authority of the male in the domestic domain, extending in extreme cases to the power of life or death over the women and children within the domestic unit, or more commonly the unilateral right to dispose of their property, the right to take decisions on behalf of the whole domestic group, and so on. Patriarchy may also be viewed however from the perspective of a male monopoly on public social discourse, political and economic decisions, and so on. Societies which are 'patriarchal' in the first sense are usually so in the second sense, since the attribution of absolute authority to the male in the domestic domain implies that the female is classed as a 'minor' or incompetent person in the public domain too. But societies that are 'patriarchal' in the second sense may not be so in the first, as women may possess some domestic authority and autonomy within societies whose political systems are nonetheless dominated by men. In any case, it is necessary to recognize that 'patriarchy' is not a unitary concept or conglomerate of features which will always coexist. Rather we should distinguish different elements or expressions of patriarchy which may coexist with expressions of matriarchy and/or of gender complementarity or equality. On the other hand, if we do not wish to extend the term as broadly as in particular some modern feminists do, we should have to reserve it for those societies in which the expression of male dominance is particularly extreme and systematic, such as those in which the legal rights of woman and children are totally subject to the authority of the male. For many feminist anthropologists, however, the term patriarchy is synonymous with male dominance in general, and thus refers not to a specific social type but to a general tendency which finds its expression in differential form in each social and historical context.

Engels, following Morgan, held that the emergence of private PROPERTY in human evolution gave rise to the overthrow of matriarchal regimes by patriarchal ones, and there is a continuing debate in modern anthropology and feminist theory about the relationship between economic systems, gender relations and social class. Some feminists follow Marxist theory in treating patriarchy as a complement and product of the CAPITALIST mode of production, which is based on the SEXUAL DIVISION OF LABOUR which assigns domestic and child-rearing tasks to an unpaid female labour force. The classification of women's work as 'non-work' (that is, as a natural and sacred role to which the woman must sacrifice herself in fulfilment of a cultural ideal of wifeliness and motherhood) disguises the real economic contribution of women which in fact sustains the capitalist system by providing essential reproductive services free of charge. In addition women constitute a reserve labour force which may be employed under less favourable terms than males. (*See* FEMINIST ANTHROPOLOGY; GENDER; WOMEN AND ANTHROPOLOGY.)

patricide. *See* PARRICIDE.

patrifocal. A form of FAMILY or DOMESTIC GROUP which is centred on the father. (*See* MATRIFOCAL.)

patrilateral. 'On the father's side'. Refers to those kin who are related to Ego through Ego's father.

patrilateral cross-cousin marriage. The rule or norm of marriage with the patrilateral cross-cousin (that is, of male Ego with his FZD) has attracted considerable anthropological attention because of its hypothetical and actual consequences for social organization. This marriage rule occurs comparatively rarely, the rule of MATRILATERAL CROSS-COUSIN MARRIAGE being empirically far more common. According to LEVI-STRAUSS' theories the ELEMENTARY STRUCTURES of kinship and marriage alliance, the system of FZD marriage is classed as one of 'delayed reciprocity' since if this pattern of marriage were consistently practised it would produce a unidirectional flow of women between groups in each generation, with the flow being reversed in the subsequent generation. Needham has argued (1962) that FZD marriage does not exist, since its consistent practice would lead to the FZD also being the MBD, and would thus merge with matrilateral cross-cousin marriage. Later students of this problem have however taken less literally the hypothetical consequences of the rigid observance of the marriage rule, regarding it rather as an ideal model which represents an ALLIANCE type but which in practice will always be modified by demographic and historical contingency and/or by the existence of competing marriage norms.

patrilineal. DESCENT which is traced through the male line. This is also referred to as AGNATIC descent. (*See* LINEAGE THEORY.)

patrilocal. In the anthropological classification of RESIDENCE patterns, patrilocal residence is the pattern in which a couple establish their residence with or near the husband's family. In order to avoid the confusion with patrilineality, since patrilineal systems are not always patrilocal and vice versa, in modern anthropology the term VIRILOCAL is often preferred.

patronage. An institution which links patrons and CLIENTS by means of DYADIC ties, and whose purposes may include ritual, economic and/or political elements. The dyadic and individualizing nature of patronage has made it an important focus of ACTION THEORY in anthropology, and patron–client relations have been extensively studied as the basis of political systems, together with other related concepts such as BROKERAGE and FACTIONS. Opponents of action theory have however pointed out that to examine the series of dyadic patron–client ties and their strategic manipulation may obscure the underlying class basis of the system as a whole and the fact that patrons as a group exercise a collective domination over clients as a group. On the other hand, a crude analysis of class dominance will also fail to do justice to the variability of institutions of patronage, which range from those situations in which patrons exercise limited control over their clients to those where the institution approaches a situation of DEBT SLAVERY or peonage.

In analysing the ritual, symbolic and ideological dimensions of patronage (for example in those cases where it appears under the guise of RITUAL KINSHIP) it is interesting to note the manner in which the ideology of patronage contributes to the maintenance of structures of politico-economic and social dominance. It does this both by dividing loyalties among the subordinate strata, encouraging competition between them in terms of the search for more favourable patronage relations, and by presenting the patron as the superior or more generous element (the one who performs 'favours' for the client) when in fact the flow of goods and services is generally objectively in favour of the patron.

pattern. The concept of pattern is employed in anthropology in a number of different ways, often without great precision. It can be used to refer to behaviour patterns or observable regularities in conduct among the members of a given group or community. But the term 'culture pattern' was used by BENEDICT (1934) to refer to common underlying attributes or 'styles' which characterize cultures as a whole as well as the psycho-social orientation of their members (*see* CULTURE AND PERSONALITY). Another use of the term is to refer to patterns or associations of CULTURAL TRAITS which display geographical or historical continuity. (*See* CULTURE HISTORY; CULTURE AREAS.)

peasant. The peasantry is a class of primary producers within a society characterized by the existence of social CLASSES and STATE formation. Some definitions of the peasantry restrict its composition to agricultural producers, while others would include fishing peoples, artisans and other productive groups whose structural position is similar to that of the agrarian peasantry. Within the category of the agrarian peasantry itself there is considerable disagreement as to the exact defining characteristics of this social type, and the term is commonly used to refer to a wide range of cultivators whose relationship to the LAND (owners, tenants, sharecroppers, and so on) and to the MARKET vary considerably. However all definitions of the peasantry agree in emphasizing the importance of the opposition or contrast between the peasant stratum and the urban elite. The peasantry and the urban centre are two opposing poles of a single socio-economic system, and this is reflected not only in their economic interdependence but also in the complex relationship which exists between peasant and urban culture (*see* GREAT/LITTLE TRADITION; FOLK-URBAN CONTINUUM).

There has been a longstanding tendency in anthropology and in the other social sciences to treat the peasantry as an intermediate category or transitional stage between the self-sufficient tribal society and modern civilization. However since the 1950s this view of the peasantry as a category somehow not suitable for serious anthropological study has given way to a new upsurge of interest in the study of peasant communities, so much so that in recent years studies of the peasantry have come to outnumber those of tribal societies in cultural and social anthropology. This rise to prominence of peasant studies has been accompanied by a general broadening of the anthropological perspective to include varying social types including URBAN studies and INDUSTRIAL anthropology, thus rejecting the earlier tendency to seek the discovery or reconstruction of 'uncontacted' societies or cultures which had characterized FUNCTIONALIST anthropology. Peasant groups provide an excellent environment for the anthropological study of inter-ethnic relations (*see* ETHNICITY), of social and economic CHANGE and DEVELOPMENT, and POLITICAL systems, all of which are prominent themes in modern anthropology. In addition the tradition of COMMUNITY STUDIES which predominated in the early studies of the peasantry within cultural anthropology has contributed a lasting influence in terms of the continuing interest in peasant culture, VALUES, and WORLD VIEW.

As mentioned above, a common feature of all attempts to define the peasantry is the central importance attached to the dual nature of peasant society and culture. This duality is expressed in a number of ways: in the peasant economy, which is linked on the one hand to subsistence needs and on the other tied in to the market by the peasantry's participation both as producers and consumers in the wider economic system; in the peasant political system, which combines elements of communal autonomy with elements of political dependence and subordination to the wider political structure; and in peasant culture, which stands in a dialectical opposition to the literate tradition of the wider society. An important aspect of peasant duality is the role of BROKERS, patrons and other intermediaries between local and supralocal levels.

Some writers emphasize the economic aspect when defining the peasantry. E. Wolf for example (1969) defines peasants as those whose surplus production is transferred to a dominant ruling group, which employs this surplus both to maintain itself and to redistribute to other non-agricultural sectors of the population. However, as has been amply debated within peasant studies, it is necessary to refine such a definition in order to take into account the fact that peasants exist within different MODES OF PRODUCTION and that their relationship to the MEANS OF PRODUCTION varies considerably. Thus within FEUDAL society as characteristically defined in its more limited sense, peasants are SERFS who are bound to the land and by a relationship of personal allegiance to the landowner. Other types of peasant may rent

their land, paying the rent in the form of part of their crops, or they may be small-scale landowners whose surpluses are extracted from them by a number of different means including taxation, patron–client relations, debt slavery and unequal participation in the regional and national market structure. Thus Wallerstein (1974) for example distinguishes between the peasant formations of European medieval feudalism and the 'coerced cash-crop labour' which exists within predominantly capitalist economies, but which is also often referred to as a 'peasant economy' by writers who do not adequately define the predominant mode of production in the society under consideration. Similarly, writers on peasant societies have often found it necessary to divide the unitary category of the peasantry into different classes or types according to economic status and relationship to the means of production. Thus within a single national or regional context peasants with differential levels of wealth and different positions may co-exist within the class structure.

Early studies of peasant communities in Mesoamerica and other regions tended to emphasize the peasant community as a self-contained and homogeneous unit, and applied many of the techniques which had previously been used for tribal societies in order to elucidate the community's cultural and social structural configuration. Typically these studies emphasized the independence of the nuclear family and household within peasant society, and indeed many authors elevated concepts such as those of 'atomism', 'familism' (*see* AMORAL FAMILISM), and DYADIC relations to the status of general or theoretical propositions about the nature of peasant society (*see* LIMITED GOOD). Modern studies of peasant society have come to stress the inadequacy of these models, however, and have demonstrated the importance of anthropological analysis of the organizational and conceptual structures mediating between the levels of family or household and community. But it is perhaps most notably in the field of economic analysis that modern peasant studies have shown the need to look beyond the individual household in order to analyse the relationship between units of production and between different social classes.

A further criticism of early peasant studies

is that they tended to isolate themselves conceptually within the local community and take the wider system for granted. Thus many features of peasant social organization, values and world view (*see* CONSERVATISM) were analysed as if they were intrinsic properties of the local community, rather than being seen as the products of the interaction between local and supralocal socioeconomic, political and cultural systems. Here the work of the Mexican sociologist Rodolfo Stavenhagen (1975) has been of pioneering importance, first of all in establishing generally the fruitfulness of the perspective which views peasant communities in terms of their interaction with regional social systems, and more particularly situating Indian peasant values and behaviour within the context of their ethnic and social class domination by the *Ladino* ruling group.

Other important developments in modern peasant studies are those which direct themselves to the analysis of the political organization and potential for political change and rebellion among peasants. It is clear when we consider the historical evidence that stereotypes of peasant FATALISM and political passivity are not applicable in very many cases, since peasant societies in fact display a tendency to political instability in many circumstances. The political philosophy of MAO TSE-TUNG is often credited with having revindicated the revolutionary potential of the peasantry which was denied by orthodox Marxism, and the theme of peasant rebellions and resistance to political domination and economic exploitation is of major importance in modern historical and social scientific studies of the peasantry. Once again, modern peasant studies have criticized earlier work for treating as cultural phenomena features of peasant life and behaviour which should be analysed in terms of their historical and political significance. Thus the tendency to autonomy, isolation and self-sufficiency of peasant communities should be interpreted not only in terms of 'peasant conservatism' and isolationist mentality, but also in terms of the bid to retain a degree of political and economic independence in the face of a regional and national system which dominates and threatens to engulf the peasant community. The applicability of models of peasant organization derived from specific historical and geographical contexts to other regions and time periods generates continuing debate. For example, Mesoamerican communities, which have often been offered as general models of peasant society, are not generally similar to those in other regions such as Asia or Africa. The status of African cultivators has been the subject of especial controversy as they do not combine the same features of economic, political and cultural dependence on the urban centre as those observed for example in Mesoamerica or in Europe. Some writers have also attempted to apply the term 'peasantry' to the rural poor in industrialized nations such as the USA, though it is debatable to what extent this confuses rather than clarifies the special features of these marginal sectors in industrial nations.

peer group. A group of persons considered to be equal because of some defining characteristic like age or occupational status. In peer group interaction the relations of dominance, equality, decision-making and so on are those established or negotiated by the persons involved, and peer groups develop norms and sanctions which influence or regulate the conduct of their members.

peon. A kind of DEBT SLAVE who may be a CLIENT, a tenant or an employee. The institution of peonage is backed up by a politico-economic system which binds the peon to his PATRON by permanent indebtedness.

people. Employed by some anthropologists in preference to terms such as TRIBE, CULTURE or SOCIETY to refer to a human group or a population unit. The use of the term implies that the group or population is considered or considers itself united by common language, residence, or other cultural and social features. The term is also employed as an equivalent to 'nation' ('the French people'). It may also be used to refer to the working class, the peasantry or the poor as opposed to the ruling class or elite.

performance. A concept employed particulary by anthropologists in the analysis of RITUAL and RELIGION, where several writers have drawn on the theory of literary and artistic criticism in order to elucidate features of cultural performance in different ethnographic contexts. (*See* AESTHETICS; ART, ANTHROPOLOGY OF; DANCE; DRAMA.)

periphery. *See* WORLD SYSTEMS.

Perry, William James (1889–1949). British social anthropologist who together with Elliot SMITH was a leading exponent of DIFFUSIONISM (e.g. 1923).

person. In cultural and social anthropology the concept of the person in the ethnographic context under study is an important element in many investigations. The study of how the person or the individual is conceived of may be approached from the perspective of the ANTHROPOLOGY OF AGE, which shows how the expectations, behaviour, norms, roles and statuses associated with the person change over the span of the individual's life. An important contribution to the study of the SYMBOLIC dimensions of the person is that of the study of RITES OF PASSAGE and RITUAL in general. Another approach is via the study of KINSHIP and MARRIAGE systems, or via the study of ETHNIC or other classificatory systems which divide persons into different categories with different role and behavioural expectations and different symbolic values.

personal culture. The individual impression of CULTURE belonging to a particular individual. The importance of personal culture has been recognized in modern anthropology since it has been demonstrated that the CONSENSUS of VALUES and uniformity of beliefs and knowledge assumed by earlier FUNCTIONALIST theory is far from being an accurate portrayal. We should approach the study of a human group not in terms of the existence of one uniform culture shared by all its members, but rather in terms of the interaction and NEGOTIATION between many different individual versions of that culture.

personal kindred. *See* KINDRED.

personality. *See* CULTURE AND PERSONALITY.

petite bourgeoisie. A social CLASS which comprises owners of small businesses (including self-employed craftsmen or artisans) and which may also be extended to cover the small farmer who is the owner of his own land. Marx believed that the process of increasing class polarization would lead to the petite BOURGEOISIE becoming absorbed into the PROLETARIAT. In fact the historical evidence is somewhat contradictory on this point, and shows considerable variability from one geographical and social context to another. In some contexts the petite bourgeoisie is linked more closely to the proletariat, in others to the large scale owners of capital, and while a process of absorption of small businesses by large ones seems to take place in some contexts, in others the small business seems to hold its own in the face of large-scale capitalism.

phenomenology. A philosophical movement which has been influential in the social sciences and in anthropology, particularly in the anthropology of systems of CLASSIFICATION and KNOWLEDGE. Its leading exponent is the philosopher Edmund Husserl, and it is concerned with the study of consciousness and the manner in which people apprehend the world and the objects within it. The aim of phenomenology is thus to describe conceptual structures and processes. A central notion is that of 'intentionality'. This refers to the fact that an object and the consciousness which apprehends it are not to be treated as two separable entities but as a single phenomenon. Thus the object in itself does not exist apart from in the manner in which it is constituted by consciousness.

phenotype. *See* GENOTYPE.

phonemics. The study or analysis of the systems of phonemes which occur in human languages. A phoneme is a minimal 'difference that makes a difference' in a language. It is a unit of sound which has no meaning in itself but which serves to differentiate meaning. Variations in sound which do not change the meaning of a word are termed 'allophones'. For example, /b/ and /v/ in English are different phonemes (there is a difference of meaning between 'vat' and 'bat') while in Spanish they are allophones or versions of the same phoneme since they do not serve to distinguish meaning. (*See* DISTINCTIVE FEATURES.)

phonetics. The study of the sound patterns in human speech. Phonetic analysis attempts to measure, describe and represent symbolically all the sounds which speakers produce. It is contrasted with PHONEMICS which is the study of significant sounds. (*See* EMIC/ETIC.)

phonology. The study of speech sounds, including both PHONEMICS and PHONETICS.

photography. *See* VISUAL ANTHROPOLOGY.

phratry. A term used in the study of KINSHIP to refer to a grouping of two or more CLANS who claim common descent from a mythological ancestor.

physical anthropology. The field of physical anthropology has largely developed as a discipline apart from cultural and social anthropology, though it has important links with theories in these fields, especially in the areas of ecological and EVOLUTIONARY theory, and with the related discipline of ARCHAEOLOGY. These links are being explored in modern BIOLOGICAL ANTHROPOLOGY, which is broadly based and interdisciplinary by nature. However, many cultural and social anthropologists resist the claims of physical or biological anthropology (or the recent version of SOCIOBIOLOGY) to provide significant explanation of human cultural and social nature and variation. In part this is due to the overtones of biological determinism and RACISM which biologically-oriented theories have acquired as a result of the more publicized and less scientific contributions in the field. Nevertheless modern advances in the field of biological anthropology are beginning to overcome this barrier, and demonstrate that it has an important contribution to make to the study of human culture and society as adaptations to given environmental and evolutionary constraints.

Early physical anthropology was dominated by ANTHROPOMETRY, or the measurement of the physical characteristics of different individuals or human groups. Later its dominant concern became the study of the evidence for human evolution. The study of hominid and early human fossil remains has vastly increased in recent years both in scope and in methodological sophistication, and physical anthropologists have developed a wide range of techniques for reconstructing information about individuals and populations from fragmentary remains of bones, teeth, and other matter. Although anthropometry began by limiting itself largely to the comparison of the characteristics of different racial groups, it gradually developed into the more sophisticated modern study of human variation. In modern physical anthropology human variation is approached not in terms of races as significant units of study but rather in terms of local populations defined in terms of the distribution of genes. The study of DEMOGRAPHIC factors, the interaction of population, disease, nutrition and environment, and the study of population genetics are all part of the conceptual tool kit of the modern biological anthropologist, who attempts to understand 'micro-evolution': the variability and evolution of local populations.

piacular. A term introduced by DURKHEIM to the study of RELIGION and RITUAL. Piacular rites are those which perform the function of expressing community solidarity in the face of crises such as the death of one of its members. (*See* MORTUARY RITES.)

Piaget, Jean (1896–1980). Swiss psychologist who was the founder of the developmental school of human psychology, and who was influential not only in the elaboration of psychological theory but also in the fields of linguistics, philosophy and the social sciences in general. Piaget's theories of cognitive development passing through a series of clearly defined stages, and his emphasis on the active construction of reality and the personality by the individual have constituted important critiques both of BEHAVIOURISM and STRUCTURALISM with their tendency to view the individual as a passive vehicle for the conditioning process or for the expression of structural tendencies.

pidgin. A simplified language used as a means of communication between two or more groups who do not share a common tongue. Pidgins typically develop out of trade languages and may evolve into CREOLE or mixed languages over time.

pilgrimage. Pilgrimages have attracted the attention of a limited number of anthropological studies, the focal point being the manner in which they confound ethnic and political boundaries. TURNER (1974) sees pilgrimage as a kind of 'normative comunitas' and as the 'ordered anti-structure of patrimonial feudal systems'. This interpretation of pilgrimage forms part of his more general theory of RITUAL and the relationship between structure and comunitas in society. M. Sallnow relates pilgrimage to the system of regional CULTS and likens it to a temporary contractual form of co-operation between communities which nevertheless retain their distinctive ritual identity. The universalism of pilgrimage cross-cuts ecclesiastical and sociogeographic boundaries and creates new ARENAS of social interaction. According to Sallnow, comunitas is not the goal of pilgrimage, which should rather be considered as a polyfaceted process of social interaction.

plantation. A large-scale single crop agricultural enterprise. Plantations have been associated historically with SLAVERY, with the use of hired free labour often under extreme conditions of poverty and instability, and on occasion with CO-OPERATIVE forms of ownership and labour under programmes of LAND REFORM or SOCIALIST economies. Plantations are a common feature of Third World economies (though they exist also in developed countries such as in the USA) where they are often controlled by overseas capital. (*See* AGRIBUSINESS; CAPITALISM; COLONIALISM.)

play, anthropology of. Play behaviour is common to mammals and humans, and primate play is in many ways similar to the play of human youngsters. Ethologists who have studied animal play have often found it difficult to define the boundaries of play behaviour precisely, since play often overlaps with other types of behaviour such as exploration, dominance and sexual activity. Children's play is often interpreted as a form of imitation of and preparation for adult life, related to the SOCIALIZATION process, and/

or as a medium for the expression of certain psychological orientations or conflicts. Within DIFFUSIONIST and FOLKLORE studies, play and games have been studied and recorded above all for their value as evidence of diffusionist theories or for the sake of 'preserving' play texts, rather than for the significance of play behaviour in culture or society. Comparative studies of play on the other hand have viewed games as expressive activities which are models of cultural patterns, and have attempted to relate the complexity or the characteristics of games to cultural factors. Thus Roberts and Sutton-Smith put forward the 'conflict-enculturation' hypothesis, according to which conflicts engendered by enculturation create certain types of game activities which embody role reversals relating to these conflicts. Play thus leads ultimately to the mastery of behaviour appropriate to social roles. Similarly the 'Six Cultures' project of Whiting and Child considered play as role-learning and studied the relationship between play and such behavioural expectations as dominance and nurture.

The theories of play which focus on its educational aspects or its function in the socialization process do not however account for imaginative play or for the structure of play itself. Huizinga in his *Homo ludens* (1949) argues that play should be studied both 'in itself' and as an aspect of many other activities such as warfare, art and law. He distinguishes play as a special and voluntary activity which is absorbing, non-productive, circumscribed by time, place and rules and characterized by 'secret' group relations (*see* GAME THEORY). BATESON (1972) on the other hand approaches play as a paradigm for METACOMMUNICATION, since play involves 'learning to learn'. C. Geertz (1972) employs the concept of 'deep play' to describe the Balinese cockfight, which he interprets as a social text embodying commentary on the hierarchical nature of Balinese society. Play according to Geertz is thus seen as a 'culturally specific reading of experience'.

A different approach to play is that taken by Goffman in his theory of ROLE (1969), which sees play as a paradigm for role enactment, and also develops Bateson's idea of metacommunication or 'frames' around different types of play interaction. Structuralist analysts such as A. Dundes have also attempted to analyse play in terms of its morphology, and Dundes attempts to locate 'motifemes' of games (1965). Developmental psychology influenced by PIAGET has studied the manner in which stages of play reflect intellectual development and concept formation.

The importance of play and games in anthropology is therefore dual: on the one hand, play has been taken as a field of study which has been employed in order to demonstrate or test certain hypotheses, particularly within diffusionist theory and within different areas of PSYCHOLOGICAL ANTHROPOLOGY, and on the other play itself has served as a paradigm and a source of theoretical models which have been applied to the interpretation of other domains of behaviour and sociocultural organization.

pluralism. Cultural or social pluralism is a very general concept which consists of the existence of multiple systems or subsystems within a single socioeconomic or political unit. We may thus refer to linguistic pluralism, ETHNIC pluralism, cultural pluralism, and so on. It is erroneous to consider that such pluralism within national or regional boundaries is abnormal or exceptional, for when the historical and ethnographic records are considered it can be seen that pluralism is the rule rather than the exception. In political theory, pluralism has a different sense, referring to the distribution of political power or decision-making among diverse groups or institutions.

plural society. This concept was originally employed by the economist J.S. Furnivall in his study of the effects of colonial rule in Burma and Indonesia (1967). The term was taken up by M.G. Smith in his study of the Caribbean islands where culturally distinct ethnic groups 'mix but do not combine'. Political domination by one ethnic group and the articulation of the different participating groups in a shared economic system, where each occupies a specific position in the DIVISION OF LABOUR are what maintain the plural society in equilibrium. Van den Berghe applies the plural society concept to the USA, where he claims ethnic groups have distinct and duplicated institutions and value systems, except in the domain of

politics and economics where there is a single common system. The plural society model thus contradicts the Chicago school of RACE RELATIONS which views inter-ethnic contact as a cycle of competition, accommodation and assimilation through which all ethnic groups must pass. Like Marxist theory, the plural society model criticizes the Chicago school notion of 'stages towards integration' which obscures both the cultural differences between ethnic groups and the structure of institutionalized RACISM in society. However, Marxist theory also differs from the plural society model in that it asserts that there is a single system of colour–class stratification which assigns different patterns of values and behaviour according to a colour–class code.

Polanyi, Karl (1886–1964). British economic anthropologist whose theories formed the basis of the substantivist school of ECONOMIC ANTHROPOLOGY (e.g. 1968).

policy and anthropology. The relationship of policy and administration to anthropology has been consistently problematic. Anthropologists sustained an uneasy co-operation with COLONIAL authorities, which continued up till the period of the Second World War, during which time several anthropologists – especially in the USA – were employed in war-related research and consultation. After this period, there was a generalized retreat both in British and US anthropology into the academic world, which in anthropology established the norm that academic research should not be related to the specific interests of any given group or client. Involvement of US anthropologists in such controversial areas as 'Project Camelot' in Vietnam and in Thailand prompted another withdrawal and renewed caution in anthropological circles about the advisability of becoming involved in government-sponsored research or applied anthropology. In general, though certain aspects of anthropological knowledge have been absorbed by policy-makers in some fields, the practising (as opposed to the academic) anthropologist is still considered marginal to the discipline. Changing circumstances, however, including the lack of employment opportunities for anthropology graduates in the academic world, are encouraging many younger professionals to seek new fields of practical application for their discipline, the most popular to date being the field of MEDICAL ANTHROPOLOGY and public health.

The interrelation between anthropology and policy may take a variety of different forms, ranging from the anthropologist who from an academic base acts as a social critic, policy analyst or political activist, to the anthropologist who undertakes contract research or is a public employee, or the applied anthropologist who combines research with involvement in a DEVELOPMENT goal at home or abroad. The visible impact of anthropology on public policy has so far however been low, even though as Van Willigen points out in his essay on this topic (1984) anthropology has always been thought of as a policy science. According to Van Willigen the main contribution of anthropology to policy is not in policy formation but in the provision of information to policy makers, and this function he states is best developed at a local level or within the context of large scale multidisciplinary teams. Van Willigen also points to the areas of confusion and contradiction between anthropological theory, policy and action, confusions which result in part from the fragmentation of academic anthropology and its separation from its practitioners in the non-academic world. (*See* APPLIED ANTHROPOLOGY.)

political anthropology. There can be as many different interpretations of political organization as there are definitions of the political domain in society. Balandier (1970) distinguishes four principal ways of defining the political sphere, which attempt to deal with the peculiarly anthropological problem of the absence or apparent absence of formal political structures in many simple or traditional societies. For some authors, following MAINE (1861) and MORGAN (1877), territorial representations are the origin and centre of political systems, which define and operate within a given territorial space. Other authors put forward functional definitions of the political sphere, usually emphasizing the conservation of the society's physical integrity and cohesion, and those of decision-making and the direction of public affairs. Another type of theory focuses on the definition of the political sphere in terms

of the modalities of political action. A fourth type of definition is the STRUCTURALIST or formal one, which focuses on the formal characteristics of political systems at an ideal rather than a practical level.

As a subdiscipline of comparatively late specialization, the field of political anthropology is still immature in its development of methodology and theoretical models appropriate to its specific concerns, though it is in the process of absorbing and modifying the considerable theoretical sophistication of political philosophy and political science, upon which it draws in order to construct its approaches to political systems and POWER in anthropological perspective. However it is true to say that while the analysis of the political dimension has formed an important part of the majority of anthropological studies, this dimension has usually been interpreted as an aspect of or as embedded in other domains such as kinship, religion, economy, and so on, and has been little analysed for the the features of a political system *per se*. One of the central issues has naturally been the definition of the political in societies without formal GOVERNMENT, without a centralized STATE, and in some cases even without formalized LEADERSHIP. The functional definition of political organization, which relates it to the norms and roles employed in society in order to maintain internal order, preserve territorial limits, and allocate power and decision-making over group action, should not obscure our vision of wider political processes which involve the tribal or peasant community in a relationship with a regional, national and international political power structure. In order to understand these wider integrations it is necessary to employ historical and processual analysis and a greater theoretical sophistication than that of the functionalist model, which postulates essentially similar human and political 'needs' as the basis for the development of political roles and functions in simple societies.

Political power is inherent in all societies, even those which do not possess formal mechanisms of government, and anthropologists have devoted much attention to the study of the manner in which societies without formal centralized AUTHORITY nevertheless manage to maintain order and cohesion. This is so not only among small populations but also among large ones such as the Nuer of the Sudan who number some 200,000 and who as EVANS-PRITCHARD's classic study showed (1940) maintain an ordered political structure based on a SEGMENTARY lineage system without an overall centralized authority. Within functionalist theory in anthropology the interpretation of political systems tended to emphasize the cohesive functions of political power and the manner in which the respect for political power and its sacralization function in order to limit conflict and competition and thus to preserve social order. Later theorists of different tendencies – notably within ACTION THEORY and MARXIST ANTHROPOLOGY have criticized this idealization of the political systems of traditional societies, pointing to the existence of conflicts of interest either at an individual or class level. Marxist theorists have pointed out that the sacralization of political power is also the mystification and legitimation of the interests of a dominant group (see IDEOLOGY). Many modern anthropologists influenced by Marxist theory seek to identify the seeds of class differentiation in the relationships of political dominance and economic exploitation which may exist in simple societies between older and younger age groups, between different lineages or kin groups or categories, between men and women, and so on. The relationship between power, COERCION and LEGITIMACY is thus essential to the field of political anthropology and to the comparative study of political systems.

Most anthropologists implicitly or explicitly employ a typology of the evolution of political systems, the predominant typology in US anthropology being that originated by STEWARD which divides societies or political systems into the following stages: BAND, TRIBE, CHIEFDOM and STATE (1955). However there is much internal differentiation within each of these categories, and there are types of society such as those characterized by the BIG MAN style of leadership which are difficult to classify in terms of this scheme. Similarly in modern nations we observe the articulation and interrelation of different sociopolitical types within a single region, and the application of an evolutionary typology obscures the fact that modern examples of these types are as much the product of contemporary interactions as they are the leftovers of previous stages of development. (See STRATIFICATION.)

political economy. In Marxist theory, the study of the interrelation between the economic process and the political system and political action.

pollution. In many parts of the world death, birth and other personal and family events entail danger and lead to the seclusion of affected persons, to prohibitions against contact and avoidance of certain foods or actions (see RITUAL; RITES OF PASSAGE). In India persons affected in this way are impure for a period of time and Indians themselves identify this impurity with the more permanent impurity of UNTOUCHABLES. In this view, organic and productive processes cause permanent or temporary pollution to those involved. Women are more impure than men, and childbirth and death cause temporary impurity to those close relatives whose natural substances are affected. In such cases purity can be restored by bathing (preferably in sacred water such as that of the river Ganges, but at least in running water), tonsuring and abstaining from dangerous foodstuffs. Permanent pollution is intrinsic to the CASTE system and to the division of labour (see JAJMANI) and is not affected by purificatory measures. Those specialists whose job it is to remove pollution from others, such as the washerman who washes soiled linen or the leather worker who removes and skins cattle carcasses, live permanently in a state of impurity. Permanent pollution, like temporary pollution, is a matter of degree. The Brahman who stays aloof from all productive and organic processes (except those pertaining to his own person and family) is purest among the living, but he is also vulnerable to pollution by any inferior.

In caste systems pollution is not primarily a matter of danger to the person. It has wider implications for the social status of individuals and groups. Since the impurity of some people is a condition for the purity of others' contacts and transactions between unequals are necessary. They are also problematic because purity is affected to varying degrees depending on the substances exchanged. Money, grain and knowledge are 'safer' than cooked food and brides (*see* HYPERGAMY). Exchanges and transactions between individuals and families provide an index of the relative purity of castes and subcastes, but the exact ranking order varies locally and is usually not agreed upon by all.

polyandry. A form of plural MARRIAGE where a woman has more than one husband. The dividing line between true polyandry and the extension of sexual services to men other than the husband is not always clear, and depends upon the definition of marriage itself. Generally the term is reserved for those systems in which paternity is assigned to more than one man. The commonest form of polyandry is adelphic or fraternal polyandry where the joint husbands are brothers. Polyandrous marriage has been reported for parts of India and especially the Himalayas, as well as in isolated cases in other parts of the world. It has been associated in some cases with shortage of women due to female INFANTICIDE, though it should be noted that in other cases female infanticide is associated with POLYGAMOUS marriage patterns. Berreman (1978) has interpreted Himalayan polyandry in terms of land shortage, as a means of limiting family expansion by assigning several males to one female. Since the woman's reproductive capacity is the same no matter how many husbands she has (unlike polygamy, which expands the male's capacity to father children according to the number of wives he has) Berreman suggests that polyandry serves to adjust the labour force to available land. Berreman also points out that polygynous and nuclear family forms coexist with polyandrous ones among the Himalayan Hindus, so that polyandry should be seen as one of a number of possible strategies which adjust human resources and family structure to land and other resources.

polygamy. Plural MARRIAGE including POLYANDRY and POLYGYNY. (*See* DOMESTIC GROUP; FAMILY; MONOGAMY.)

polygyny. A form of plural MARRIAGE in which the husband is permitted more than one wife. Where the co-wives are customarily sisters this is called SORORAL POLYGYNY. Polygyny is the normal form of marriage in many ethnographic regions, and is far more common than the POLYANDROUS form. Polygyny in LINEAGE systems has been examined in terms of the manner in which conflicts of interests between co-wives and their children reproduce the segmentary tendencies of the lineage system within the family itself. Polygyny is generally reserved for older and more powerful men, and in some cases may be the exclusive privilege of leaders or chiefs, as in some native Amazonian societies where the leader's multiple spouses are both a sign of his power and an important element in building and maintaining his power base. Polygyny not only permits a man to have more children and more affines, thus giving him the possibility of strategic manipulation of factional and/or kin group ties, it also provides him with a broader economic base since he controls to some extent the labour of his wives and children. Polygyny is often correlated with age asymmetry in the marriage relationship, such that older men marry very young girls and younger men are obliged to remain celibate for an extended period of time or alternatively to marry the widows of older men. We may thus interpret polygyny in these cases as part of a system of age-gender stratification, where older men control human resources and thus control productive and reproductive activities.

Polygynous marriage is correlated with those economic and political systems where the most important resources are human resources. Where resources such as land or forms of private property predominate, monogamous nuclear family forms tend to be the rule. (*See* DOMESTIC GROUP; FAMILY; MARRIAGE PAYMENTS; MONOGAMY.)

polysemy. Used to describe the effects of morphemes which appear to be identical but have distinct meanings: for example, the 'bark' of a tree and the 'bark' of a dog.

polytheism. Polytheistic religions are those which posit the existence of a number of deities or spiritual beings, with no overall high god. (*See* MONOTHEISM.)

Popper, Sir **Karl Raimund** (1902–). Viennese-born philosopher and student of scientific method. Important aspects of his work, which has had widespread influence, directly and indirectly, on theory and method in the social sciences, include his distinction of true and pseudo-science by the criterion of refutability, his criticism of HISTORICISM and his advocacy of METHODO-LOGICAL individualism (e.g. 1957).

population. *See* DEMOGRAPHY.

population control. *See* CONTRACEPTION AND ABORTION; DEMOGRAPHY.

populism. A political movement which makes its appeal to the mass of ordinary people, though in government the actual policy decisions of its parties are often not in accord with their rhetoric. Populism is a feature of many political movements characterized by NATIONALIST and FASCIST tendencies.

possession. A form of ALTERED STATE OF CONSCIOUSNESS in which the person, under the influence of DRUGS or some other exceptional physical or mental state, appears to be possessed by spirits which may speak and act through his or her body. Experiences of possession may be culturally conceived of as illnesses or as potentially curative or spiritually valuable, depending upon the history of the individual, the social context, and the cultural interpretation of his or her specific possession experience. I.M. Lewis (1971) has interpreted possession cults as a form of self-expression and self-assertion permitted to subordinate groups within the social structure, such as women in North Africa. (*See* HALLUCINOGENS; RELIGION; RITUAL; SHAMANISM.)

potlatch. A form of ceremonial EXCHANGE of gifts which was employed on the Northwest Coast of Canada and which was related to the distribution and display of RANK and TITLE among the indigenous population. In the potlatch individuals, supported by their kin, held feasts in connection with events in the life cycle. At these feasts they took names which were the property of *numayms* ('houses') or name corporations. In return for the recognition of their status they gave away food and wealth. Name corporations also controlled property and resources, and were 'owned' by the chiefs. Analysis of the political functions of potlatching show that

there are two principal aspects: the competitive use of potlatching by aspiring leaders in order to move up the system, and the oligarchic use by which the chiefs of different communities unite to employ the potlatch in order to reinforce their collective dominance. The extreme manifestations of potlatching, such as the burning or throwing away of great quantities of goods, were results of social, economic and political changes brought about by colonial rule. Codere has suggested (1950) that this form of potlatch was a substitute for war under colonial rule, though this interpretation has been contested.

Ecological anthropologists such as P. Vayda (1969) have argued that the potlatch functions to redistribute resources (wealth and food) in an uncertain environment. Adams on the other hand argues (1981) that the potlatch serves to redistribute people to resources (not resources to people), since people move around in the potlatching system in order to fill empty positions or shift from one corporation to another.

poverty. In spite of the fact that anthropology devotes the greater part of its attention to peoples who would commonly be classified as 'poor', little attention has been paid in anthropology to the concept of poverty itself. While in sociology the definition and study of poverty have been of central importance, anthropologists have tended to carry on their debates in terms of concepts such as MARGINALITY, DEVELOPMENT and so on. This avoids the difficulty inherent in the concept of poverty, which is the distinction between and definition of absolute poverty as measured in terms of human needs, and relative poverty or poverty as it is perceived according to the categories employed by a given population. Many would reserve the term for the lower strata of a class-based society, since in pre-class societies the consciousness of poverty is absent, even though material levels may appear low to an outside observer. Together with inter-ethnic contact and the processes of colonization and absorption of ethnic minorities comes a new consciousness of poverty, and 'the poor' may be considered in many contexts almost as a new ethnic classification which replaces older 'tribal' distinctions. (*See* CULTURE OF POVERTY.)

power. Power is invoked as an explanation of many different types of event and phenomenon, ranging from the power of a politician to that of a SHAMAN or to a concept such as MANA. In recent years an emerging anthropology of power has attempted to synthesize these different senses of the term and analyse what they have in common from an anthropological perspective. Adams, who has pioneered this field (1977), defines power in anthropological terms as 'the ability of a person or social unit to influence the conduct and decision-making of another through the control over energetic forms in the latter's environment (in the broadest sense of that term)'. WEBER on the other hand had defined power as 'the probability that one actor within a social relationship will be in a position to carry out his will despite resistance regardless of the basis on which this probability rests' (1948). In this definition Weber avoided specifying the origin or basis of power, since this may rest on control over a very wide range of resources, both material and immaterial. Power is distinguished from AUTHORITY, the socially acknowledged right to take decisions or to exercise power, and from COERCION, the application of power in spite of resistance. Power similarly differs from constraint, in that constraints are limiting conditions which are always present in social interaction but do not necessarily imply the existence of a power relationship, though they may be employed in order to create such a relationship.

Adams also distinguishes dependent from independent power. Independent power is a quality ascribed to people or social groups and which manifests itself not only by its practical effects but also in certain special spiritual or ceremonial signs. A person's individual or independent power is the sum of his inherited and acquired capabilities, and in every society there are rules and codes for expressing and measuring this individual power and for the negotiation of relationships between persons with different kinds or degrees of power. Adams points out that many native ideologies of power operate with the central distinction of control/out of control, often linked to other binary oppositions (safety/danger, nature/culture). STRUCTURAL analysis is a useful tool for elucidating features of native models of power and their linkage to social organization.

More complex societies tend to have more complex mechanisms of control and more varieties of dependent power, that is, power which is not inherent to persons or groups but which is delegated, allocated or granted from a power holder at another level. Adams claims that as societies expand or evolve demographically and techno-economically there is an overall increase in power (and energy), but there is also an increase in the concentration of power in the hands of ruling elites or classes, to such an extent that while the lower strata have more power in absolute terms they have less power in relative terms, and the increasing complexity of structures of dependent power means their decisions have much less power in the total system. It is debatably true to say that the lower strata of a complex society have more power in absolute terms than the members of a simple society, as historical tendencies towards over-exploitation and polarization of social classes may reduce the lower strata to conditions of greater absolute poverty and powerlessness.

Many ethnographers have focused on the ambiguity of power, especially those who have analysed folk or native models of power and its spiritual, cognitive or normative dimensions. This approach contrasts with analyses of political and legal power which emphasize exchange theory and NEGOTIATION, seeing power as a relationship between persons with different resources, attributes and goals. This 'free market' concept of power is however less appropriate, for the analysis of situations in which actors are heavily constrained by normative or ideal factors or by institutionalized power. It is however necessary to combine these different approaches to the study of power, since there is in any given social context a constant interplay between ideal models and the margin which these leave for interpretation and strategic manipulation. The theories of Adams and other modern anthropologists working in this field attempt to synthesize the two prevailing conceptions of power in anthropology, the SYMBOLIC and the material, by examining the strategic management of power relations within a given ecological context and within given cognitive-symbolic constraints. (*See*

prestation 231

IDEOLOGY; POLITICAL ANTHROPOLOGY; RELIGION; RITUAL.)

praxis. A Greek word meaning 'doing' or action. In Marxist theory the word is used to denote the primacy of practical action in the discovery of knowledge. Such practical action relates to the material base of society, and is undertaken on a class rather than individual basis. Praxis represents the movement towards the discovery of objective knowledge and away from false consciousness based on IDEOLOGICAL distortions.

preferential marriage. See PRESCRIPTION/PREFERENCE; MARRIAGE.

prehistory. See ARCHAEOLOGY.

prejudice. A preconceived negative judgment of persons or groups, based not on knowledge of their actual behaviour but on STEREOTYPED images. Prejudice in terms of RACE, ETHNICITY and GENDER are common examples, though prejudice exists also in a very wide range of other cases embracing almost any form of identifiable difference (prejudice against homosexuals, against the disabled, class prejudice, for example). Prejudice translated into actions or behaviour (as opposed simply to attitude) becomes DISCRIMINATION.

prescription/preference. In the study of MARRIAGE and of the ELEMENTARY STRUCTURES of kinship, the question of prescriptive and preferential marriage rules was a focus of debate during the 1960s, a debate which revealed many of the fundamental differences between the basic orientations of STRUCTURALIST theory as propounded by LEVI-STRAUSS and the more empirically-oriented interpretation of structuralism developed by British and US anthropologists. In his first edition of *The Elementary Structures of Kinship* (1949) Levi-Strauss deals with 'preferential' marriages but does not clarify unequivocally the distinction (if any) between prescription and preference. He speaks of cross-cousin marriage as preferential or 'privileged' in the sense of being the most elementary product of a system of exchange of women between men. R. Need-

ham (1962) however interprets 'preferential' as a reference to statistical patterns of marriage choice, and distinguishes preferential systems which allow a choice among several categories of marriageable persons from prescriptive ones which allow no choice. In Needham's view, Levi-Strauss' theory of elementary structures is concerned only with prescriptive systems as so defined. Levi-Strauss (1965) refutes this distinction between preference and prescription which had been developed by Needham and LEACH (1962). He reiterates that his concern is with structural principles of marriage exchange which may or may not be fully realized at the level of actual marriages due to the influence of demographic, psychological or other contingent factors. According to Levi-Strauss, preferential systems in Needham's sense are prescriptive at the level of the model, while prescriptive systems are preferential at the level of actual practice. So the important distinction for Levi-Strauss is not that between prescription and preference, but rather between elementary and complex structures: that is to say, between systems which define the spouse category as a kinship or alliance category and those which define the spouse in terms of subjective inclination or other non-kin considerations.

D. Maybury-Lewis (1965) formulates what has been generally accepted in modern anthropology as the defining criterion of a prescriptive marriage system. He points out that definitions in terms of marriageable categories are deficient since marriage in any system is with a marriageable category and thus 'prescriptive'. Maybury-Lewis suggests that prescriptive systems should be regarded as those which classify (or reclassify) terminologically all marriages as if they were with the prescribed category, while preferential systems are those in which marriages not following the rule are not reclassified or corrected terminologically.

prestation. A term employed by MAUSS (1925; trans. 1954) to refer to the 'total social phenomenon' constituted by GIFT-giving and RECIPROCITY. In the prestation, according to Mauss, 'all kinds of institutions find simultaneous expression'. Prestation thus differs from gift or EXCHANGE in that it refers to the total social context or relationship in which the exchange is embedded.

prestige. A term which may be used in two rather different senses: to refer to an individual's ability to command esteem or positive evaluation from others, or to the positive valuation or respect accorded to a social position, RANK or OFFICE. Personal prestige may be achieved on the basis of individual behaviour or attributes by persons regardless of their rank or STATUS, while on the other hand certain social positions automatically confer prestige on those who occupy them. In different types of political system the attribution, distribution and significance of prestige vary widely. For example, in BIG MAN-type political systems or in the Northwest Coast CHIEFDOMS during the height of the competitive POTLATCH, the competition for prestige had important implications for political action and organization. (*See* POLITICAL ANTHROPOLOGY.)

priest. In the anthropology of RELIGION a distinction is drawn between two types of religious specialist, the SHAMAN and the priest. The priesthood is characterized by the existence of an OFFICE which may be hereditary and/or conditional upon a period of formal training or education for the position. It is the office and the institution of priesthood which confer AUTHORITY and POWER upon the priest, and not, as in the case of the shaman, his personal CHARISMA. Priesthoods are generally more developed in complex class-based societies, though in less differentiated or technologically advanced societies we may also observe the existence of priestly office, though generally in a less hierarchical or formally institutionalized manner. In complex societies where the priesthood is formally organized into a hierarchical institution, it often has important political and IDEOLOGICAL functions as well as its overt religious or spiritual ones.

primary/secondary institutions. A distinction employed by the anthropologist A. Kardiner in his theory of CULTURE AND PERSONALITY (1945). Primary institutions are those which form the 'basic personality' of the members of a given social group. This basic personality in turn shapes the form of the secondary institutions, which are seen as expressions or projections of the collective psychology.

primary process. In PSYCHOANALYTIC theory, a form of thinking which is characteristic of infants, of the dream state, and of states of mental illness or ALTERED STATES OF CONSCIOUSNESS in the adult. Primary process thinking is governed by the ID and does not distinguish fantasy from reality.

primitive. Anthropology was identified until fairly recently as the study of 'primitive peoples', and was distinguished from other disciplines such as sociology, political science and economics because its focus was 'primitive society', 'primitive government' or 'primitive economy'. However during the 1960s and 1970s increasing debate and questioning of the concept of primitiveness led to the gradual abandonment of the term by most practitioners of cultural and social anthropology, and the search for terms which would avoid the pejorative connotations of the label 'primitive'. The word's falling out of favour reflects also the fact that many anthropologists no longer define their field of study as limited to or even as principally directed towards 'simple' societies, but have broadened the scope of their enquiries and investigations to include the study of complex INDUSTRIAL societies as well. The term 'primitive' had itself replaced the earlier term 'SAVAGE' which was employed in 19th- and early 20th-century social science to refer to less technologically developed cultures. One of the principal criticisms of the use of 'primitive' is that it implies that the peoples so designated represent an earlier or older stage or an evolutionary SURVIVAL thus denying that all human societies, including the technologically simpler ones, participate in processes of historical change and development. However by avoiding the term and substituting some other one like SIMPLE, TRIBAL or 'non-literate', we are not resolving the underlying problem associated with the use of any dichotomy which implicitly or explicitly contrasts peoples seen as CIVILIZED with those seen as 'uncivilized'. If we feel uncomfortable calling peoples 'primitive', the solution is not to seek a euphemism to replace it but to undertake instead an anthropological study which explores and demonstrates the historical development of given human groups and their relationship to other groups with differing technological levels or MODES OF PRODUCTION. In CRITICAL ANTHROPOLOGY and in MARXIST ANTHROPOLOGY we can see the attempt made by anthropologists to develop a critical consciousness of the profession's own classificatory systems. (*See* HISTORY AND ANTHROPOLOGY; LITERACY.)

primitive capitalism. *See* CAPITALISM, PRIMITIVE.

primitive mentality. The notion that primitive mentality differs qualitatively from the mentality of 'advanced' or 'civilized' peoples is associated with LEVY-BRUHL who argued that primitive mentality was prelogical and dominated by the belief in supernatural forces which distorted rational thought processes (1923). Levy-Bruhl's theories generated much debate and different critical responses from anthropologists ranging from DURKHEIM and MALINOWSKI to EVANS-PRITCHARD and LEVI-STRAUSS, though in modern anthropology he has also found his defenders, who stress above all that his arguments are not as unsophisticated or simplistic as they are often portrayed by his detractors. Indeed it is true to say that while rejecting Levy-Bruhl's dichotomy of prelogical–logical thought many anthropologists have merely substituted other dichotomies equally pernicious. As J. Goody points out (1977) all these dichotomies, whether that of Levy-Bruhl or proposed by later anthropologists as 'value-free' – as savage–domesticated, closed–open, pre-scientific–scientific and so on – inhibit a developmental view of the question of how modes of thought or reasoning have changed over time. Levi-Strauss in his work (1966) stresses not only continuity, because CLASSIFICATION is basic to all thought whether 'savage' or 'domesticated', and because of the intellectual complexity which characterizes thought in all human groups, but also discontinuity in terms of the kind of relationships which exist between thought, action and the world. Thus in 'savage' thought there is a scientific tradition which is characterized as the 'science of the concrete', characteristic of the Neolithic phase of human evolution, while in 'domesticated' thought there is a tradition of

abstract science and of historical (rather than mythical) consciousness.

Goody emphasizes changes in COMMUNICATION and especially the development of LITERACY as vital elements in producing many of the transformations which characterize the dichotomy of 'primitive' and 'advanced' thinking, and raises the question of whether literacy itself transforms cognition. Many anthropologists have focused on the development of RELIGION and religious beliefs as indicators of mentality or thought processes, though some of these theorists fail to take into account that magical and religious thinking continue to exist in modern society side by side with the advancement of science and scientific knowledge. The contrast between primitive MAGIC and religion and modern science as modes of cognition is thus perhaps misplaced: instead we should contrast primitive science with modern science and primitive religion with religion in modern societies, or the religious and the scientific modes of thinking within each culture. This criticism has been levelled at the NEO-TYLORIAN approach pioneered by R. Horton (1967) who argued that African religion consists of explanatory models relating to events in the observable world in a manner fundamentally similar to Western science. Horton applies POPPER's notion of the 'closed' and 'open' predicaments (1966), defined by the existence or non-existence of awareness of alternative modes of thinking, to primitive and modern societies on the basis of the contrast between primitive religion and modern science. But it is probable that within any society, whatever its technological level, we could discover the existence of both open and closed modes in the context of different kinds of cognitive process or different institutional and psychological frameworks.

The question of the fundamental similarity or difference in cognitive modes between technologically more or less advanced cultures is one which is by no means closed, and there continue to be fundamental differences of opinion between different anthropologists and different theoretical schools. These differences of opinion may themselves relate to ideological stances on the relationship which should exist between dominant and minority groups. Those who argue for fundamental or qualitative differences in mentality may be implicitly arguing for a policy of 'protection' or 'segregation' of minority ethnic groups, while those who argue for fundamental similarities may be broadly interpreted as pursuing an 'integrationist' policy. Thus the question of 'primitive mentality' should be examined not only in terms of its scientific or theoretical interest but also in terms of its practical applications to inter-ethnic politics.

primitive promiscuity. The theory that the original state of human society was characterized by the absence of INCEST TABOOS, or rules regarding sexual relations or MARRIAGE. Early anthropologists such as MORGAN, MCLENNAN, BACHOFEN and FRAZER held this view. It was opposed on the other hand by those who like FREUD argued that the original form of society was the primal patriarchal horde or like WESTERMARCK and MAINE that it was the paternal monogamous family.

primogeniture. The rule of INHERITANCE or SUCCESSION which favours the eldest child (or the eldest son, in societies where inheritance or succession is solely or preferentially in the male line).

procreation. *See* CONCEPTION; KINSHIP.

production. *See* MODE OF PRODUCTION.

profane. According to DURKHEIM's theories of RELIGION and of social structure there is a fundamental dichotomy between two basic domains or states which he terms the SACRED and the profane. The profane or ordinary is divided and marked off from the sacred by a series of special RITUAL and SYMBOLIC observances and attributes.

projection. In PSYCHOANALYTIC theory this is a mechanism whereby the individual, in response to some internal psychological conflict, 'projects' his or her wishes, desires, fears, emotions or attitudes, attributing them to other persons or to individual or collective fantasy images such as gods and spirits. The notion of projection has been employed by some psychoanalytically-oriented anthropologists in order to explain the nature of religious or belief systems. (*See*

CULTURE AND PERSONALITY; PSYCHOLOGICAL ANTHROPOLOGY; RELIGION.)

property. In modern capitalist society the popular conception of property is that of a relationship between a person (the owner) and a thing (that which is owned, or the property). In fact the extreme development of private property and 'absolute property', the right to dispose of property in the manner in which the owner decides, have obscured the true nature of property in all human societies. It is not in fact a relationship between a person and a thing or things but a relationship between persons which is expressed in terms of rights over things. Property itself has no meaning except as the right of an individual or group to exclude others from access to, use of or control over certain items or commodities. In this sense, and viewed in comparative perspective, property rights are extremely variable and take many different forms. In fact absolute property is rare even in modern society, as there always exist certain legal and administrative limitations as to the manner in which the owner may employ or dispose of that which is owned. Thus I may 'own' a piece of land in the sense that I have the right to forbid access to other persons to that land under normal circumstances, but there are often many legal restrictions as to the uses that I may make of the land (for housing, for industry, or for illegal activities for instance) which place limits on my rights or subject them to bureaucratic or legal control.

In pre-capitalist society the relational and social nature of property is more apparent, due to the lesser development of legal categories and reglementation of different types of property. In some less technologically advanced societies, property rights are defined almost entirely in an informal fashion and according to the criterion of use, and in these contexts it is appropriate to speak of the existence of personal property but not of the type of private property which involves control over critical resources and the right to exclude others from these resources. In many pre-capitalist societies significant property is held not by individuals but by CORPORATE groups which may be based on KINSHIP, MARRIAGE, co-residence or a combination of these factors. The development of private property in the sense of individual ownership of the MEANS OF PRODUCTION is linked to the emergence of social CLASSES and the STATE, and includes the development of a series of legal and ideological structures which uphold and justify the exclusion of the primary producer from control over the means of production. (See ECONOMIC ANTHROPOLOGY; INHERITANCE; LAND.)

prostitution. Generally defined as the exchange of women's or men's sexual services for payment. In fact the mere existence of such an exchange is not the only element: prostitution is an institution which involves the creation of a special STATUS and ROLE which is characterized by a multiplicity of special features apart from this exchange. The prostitute symbolizes 'abnormal' sex role behaviour, which may under certain circumstances and in certain cultures be SACRED but is more likely to be subject to social STIGMA. The features of this stigma vary according to the nature of sex-role socialization in each culture, and the analysis of the SUBCULTURE of prostitution reveals important features of the accepted image of 'normal' sexual and GENDER-related conduct.

Protestant ethic. A phrase associated with WEBER's theories on the rise of CAPITALISM (1958). Weber challenged the Marxist view that infrastructures were the main generators of social change, claiming that under certain circumstances changes in value systems could definitively determine economic changes. He did not however, as has sometimes been suggested, assert that Protestantism caused capitalism, but rather that there was an affinity between Puritan protestant values and the attitudes towards work, consumption, investment and profit which were necessary conditions for the development of a rational capitalist economy. Much of the debate about Weber's thesis has centred on this question of the relative importance or priority of the economic and the ideological changes which contributed to the rise of European capitalism.

proxemics. A field of anthropological investigation associated with E.T. Hall (1974) which investigates the cultural and social use of space. (See VISUAL ANTHROPOLOGY.)

psychoanalysis. The theories of human psychology developed by FREUD are referred to in their totality as psychoanalysis, and the term is also employed to refer to a broader group of theories influenced by Freud but diverging from his work in different ways, such as the schools of thought associated with Jung, Adler and other later theorists. Psychoanalysis includes theories of the functioning and nature of the human personality, methods for the investigation of the personality, and therapeutic techniques relating to abnormal personalities or mental illness. Freudian theories have been influential in many areas of anthropological thought, including in particular the field of KINSHIP studies, the anthropology of RELIGION and RITUAL, CULTURE AND PERSONALITY theory and PSYCHOLOGICAL ANTHROPOLOGY.

psychological anthropology. This field includes the study of the individual's relationship to culture and society (see CULTURE AND PERSONALITY) as well as the broader area of interrelationship between psychology and anthropology, an area with many different dimensions. In general, two kinds of study have prevailed in psychological anthropology, as Keefer points out when reviewing the topic (1977). There is the generalizing or survey type of research into such topics as child rearing or SOCIALIZATION, subsistence patterns, perception, cognition, and so on. These studies divide behaviour conceptually into discrete variables, and elaborate 'group profiles' which summarize individual behaviours. They then attempt to relate these patterns of behaviour to wider factors which may be biological, biosocial, ecological, historical or social structural, depending on the theoretical orientation of the writer. On the other hand we have what Keefer sees as the particularizing type of study, which attempts to understand and interpret complex individual/social situations. These studies, influenced by CULTURAL RELATIVISM, CONFIGURATIONALISM and INTERACTIONISM focus especially on the personality, on the relationship between personality traits and culture CHANGE, on the cross-cultural study of developmental change throughout the life cycle, and on the concept of IDENTITY. Such studies have shown that the sense of self and of identification with an ETHNIC or cultural group is particularly problematic in situations of change, where ethnic or cultural self-identifications may have both positive and negative attributes or consequences.

The culture and personality school which was the first manifestation in systematic form of psychological anthropology was dominated by two important theoretical orientations: the PSYCHOANALYTIC theory of personality and the learning or BEHAVIOURIST, theory. An important pioneering study within the field of socialization was that of Whiting and Child (1953), who studied the relationship between child-rearing patterns and 'custom complexes' in cross-cultural perspective. As anthropology itself has moved towards greater recognition of intracultural diversity, so models of 'modal personality' and monolithic systems of norms have given way in psychological anthropology to approaches which take into account two new areas: cognition and interaction. The concept of personality itself has been criticized for its individualistic and static connotations, and in psychology today situational and interactionist views of personality have gained ground. Indeed it has been suggested that the concept of personality, while it may be appropriate to or consonant with our own culture, may be less so in other cultures which place less emphasis on subjective individual experience and more on experience organized around relationships to groups.

According to A. Howard (1982) the task of psychological anthropology as defined in the light of the advances of modern interactional psychology is the study of how situations are structured by what he calls 'person-centred variables', including motives, cognition and learned dispositions, and conversely of how cultural variables may select or influence these person-centred variables in the context of the public domain and/or the personal intra-psychic domain. Howard argues that if the problems are defined in this way, we may avoid the problems either of psychological reductionism or CULTURAL DETERMINISM.

There are important links between psychological anthropology and COGNITIVE ANTHROPOLOGY on the one hand and SYMBOLIC ANTHROPOLOGY on the other. Psychological anthropology, like these two related fields, addresses itself to the problem of the relationship between symbols, thought and social ACTION. In psychological anthropology as in anthropology generally, linguistic models and particularly structural linguistics have been important influences in the formation of interpretative and analytical models. Influenced too by modern trends in philosophy, psychological anthropology is today moving towards a new view of symbols as extremely plastic and variable in their relationship to thought and action.

There are also close links between psychological anthropology and biological or PHYSICAL ANTHROPOLOGY, in the sense that both these disciplines attempt to discover the biological basis or shaping of human behaviour. In modern physical and psychological anthropology most writers have abandoned crude deterministic positions and would argue, as Spiro does (1978), for an interactionist view which sees personality and behaviour as the result of the interplay between biological predispositions and experience. He contends that below cultural and individual behaviour differences there are universal behavioural predispositions or repertoires of emotions and responses which may be differentially channelled or developed by different cultures but which cannot be totally eliminated or reformed. Basic human tendencies and emotions, Spiro argues, may be encouraged in different ways or expressed according to the different styles prescribed by given cultural codes, but can never be totally denied. However it is important to remember both that there are considerable differences of temperament and behaviour between different members of a single culture, and that human behavioural predispositions exist at a very general level and do not consist in specific programmed behaviour patterns or INSTINCTS but rather in open-ended propensities which will find their expression through cultural learning in a specific context and will thus vary considerably in their manifestations.

Another important aspect of psychological anthropology is the study of mental illness in cross-cultural perspective, or ETHNOPSYCHIATRY. Some of the research in this field has been devoted to the study of specific culture-bound syndromes and the variability or invariability of types and syndromes of mental illness in different cultures. The interpretation of mental illness in other cultures has shown clearly that the content of mental disorders, the 'career' of the mentally ill person and the interpretation of his or her disorder are widely variable and dependent in a very large part on the cultural and social context. Thus what is considered mental illness in one cultural context may be accorded no importance in another, or regarded in yet another as a sign of special spiritual or religious power. Similarly the content and form of mental illnesses reflects the content and form of normal behaviour in the culture concerned, with certain typical distortions or exaggerations.

The studies of WALLACE (1970) and his students have broken important new ground in the study of culture-bound syndromes such as Arctic hysteria or Windigo psychosis which are highly conventionalized responses to psychological stress. Wallace and his followers have investigated the possibility that these and other types of behavioural pattern – including such traits as aggression – may be related not only to cultural learning but also to imbalances in body chemistry due to deficiencies in the diet and other factors.

One of the principal theoretical influences in psychological anthropology has been Freudian or psychoanalytic theory, which has also generated considerable controversy not only in the field of psychological anthropology as narrowly conceived but also in other fields where psychoanalytically-oriented anthropologists have attempted to apply it. Many major modern anthropologists have been considerably inflenced by such theories, as we may appreciate for example in the fields of KINSHIP studies or the anthropology of RELIGION. The interchange between psychoanalysis and anthropology which has taken place over the years has focused both on the broadening of psychoanalytic theory, attempting to rid it of many culture-bound or ethnocentric elements, and on the possible uses of the theory to illuminate the significance of behaviour and beliefs in non-Western cultures. However it is true to say that psychoanalytic anthropology in the narrow sense has remained rather isolated from the mainstream of anthropological thought. For example, in the study of symbolism many anthropologists would reject the Freudian emphasis on the primacy of the physical and sexual meanings of symbols and their interpretation in terms of 'classic' complexes such as the Oedipus complex, in favour of an analysis in terms of the interplay of cultural, social and physical referents of symbols which does not prejudge their psychological significance.

puberty. *See* AGE, ANTHROPOLOGY OF; INITIATION; RITES OF PASSAGE.

R

race. The common use of the word in English is to refer to a group of persons who share common physical characteristics and form a discrete and separable population unit has no scientific validity, since evolutionary theory and PHYSICAL ANTHROPOLOGY have long since demonstrated that there are no fixed or discrete racial groups in human populations. Instead, human groups constantly change and interact, to such an extent that modern population genetics focuses on CLINES or patterns of the distribution of specific genes rather than on artificially created racial categories. However as a folk concept in Western and non-Western societies the concept of race is a powerful and important one, which is employed in order to classify and systematically exclude members of given groups from full participation in the social system controlled by the dominant group. As a folk concept, race is employed to attribute not only physical characteristics but also psychological and moral ones to members of given categories, thus justifying or naturalizing a discriminatory socal system. (*See* RACISM.)

race relations. The relations between persons and groups conceived of according to folk categories as being of different RACES. There is not always a clear distinction between race relations and ETHNIC relations, since groups conceived of as racially separate often also possess an ethnic identity (or may be divided internally into different ethnic minorities) which confuses this distinction. The first major contribution to the theory of race relations in the social sciences was that of Park and the Chicago school. He held that race relations were the product of racial consciousness created by competition between populations attempting to occupy the same ecological niche (1950). The Chicago school tended to view racial conflicts as stages in the process of integration which would eventually result from population migration and contact. This view was challenged by social stratification theory which argued that race was an expression or extension of social CLASS, and should be analysed as an aspect of social stratification in general. According to stratificationists, the Chicago school's emphasis on a movement towards integration disguised the fundamental nature of race relations, which are the product not of competition but of the exploitation of non-European by European races. (*See* PLURAL SOCIETY.)

racism, racialism. Doctrines of or beliefs in racial superiority, including the belief that race determines intelligence, cultural characteristics and moral attributes. Racism includes both racial PREJUDICE and racial discrimination, and thus is also employed describe social systems which systematically discriminate against given racial categories. Many writers employ the term 'institutionalized racism' to refer to the social structural aspect of racism and the manner in which specific racial prejudices and stereotypes are incorporated into legal, administrative and social systems. Institutionalized racism may be analysed as a product of class interests and class ideology, as well as at an international level as a product of COLONIALIST and IMPERIALIST strategies employing racism as an important element in the justification and maintenance of relations of exploitation and unequal exchange with subordinate populations who happen to be physically different. Students of racism have pointed out how the rise and fall of racial stereotypes and racial prejudice is closely related to the changing historical relations between different populations and above all to the interests of dominant groups (*see* APARTHEID; SLAVERY). However there has been little systematic anthropological study of racism and the forms which it takes in colonial and post-colonial societies, in spite of the fact that many Third World nations are stratified like those of the West according to a race-class categorization of their population.

Radcliffe-Brown, Alfred Reginald (1881–1955). Major figure in British social anthropology and in the development of the STRUCTURAL FUNCTIONALIST perspective. Radcliffe-Brown was born in England and educated at Cambridge, where as a post-graduate student he turned his attention to the study of anthropology. His work was influenced above all by DURKHEIM and also by the theories of COMTE and FRAZER. He went on to carry out fieldwork in the Andaman Islands from 1906–08 and in Australia from 1910–12. Like MALINOWSKI, Radcliffe-Brown argued against EVOLUTIONARY perspectives in anthropology, and advocated a synchronic or FUNCTIONAL approach to the laws of social life. He regarded the concept of CULTURE as an abstraction of little analytical value, preferring to analyse the SOCIAL STRUCTURE, a preference which was to be profoundly influential in shaping the nature of British social anthropology. He adopted many key concepts from Durkheim, including the concept of SOCIAL FACTS and a Durkheimian functionalist model of society. Major works include *The Andaman Islanders* (1948), *Method in Social Anthropology* (1958) and *Structure and Function in Primitive Society* (1965).

Radin, Paul (1883–1959). US anthropologist who was a student of BOAS and who devoted his attention to the study of the ethnology of the Winnebago Indians and especially to aspects of their religion and mythology. In his *Method and Theory of Ethnology* (1933) he advocated the case history method, focusing on the individual as a means of studying historical and cultural regularities. Other major works include *Primitive Man as Philosopher* (1927) and *Primitive Religion* (1937).

raiding. *See* WARFARE; FEUD.

ramage. According to the usage established by MURDOCK, this is an ancestor-focused bilateral descent group. (*See* NON-UNILINEAL DESCENT.)

rank. Ranking, the ordering of persons and groups according to a hierarchical classification in terms of differential position, POWER or PRESTIGE, is a universal feature of human society. The behavioural expression of ranking is social inequality, which is also a universal feature of human society. Where ranking is translated into institutional terms in such a manner as to systematically exclude lower ranking persons and groups from control over the MEANS OF PRODUCTION, political decision-making, and other socially important functions, it is referred to as social STRATIFICATION. (*See* POLITICAL ANTHROPOLOGY.)

rationality. Thoughts, actions or patterns of organization which are held to follow the rules of logic or to consistently pursue the maximum benefit for the minimum input of resources. The capacity for rational thought and for problem-solving and decision-making is an integral part of the human behavioural heritage, linked to the universal human tendency to elaborate rules and systems of CLASSIFICATION and also to human CREATIVITY. Anthropologists have often pointed out however that the factors which are taken into account when making a rational decision are not only physical and material needs and satisfactions, but also psychological and SYMBOLIC ones. Modern capitalist society privileges one form or expression of rationality – economic rationality – while pre-capitalist societies privilege other domains such as KINSHIP or RELIGION. Thus in making a decision which places priority on the demands of the kinship system or the religious system at the expense of economic rationality as we would conceive of it in our society, the member of a pre-capitalist society is acting not irrationally but rationally in terms of the dominant mode of social organization in his or her community.

Discussions about rationality and the universality of criteria of rational thought in anthropology have been particularly evident in the fields of ECONOMIC ANTHROPOLOGY and also in the still unresolved controversies about PRIMITIVE MENTALITY. While the logical extension of CULTURAL RELATIVISM would lead us to suppose that each culture creates its own rationality, not necessarily translatable in terms of another, critics of this position have argued that there are fundamental universal criteria of rationality which are linked to the very need for survival and which ensure the mutual intelligibility of cultures.

Much of the confusion surrounding rationality from the cross-cultural perspective stems from the failure to distinguish between individual or group decision-making and to assess the overall evolutionary or ecological rationality of a given strategy or action. Actions and decisions which are rational in terms of the knowledge available to the decision-maker and his or her material and symbolic priorities may or may not be rational in their ultimate evolutionary advantage or ecological effects. In FUNCTIONALIST theory and cultural ecology writers often fail to make this distinction, confusing individual or micro-rationality with functional, evolutionary or ecological macrorationality.

As pointed out by WEBER in his study of the rise of CAPITALISM and BUREAUCRACY (1958), modern society is characterized by the erosion of traditional social institutions and their progressive replacement by formally rational organizations. This rational–legal mode of social organization, however, as Weber himself pointed out, may ultimately lead to a social system which is totally irrational or devoid of meaning, imprisoned in its own apparently rational forms. Precapitalist society may in this sense turn out to be more rational than capitalist society, though its social institutions are apparently integrated or organized by non-rational principles such as symbolic or religious ones.

rebellion. Usually defined as a revolt against existing power holders by a competing group, while a REVOLUTION implies not only competition for power but also the overthrow of existing power structures and their replacement by new forms of economic, political and social organization. However the distinction between a rebellion and a revolution is not always clear cut, since what begins as a rebellion may become a revolution if the conditions exist for the structural transformation of society, while what begins as a revolution may turn out to have been merely a rebellion, as promised changes are forgotten and the overall outcome is simply a change in the members of the ruling ELITE.

The historical and anthropological study of rebellions is a fascinating area of enquiry, because rebellions are moments of crisis and tension in which the· underlying strengths and weaknesses as well as the points of fusion and fission of a sociopolitical system are clearly displayed.

Conventional assumptions of conservatism and fatalism in traditional and peasant societies are belied by the study of rebellions in the history of Western and non-Western society. Tribal and peasant peoples have consistently displayed a potential for organized political rebellion and opposition, sometimes expressed in a religious idiom (*see* MESSIANISM; MILLENARIANISM) and sometimes in the form of purely military and/or political movements which are directed with more or less spontaneity to the overthrow of an oppressive dominant group. However the greater military, economic and political power of the dominant group combined with the localized nature of many of these rebellions has doomed them to failure. Peasant rebellions have rarely turned into successful revolutions, for example, without the assistance of a leadership from urban centres which orchestrates and combines their efforts and provides them with strategic orientation. (*See also* RITUAL REBELLION.)

reciprocity. Reciprocity, or the return of a GIFT or PRESTATION, has been an important topic of anthropological study since the works of DURKHEIM and MAUSS established the centrality of reciprocity to the organization of social life. Reciprocity is the basis of EXCHANGE, and as such is a key concept in the areas of ECONOMIC ANTHROPOLOGY, KINSHIP and MARRIAGE. Reciprocity as a relationship between persons or social units both unites them by the relationship of exchange and divides them as separate members of the exchange relationship. This double function of setting apart and uniting makes reciprocity a particularly appropriate means for the expression and manipulation of social relationships and social identity.

In his discussion of anthropological economics POLANYI (1968) divided economies into three types according to the dominant mode of DISTRIBUTION: economies where the dominant mode is reciprocity, those where it is REDISTRIBUTION and those where it is MARKET exchange. Sahlins, in a discussion of reciprocity in primitive economies (1972), further elaborates the significance of reciprocity and the links between material flow and social relations. He elaborates a scheme of three types of reciprocity, each of which is correlated with social distance: generalized reciprocity, balanced reciprocity and negative reciprocity. Generalized reciprocity is the solidary extreme and characterizes interactions between close kinsmen or within a restricted and intimate social group. In generalized reciprocity the 'free gift' or the sharing of resources without strict measurement or obligation to repay are the norm. Thus close kinsmen often assist one another and interchange food and other goods without any strict expectation of return, other than the existence of a diffuse obligation of a moral rather than economic nature to reciprocate or to assist when needed. Balanced reciprocity is the midpoint and is the form of exchange between structural equals who trade or exchange goods or services. Balanced reciprocity is less personal and moral and more economic in type. The third type, negative reciprocity, is characteristic of interactions between enemy or distant groups and is the attempt to maximize utility at the expense of the other party. Negative reciprocity ranges from haggling to theft and raiding or WARFARE. Sahlins suggests that these types of reciprocity form a continuum which correlates with kinship and social distance.

Redfield, Robert (1897–1958). US anthropologist who was initially trained in law and turned to anthropology as a graduate student. Redfield was one of the leading theorists who influenced the growing anthropological interest in the study of PEASANT society and the comparative study of forms other than the 'primitive societies' which had been the major focus of anthropological enquiry until the 1940s. He made important contributions to Mesoamerican anthropology. Influenced by DURKHEIM's theories of the DIVISION OF LABOUR and by TONNIES' concept of GEMEINSCHAFT/ GESELLSCHAFT, Redfield developed the concept of the FOLK-URBAN CONTINUUM. He is usually seen as a cultural idealist much influenced by the CULTURAL RELATIVISM and HISTORICAL PARTICULARISM of the BOASIAN school, and he has been criticized

for viewing ideas as the motive force in CHANGE and DEVELOPMENT and for concentrating on goals and VALUES rather than actual behaviour in his ethnographic studies. Major works include *The Folk Culture of Yucatan* (1941) and *Peasant Society and Culture* (1956).

redistribution. One of the three major modes of EXCHANGE proposed by Polanyi (1968) in his typology of economic systems, the other two being RECIPROCITY and MARKET exchange. Redistribution in its simplest form is the pooling of goods by producers for the common use of the group and its members (for example, the pooling of food produced by members of a household). In its more complex and institutionalized form it is the movement of goods towards a political or administrative centre, from which the goods are then redistributed outwards to the consumer. Some form of redistribution is apparent in all economic systems, but redistribution is the dominant mode in, for example, FEUDAL societies and traditional CHIEFDOMS. Redistributive systems permit those at the centre to accumulate goods and to redeploy them strategically in order to maintain specialists such as craftsmen, military personnel, priests and others – a possibility which is absent in systems where reciprocity is the dominant mode. The rise of a redistributive economy thus lays the foundations for the future development of social CLASSES and the STATE. As Sahlins points out (1972), redistribution is also a form of exchange with more integrative potential, since redistribution is a relationship within the group while reciprocity always divides as it is a relationship between. Within the primitive economy, according to Sahlins, the concomitants of pooling or redistribution are co-operative food production, rank and chieftainship and collective political and ceremonial action. In traditional chieftainships there is often a conflict of interest between the relationship of reciprocity held among chief and people, the obligations of kinship and morality which bind the chief to use the resources collected for the good of the whole community, and the tendency towards chiefly accumulation and the deployment of resources to display rank and to enlarge the chief's power base.

refugees. Persons who in response to physical, economic, military or political pressures leave their region or country of origin and move to another. Refugee movements can consequently arise in response to situations of FAMINE, to political persecution of specific ethnic or other groups, in times of war, and so on. The problems of refugees, in addition to those created by ordinary MIGRATION, include the involuntary nature of their movement and the special circumstances of social and politico-economic crisis which generally accompany the creation of a refugee problem. The anthropological perspective has important applications in POLICY decisions regarding refugees, since problems of inter-ethnic conflict are often an important feature of the refugee situation.

regional analysis, regional social system. In response to critiques of traditional ethnographic practice within cultural and social anthropology, some modern anthropologists are exploring the possibilities of regional analysis. Traditional ethnography often tended to assume that it was possible to isolate for the purposes of anthropological enquiry a TRIBE, a CULTURE or a SOCIETY, attempting to reconstruct a self-contained traditional sociocultural system and virtually ignoring contacts and interrelationships both with neighbouring groups and with the dominant regional, national and international power structure. Regional analysis attempts instead to elucidate the features of a regional social system which may embrace members of different ethnolinguistic groups involved in networks of trade, intermarriage and political relations, and which in turn is connected to a larger dominant politico-economic and social system.

Reichel-Dolmatoff, Gerardo (1912–). Colombian anthropologist of Austrian origin who has made important contributions to Amazonian anthropology and to the study of SHAMANISM.

reification. This term, which means 'making a thing', is employed to describe what Marx called COMMODITY FETISHISM, a notion which is extended by some neo-Marxist and CRITICAL THEORISTS to include the general tendency to artificially isolate moments or aspects of a totality, falsely attributing a concrete status to them.

relations of production. According to Marxist theory, the MATERIAL FORCES OF PRODUCTION together with the social relations of production constitute the MODE OF PRODUCTION. Because productive forces constantly tend to expand and evolve and so outgrow the social relations of production, they generate tensions and contradictions which will ultimately culminate in REVOLUTION or the overthrow of the old productive relations in favour of new ones in accordance with the development of the productive forces.

religion, anthropology of. Like many important areas of anthropological enquiry, the anthropology of religion does not possess a fixed and universally accepted definition of its central focus, in this case the phenomenon of religion. While we may have an intuitive idea of which behaviours should be labelled 'religious', it is extremely difficult to delimit and define religion for anthropological purposes. Substantive definitions of religion in terms of its content date back to Tylor who defined religion as the 'belief in spiritual beings' (1871). This definition has however been questioned, since it is not always clear whether a given phenomenon is believed to be spiritual or natural, and this judgement may be different from the observer's point of view than from the believer's. Most modern anthropologists would not agree that beliefs in spiritual beings or the supernatural are substantively different from those in natural phenomena, since both kinds of belief are acquired by means of the same socialization and educational process and are accepted on the authority of others.

Other anthropologists have preferred FUNCTIONAL definitions of religion – in terms of what it does – a view influenced by DURKHEIM's theories of the sociological functions of religious beliefs and religious action. Developing another strand of Durkheim's work others have sought to isolate the special symbolic features of religion which demarcate the SACRED from the PROFANE.

In the 19th century, studies of comparative religion were mainly concerned with the question of the origin and evolution of religious forms, and in this field as in other areas of anthropological enquiry debate as to the earliest form and its development into modern forms predominated. Tylor proposed ANIMISM as the earliest form of human religion. He thought that it had developed out of the experiences of early humans and their reflections upon sleep and waking, dreams, death and so forth, which had led to a belief in the soul as a separable entity from the body. Tylor thought that this first religious form had then developed into ANCESTOR WORSHIP, which in turn gave way to POLYHEISM and ultimately to MONOTHEISM. FRAZER (1890), who shared Tylor's rationalist vision of the origins of religion in the sense that he also argued that religion had originated in the attempts of early humans to make sense of or explain their experience of their environment and their life process, proposed a different kind of typology. He argued that there were three basic stages of intellectual development in human culture: MAGIC, religion and SCIENCE. Each stage is characterized by a different kind of theory of causality and of how humans may affect the outcome of events.

Opposed to these rationalist theories of religion were other schemes which stressed the nonrational aspects or functions of religious beliefs. Thus MARRETT (1900) argued that the origin of religion was to be found in ANIMATISM, or a belief in a diffuse impersonal power which stemmed from the early human's sense of awe and wonder at the contemplation of the natural world. FREUD (1913) on the other hand advanced a theory of religion which related it to his model of human psychodynamics, arguing that religious beliefs are PROJECTIONS of psychic tensions, conflicts and complexes. Thus deities or spirits are collective fantasies, to be generally interpreted as parental figures towards which we have ambivalent feelings, and religion is regarded as a kind of collective neurosis.

Durkheim however viewed religion as a social creation which expresses and reinforces social SOLIDARITY, such that religious beliefs are in a sense metaphors for society itself and the sacred nature of social obligations and social cohesion. He proposed TOTEMISM as the earliest form of human religion, and he rejected Tylor's criterion of the belief in spiritual beings in favour of the criterion of the sacred as the defining characteristic of religion. It is the functional aspect of Durkheim's work which was developed in British social anthropology and in the STRUCTURAL FUNCTIONALIST view of religion as a reflection of social structure. In French STRUCTURALISM and in other areas of SYMBOLIC ANTHROPOLOGY however, another aspect of Durkheim's work has been emphasized: his focus on the symbolic dimensions of religion and the demarcation of the sacred and the profane.

Another major theory of religion which has influenced modern anthropology is that of MARX, who viewed religion as a product of the IDEOLOGY of a dominant class, which served to justify and naturalize their dominance and at the same time to neutralize the revolutionary potential of the oppressed by substituting an illusory liberation in the other world for real liberation in this one. So while Durkheim viewed religion as a true and positively functional reflection of social structure, Marx proposed on the contrary that it was a distorted or ideological reflection created by the interests of a given social class.

These 19th-century debates and theories are still carried on, albeit in modified form, in the anthropology of religion today. Many modern anthropologists still adhere to Tylor's definition of religion in terms of the belief in spiritual beings. Spiro (1966), while acknowledging the difficulties in defining 'spiritual' (or 'superhuman') beings, and also the existence of religions which – like some Buddhist philosophies – are atheistic, concludes that the best definition of religion is still 'an institution consisting of culturally patterned interaction with culturally postulated superhuman beings'. One of the principal modern theorists within the anthropology of religion is C. Geertz, who defines religion as 'a system of symbols which acts to establish powerful, pervasive and long-lasting moods and motivations in men by formulating conceptions of a general order of existence and clothing these conceptions with such an aura of factuality that the moods and motivations seem uniquely realistic' (1966). The approach put forward by Geertz combines features of many of the theories already mentioned, all of which in reality refer to aspects of the religious phenomenon but none of which is sufficient alone to describe and define this complex totality. Geertz agrees with WEBER (1958) that religion confronts the problem of meaning or understanding (*Verstehen*) and the problems of evil and suffering, by relating them to a wider framework which depends upon the acceptance of AUTHORITY or faith. Religion, unlike common sense, moves beyond everyday reality or 'naïve realism', not in terms of scientific action or analysis but in terms of faith and authority. In RITUAL, this fusion of everyday and sacred reality is demonstrated and affirmed.

The emphasis on religion as a response to the facts of suffering and stress was also important to the work of MALINOWSKI (1948), who proposed that religion, magic and ritual provided sociopsychological mechanisms for coping by opening up ritual and spiritual 'escapes' for tension. Malinowski emphasized the fact that religion, ritual and MYTH all serve to explain and justify the existing order of things and act as safety valves for the expression of tensions and unresolved contradictions. LEVI-STRAUSS' theory of religion and mythic thought is in a sense somewhat similar (1969), since he too postulates that symbolic and mythic thought constitute a process of constant working and reworking of basic philosophical, existential and social contradictions and oppositions.

The interest in the evolution of religion and in the comparative study of the features of religious systems in different kinds of society is also one which has persisted in modern anthropology, though few would advance simplistic universal evolutionary schemes like the ones prevalent in the 19th century. Some overall generalizations about correlations between religious and social systems have however emerged from the comparative study of religions. G. Obeyesekere points out (1981), that 'ethicization' is a general feature of religious evolution. Preliterate religions are generally without ethics, in the sense that they do not contain a systematic theory of sin, merit and MORALITY. In the religions of the great literate traditions however there are more developed ideas of relgious ethics, linked to a belief in the possibility of a religious salvation. A salvation religion such as Christianity or Islam poses the problem of evil and suffering and of the justification of God in the face of the existence of evil, and proposes the

overcoming of this problem by the religious means of salvation. Salvation is a RITE OF PASSAGE which carries the individual to a final status beyond suffering. Preliterate religions generally, but not always, lack this concept of salvation, and the ideas of the other world in such religions are as a rule either hazy and indeterminate or else consist of reflections or transformations of aspects of everyday social structure without the notion of the elimination of suffering. Similarly, the reincarnation beliefs of preliterate religions are not generally linked to ethical notions but instead to the reincarnation of ancestors or the 'recycling' of souls, names, and so on. In ethical reincarnation religions such as Hinduism and Buddhism, however, there is a differential destiny of reincarnation which depends upon ethical or moral considerations. Other kinds of salvation religion designate two afterworlds, one for the sinners and one for the saved – as Christianity does, for example.

The anthropology of religion has paid considerable attention not only to the contrast in evolutionary terms between literate and preliterate religious traditions but also to what has been termed the 'dialectic of practical religion', that is to say the dialectical relationship which exists between the literate tradition of the great world religions and the local practice of these religions. Philosophical or doctrinal and practical religion modify one another constantly through the social relationships which exist between theologians, priests and practical 'believers'. The lay practitioner is faced with a series of contradictions between religious precept, local practice and non-religious needs and demands. For example, the Buddhist monk who is an ascetic ideal of holiness is supposed to be a model for ordinary men, but he is in practice an unattainable one. In reality the ordinary person and the monk enter into a series of transactions whereby the layman may obtain some merit in return for practical gifts and certain forms of behaviour not incompatible with everyday lifestyle. Other studies in this same field have shown how the great world religions are adapted at local level to express features of social organization and local loyalties and oppositions in the organization of rituals, regional CULTS and PILGRIMAGES.

There is no generally agreed typology of

religions, and certainly none which would exclude the existence of mixed types. One of the more commonly accepted typologies however divides religions into two major classes according to the kind of religious specialist: SHAMAN or PRIEST. Writers like Weston LaBarre (1970), who have made extensive studies of shamanism, claim that shamanism or direct visionary experience is the universal origin of religion, and that such direct experience becomes institutionalized over time in the priestly religions characteristic of more advanced and stratified societies.

reproduction. The concept of reproduction in the social sciences is sometimes employed in the sense of the physical or biological reproduction of the population. More often however it is employed in the sense of SOCIAL REPRODUCTION, a concept developed within Marxist thought and applied to all mechanisms and processes through which a system of production is sustained and maintained over time. This includes not only the reproduction of the labour force, the technology, tools and knowledge necessary for production, but also the reproduction of the social organization and ideological structures which serve to structure the relationships of production and justify the distribution of control over the MEANS OF PRODUCTION. The reproduction of social and productive systems is problematic, and is not the perfectly orchestrated process that synchronistic FUNCTIONALIST social theory sometimes portrays it as being. Rather all societies are caught up in historical processes of change and transformation, so that at any one moment we may examine the tensions and crises which emerge in the process of social reproduction and which may lead under certain conditions to the transformation of productive and social structures. (*See* MARXIST ANTHROPOLOGY.)

research design. An investigation's organizing and directing plan. The stage of research design is in a sense the most important one in the investigation since it is this stage which will determine and orient it, though it is also necessary to incorporate mechanisms into the research design which allow for the modification of the research to take into account new and unexpected findings. This is particularly necessary in anthropological research because so many unknown factors may be involved, both in the field situation and the fieldworker's response. At the very least the research design should delimit the area of investigation, the stages of research (fieldwork, analysis of data, evaluation), the methods of data collection (PARTICIPANT OBSERVATION, survey, interview), the hypotheses to be tested and by what means. (*See* RESEARCH METHODS.)

research methods. In anthropology these include methods for RESEARCH DESIGN, for the carrying out of ethnographic FIELDWORK and for the analysis and evaluation of data. In the 19th century, anthropological research methods had been little developed, and many writers limited themselves to the collection of odd fragments of data from different areas or within a given geographical region, fragments which were then pieced together according to the particular EVOLUTIONARY or DIFFUSIONIST theory being advanced. 20th-century anthropology, under the influence of BOAS and MALINOWSKI among others, turned away from the piecemeal use of ethnographic data to justify preconceived schemes and towards the advocacy of thorough and holistic investigation of non-Western cultures. The Boasian insistence on cultural particularism and methodical and complete data collection, together with Malinowski's method of PARTICIPANT OBSERVATION became an integral part of the anthropological tradition, which moved towards holistic COMMUNITY STUDIES and studies of SOCIAL STRUCTURE or CULTURE influenced in many cases by FUNCTIONALIST social theory.

Participant observation is supplemented in modern anthropology by a number of different techniques, which depend in part on the area of study and the subdiscipline or field of enquiry. Since modern research tends to be more problem-oriented and less general or holistic in its focus, a number of specialized research techniques have been developed which relate to fields as diverse as ecological anthropology, KINSHIP studies, and APPLIED ANTHROPOLOGY. Commonly employed methods include the interview (the structured interview or questionnaire on the one hand, and the in-depth interview on the other), the CASE STUDY, surveys and mapping, the use of historical and archival material to provide time depth, the use of statistical or census material, etc. To aid in data collecting, photographic and sound recording methods are employed. In the field of VISUAL ANTHROPOLOGY and that of ETHNOGRAPHIC FILM increasingly sophisticated methods are being developed in order to incorporate these methods into research design and data analysis.

In recent years the use of COMPUTERS, MATHEMATICAL MODELS and statistical models in anthropology has increased in scope and sophistication, so that modern anthropologists now have a vast array of computer techniques, mathematical and statistical models available which may aid them in the formulation and testing of data and in the interrogation of their material in order to generate new and meaningful results. One of the major challenges in modern anthropology is to absorb these new methods and link this increasing mathematical sophistication to the interpretative aspects of anthropology, in order to avoid a predominance of sterile FORMAL ANALYSIS while at the same time taking advantage of methodological advances. Advances in anthropological reflection upon and sophistication of the philosophical and ideological implications of research methods have been notable in CRITICAL ANTHROPOLOGY. (*See* ETHNOGRAPHIC WRITING).

revitalization. Defined by A.F.C. Wallace as deliberate and organized movement by some members of a society to create a more satisfying culture. According to Wallace's classic account (1958) these movements occur under conditions of extreme stress, social disruption and cultural disintegration. Such conditions may be caused by situations of culture contact and forced ACCULTURATION, by natural disasters or by any other factor which creates rapid change which a culture is unable to assimilate. The revitalization movement, which is generally religious in character but may also be predominantly political or social, is characterized by the sudden emergence and acceptance of a new cultural 'blueprint' or a series of innovations. The new blueprint is often the creation of single individual (a prophet

or CHARISMATIC leader) or a small group, and is utopian in character. Members and converts to the movement undergo a 'mazeway transformation': a revelatory conversion to the new way of thinking and pattern of attitudes and behaviour.

Many revitalization movements, like REBELLIONS in general, are doomed to failure, and it is only the occasional one which encounters the necessary and sufficient conditions in a wider regional or national context and becomes a widespread and successful social movement. In these cases the very success of the movement produces radical changes in its form and structure, and what began as a revolutionary and utopian movement becomes institutionalized and ROUTINIZED. A revitalization movement may thus eventually become an established orthodox religion, and new revitalization movements may emerge over time to challenge it.

Kopytoff (1964) proposes that religious movements should not be analysed in terms of fixed types, which may obscure both the internal differences between members of a type and the similarities between different types, but instead that we should characterize each movement in terms of an analytical approach, as a cluster of variables. Thus each particular religious movement possesses a unique profile in terms of a set of multiple dimensions. (*See* CULTS; MESSIANISM; MILLENARIANSIM.)

revolution. A term with several distinct, though related, senses. It is sometimes used to refer to the overthrow of one ruling group by another, though more commonly this is termed a *coup d'état* since 'revolution' is more commonly used for those historical events where a political system (not just a political ruling group or ELITE) is overthrown. A third meaning is that of radical changes in the economic, political and social order, whether or not these are accompanied by or include at some point a revolution in the strictest sense. Thus the adoption of AGRICULTURE and the profound changes which this wrought in human social and cultural organization are referred to as the 'neolithic revolution', and other periods of complex and radical sociocultural change are also called 'revolutions': the industrial revolution, the cultural revolution, and so on.

The study of revolutions and of the concept of revolution is most developed within Marxist thought (*see* MARXIST ANTHROPOLOGY). According to Marx, the key or determining feature of a revolution is the transition from one MODE OF PRODUCTION to another. This transition in class-based societies is expressed as the passing of control over the MEANS OF PRODUCTION from one social class to another, and requires organized political action in order to achieve this transition against the will of the current ruling group. But according to the Marxist MATERIALIST conception of history, revolutions are inevitable, since they are the product of the universal tendency for the FORCES OF PRODUCTION to develop and thus outgrow the RELATIONS OF PRODUCTION. The ruling class, which represents the social organization appropriate to an earlier stage of development of the productive forces, is thus doomed to be ousted by a new dominant order which represents the social organization appropriate to the new relations of production established by the developing productive forces. The revolution which most concerned Marx was the socialist revolution, which he held to be inevitable as the socialized nature of industrial production made private ownership of the means of production an anachronism. According to Marx the progressive polarization of social classes (labour and capital) in capitalism would lead to increasing misery among the proletariat, until eventually at the point when it had 'nothing to lose but its chains' the proletariat would revolt and effect the necessary transition from private to socialized ownership of the means of production. Marx's account of the revolutionary process and the debates and differing interpretations which it has generated among Marxist and non-Marxist historians and social scientists are of course extremely complex. The major points of controversy have been the theory of increasing class polarization, the proletarian nature of the revolution, and the historical determinism implied in Marx's analysis. Several commentators have argued that revolutions occur not in moments of extreme and absolute poverty, when the masses are actually politically passive, but in moments of overall economic and social improvement. An important factor in creating revolutionary potential may therefore be the failure of the economic system to keep up with the expectations of some or all of its members as to growth and increased prosperity. It has been pointed out along the same lines that not all modern revolutions are predominantly proletarian, and that Marx had underestimated both the revolutionary potential of PEASANTS and the strategic role played by certain sectors of the bourgeoisie in the organization and direction of revolutionary movements. The implications of Marx's historical determinism and his thesis of the inevitability of revolution have also been amply debated within Marxist political and social thought. Much of this debate rests on a fundamental confusion or failure to distinguish between the revolution in the sense of a political movement or political moment, and the revolution in the sense of a social transformation. Many revolutionary moments in history do not in fact correspond to revolutions in the more profound sense of social transformation or of a shift in control over the means of production from one social class to another. Whether we interpret this as evidence that the revolution is a MILLENARIAN or utopian concept which can never exist in reality, or as evidence of the need to persist in revolutionary PRAXIS until the necessary conditions exist for social and economic transformation, depends upon our underlying political philosophy and our acceptance or rejection of the materialist theory of history.

In a Third World context the political economy of revolutions must be considered in the light of the relationships of COLONIAL and neo-colonial domination and DEPENDENCY which have increasingly become the focus of modern anthropology. Third World nations are caught up in the extremely complex worldwide system of international dependency, interpreted by some authors as a manifestation of a single WORLD SYSTEM and by others as a product of the ARTICULATION OF MODES OF PRODUCTION as capitalist economies of the developed world extend their domination over pre-capitalist societies of the Third World. If the interpretation of revolutions in the context of national history and national class relations is complex, their interpretation in terms of the play between international political and economic forces is doubly so. The rhetoric of national liberation in Third World revolutions is sometimes employed to disguise what is simply the ousting of one elite by another, and the force of internal transformations or shifts in control over the means of production may be insignificant in the face of movements in the world market or manipulation of political and economic control by the more powerful nations on an international level.

Richards, Audrey Isabell (1899–1984). British social anthropologist who carried out important ethnographic research among the Bemba of Northern Rhodesia. Her *Land, Labour and Diet in Northern Rhodesia* (1939) and *Chisungu: A Girl's Initiation Ceremony among the Bemba of Northern Rhodesia* (1956) are two major works among her many writings, all of which have constituted important contributions to African anthropology. Her major theoretical interests included economic and political systems, the study of colonial rule and anthropological participation, social change and the study of ritual.

ridicule. One form of SOCIAL CONTROL which may be employed in small-scale societies or small groups in order to exert pressure upon an individual. It is also a mechanism of asserting social distance, as when the attributes (or supposed attributes) of another group are ridiculed.

rite. *See* CEREMONY; RITUAL.

rites of passage. A term employed by VAN GENNEP in his classic and pioneering cross-cultural study of status changes and the associated RITUAL (1909; trans. 1960). Van Gennep noted that many rituals follow the same conceptual pattern as INITIATION rites. This includes three separate ritual stages, that of separation, that of transition or liminality and that of reincorporation. The anthropological study of ritual has been greatly influenced by Van Gennep's scheme and by his interpretation of the SYMBOLISM of rites of passage.

ritual. It is extremely difficult and perhaps ultimately unnecessary to define ritual, or to delimit it from CEREMONY on the one hand or from instrumental or practical action on the other. It is regarded by some anthropologists as a category of behaviour, in which

case it may be defined as a form of ceremony characterized by its religious nature or purpose. Thus GLUCKMAN (1962) distinguished ritual from ceremonial by defining ceremonial as 'any complex organization of human activity which is not specifically technical or recreational and which involves the use of modes of behaviour which are expressive of social relationships', while ritual is a more limited category characterized by its reference to mystical or religious notions, ends or agencies. Ritual is thus regarded as being symbolically more complex and involving more deep social and sociopsychological concerns. Goody on the other hand (1961) defines ritual as 'a category of standardized behaviour (custom) in which the relationship between the means and the end is not 'intrinsic' (i.e. is either irrational or non-rational). Other anthropologists such as LEACH (1954) regard ritual not as a category of behaviour but as an aspect of behaviour: that is to say, as the aspect of behaviour related to its symbolic value rather than to its practical utility. He points out that even the most practical or technical act is performed in such a way as to express the particular cultural identity or values of the actor, so that it has a symbolic or ritual dimension. He proposes the existence of a continuum between acts whose technical or practical aspects predominate and those where ritual and symbolic ones predominate, without excluding the possibility of analysing the technical aspect of predominantly ritual acts or the ritual aspect of predominantly technical ones. It is clear therefore that the categories of technical, ritual and ceremonial are arbitrary distinctions among phenomena which are not always in themselves neatly classifiable.

Another area of difficulty and ambiguity has been that of the relationship which exists among the categories of ritual, MYTH and BELIEF. For a time anthropological studies of ritual and myth were dominated by sterile controversies as to which should be accorded primacy: myth as a codification or recording of ritual, or ritual as an expression or enactment of myth. However in modern anthropology this controversy has been largely abandoned, since ritual and myth are generally viewed as two forms of expression of the human symbolic and expressive facility, neither one of which should be accorded primacy over the other. Myth may be a commentary on ritual and ritual on myth, and there is no need to posit any overall dependency or determination. As far as the relationship between ritual and belief is concerned , it was also widely assumed in the past that there was a close enough relationship between the two for rituals to be held to express or reinforce beliefs and beliefs to underlie or justify rituals. But modern anthropology has increasingly demonstrated that there is considerable intra-cultural diversity in attitudes, feelings and beliefs, and that an accepted social form of expression or action like those embodied in ritual do not imply that the actors concerned share the same beliefs or feelings about the ritual. Modern studies of ritual and SYMBOLISM consequently proceed with great caution when they deal with the question of belief, recognizing that there is a complex and dialectical relationship between individual psychology and experience on the one hand and social and cultural forms on the other.

To turn to the way in which ritual has been analysed in anthropology, we should first of all mention the pioneering studies of Durkheim (1912), whose theories have influenced many writers in this field. Durkheim's work contained many different strands. On the one hand his FUNCTIONALIST theory of RELIGION and ritual as reinforcing collective sentiment and social integration was developed by RADCLIFFE-BROWN (1952) and other British social anthropologists who elaborated the study of what ritual does and how it expresses features of the social structure. On the other hand Durkheim's theories of the formation and transformation of COLLECTIVE REPRESENTATIONS influenced the development of another kind of analysis: the analysis of the content of ritual or what ritual says. The works of MAUSS (1925) and VAN GENNEP (1909) were also of great importance in influencing both the development of the British social structural interpretation of ritual and the French STRUCTURALIST approach to ritual and symbolism.

The British social structural approach, which examined ritual categories and actions as expressions of and forces within the social order, paid little or no attention to the symbolic content of ritual or the language which ritual employed to express symbolic oppositions, conjunctions and disjunctions. Structuralist theory was extremely important in arguing for the study of the systematic nature of the content of cultural systems, as was COGNITIVE ANTHROPOLOGY, among other approaches which contributed advances to the study of symbolism and systems of CLASSIFICATION. Most modern students of ritual and of religion and symbolism in general are in agreement that it is necessary to study both what ritual does and what it says, since these are interdependent and mutually reinforcing aspects of the religious and symbolic phenomena in human society. Ritual action depends upon ritual language for its effectiveness, though different analysts place different degrees of emphasis on the sociological and the symbolic aspects of their interpretation. INITIATION rites have attracted particular attention from anthropologists, in part because of the continuing compulsion exercised by Van Gennep's model of the RITES OF PASSAGE and in part because they are often occasions for especially highly-developed expressions of the symbolic systems of society and the manner in which these relate to the regulation of the individual life cycle.

An important contribution to the study of ritual is that of TURNER, who has described a rich system of ritual symbolism among the Ndembu (1967) and has also contributed important theoretical orientations in the field (1969; 1975). Ritual symbolism among the Ndembu of Zambia is dominated by the existence of a set of key symbolic objects and qualities (for example colours) which consistently recur in ritual acts and settings. Each symbolic object or quality possesses a broad fan of meanings ranging from physiological and psychological referents to social and abstract ones. The 'meaning' of a ritual is thus complex and ambiguous, since ritual acts manipulate symbolic values which are in turn complex and ambiguous. So a ritual has many levels of meaning and many possible ambiguities, but serves ultimately to relate abstract principles and social relations to physiological and psychological realities, though not in a simplistic or deterministic fashion.

M. Bloch has suggested (1975) that some of the sophisticated analysis of the content of ritual symbolism misses an essential point about the social use of such symbolism, which is that it is employed in order to express relations of authority. The use of stylized ritual formulae, he argues, may be important not in terms of the content of these ritual forms but rather in the sense that, by eliminating the possibility of discrepant or original responses, it binds the members of the group to the acceptance of the authority of ritual elders who represent the dominant group in society. F. Barth has also examined the manner in which the manipulation of ritual knowledge and successive levels of secrecy in initiation cults is a form of social and political domination of younger by elder men (1975). The examination of the manipulation of ritual as a means of mystifying specific exploitative or unequal social systems is an important area for further investigation, though we should not fall into the trap of equating ritual statements of authority with real authority in non-ritual contexts, which may be a quite separate issue.

ritual homosexuality. *See* HOMOSEXUALITY; INITIATION; RITUAL SEXUAL SYMMETRY.

ritual kinship. Ritual or spiritual kinship is the anthropological term employed to describe the complex of rituals and relationships associated with baptism and godparenthood (*see* COMPADRAZGO). The ritual of baptism and the social relationships which it creates have been examined from different points of view, the two dominant trends being the analysis of the symbolism of ritual kinship and the statements which it makes about personal, spiritual and social identity, and the examination of the network of social relationships created by ritual kinship and the manner in which these function as relations of solidarity, mutual aid and/or PATRONAGE. Few analyses however combine these two perspectives to show how the symbolic attributes of ritual kinship are manipulated strategically by social actors. Another interesting dimension which has yet to be developed is the study of ritual kinship in comparative perspective and its similarities to or differences from rituals of naming and INITIATION in societies with a non-Christian religious tradition.

ritual rebellion, ritual reversal. GLUCKMAN (1963) argues that the role reversal in rituals

of rebellion functions as a mechanism of psychological catharsis which ultimately reinforces the social order: ritual rebellions against the king function to release tensions and therefore strengthen the institution of kingship. His interpretation of these rituals is thus sociopsychological, for he contends that the rituals represent and discharge real social tensions associated with hierarchical relations, and as a symbolic protest they reduce the possibility of real conflict. LEACH (1962) puts forward a more general symbolic interpretation of role reversal. He argues that role reversals are generally associated with RITES OF PASSAGE and are a characteristic element of the symbolic representation of time. (*See* RITUAL; SYMBOLISM.)

ritual sexual symmetry. Ritual expressions of sexual symmetry or the imitation of characteristics associated with one sex by the other include acts of ritual homosexuality, genital mutilations, and imitations by men of the reproductive role of women. These are found as features of INITIATION rites in many societies. They have received psychoanalytic interpretation as expressions of 'womb envy' by men, as in Bettelheim's study of male intiation rites (1954). They have also been interpreted by authors like Mary Douglas (1975) as expressions of social morphology. P. Hage interprets ritual sexual symmetry in New Guinea (1981) as part of magical acts which are held to influence male growth by analogy with female reproductive power, and which express the symmetry of social divisions in societies characterized by DUAL ORGANIZATION. They have also been interpreted as ritual acts which reinforce male dominance by asserting male control over male and female sexual powers.

Rivers, William Halse (1864–1922). British anthropologist who carried out research into Melanesian culture and who was associated with the DIFFUSIONIST school of SMITH and PERRY (e.g. 1924).

Robertson-Smith, William (1846–94). A student of comparative religion who was one of the pioneers in Britain of the anthropological approach to religion, in the sense that he argued for the social and functional interpretation of religious beliefs and practices rather than the purely theological or philosophical one. His best known work is *The Religion of the Semites* (1894).

role. The classic definition of role, formulated by LINTON (1936) is 'the dynamic aspect of status'. While STATUS is a social position which has a determined set of associated rights and duties, a role involves the acting out of status and 'role expectations' in the expected conduct associated with a given status. This approach to role was developed in FUNCTIONALIST sociology and anthropology, and MERTON (1949) added the further categories of 'role set' (the set of role relationships associated with a given social status) and 'role conflict' (where incompatible expectations or demands are placed on the individual). The functional theory of role has been criticized as overly static and passive, assuming as it does that there is a CONSENSUS in society over a uniform set of expectations, and that the individual merely passively receives or learns these expectations. ACTION THEORY and other modern approaches to anthropology do not however assume consensus over role expectations, and emphasize instead the active participation of individuals and groups in creating roles during social interaction (*see* ETHNOMETHODOLOGY). In taking up roles we also comment upon these roles and create new variations, so that the static conception of role is now generally regarded as inappropriate.

I. Goffman's sociological theories of status and role have also been of considerable influence in the anthropological treatment of the topic. Goffman (1969) emphasizes the manner in which individuals distance themselves from roles, adopt them more or less consciously, or are coerced into adopting them by the pressure of others' labelling or as a result of the dynamics of group and interpersonal relations.

Rorschach test. A type of psychological test referred to as 'projective' since it encourages and permits the subject to project his or her psychological attributes, fantasies and tensions. In the Rorschach test the subject is asked to state what he or she sees in a series of inkblots which are ambiguous in form. CULTURE AND PERSONALITY research has employed the Rorschach test widely in the past in order to obtain data on personality traits which was then related to cultural patterning.

Rousseau, Jean-Jacques (1712-78). French philosopher of the ENLIGHTENMENT who is regarded as an important precursor of anthropology because of his emphasis on the inherently social and cultural nature of human life and human history. In his *Le Contrat social* (1761) Rousseau formulated the theory that the nature of the social collectivity, which was later to influence DURKHEIM was the expression of the 'general will'. Rousseau is often cited for his notion of the 'noble savage', and his argument that with the progress of civilization and the accompanying economic inequality man's moral nature degenerates, a situation which he believed could be remedied through the implementation of enlightened educational policies and the political application of the principles of the social contract.

routinization. A concept introduced by WEBER to refer to the transformation of CHARISMATIC leadership into INSTITUTIONALIZED leadership. This concept has been applied to the study of the history and development of CULTS and SECTS as well as political movements.

rural-urban continuum. *See* FOLK-URBAN CONTINUUM.

rural-urban migration. *See* MIGRATION.

S

sacralization. The process of transition or transformation from the profane to the SACRED state.

sacred. An idea regarded by DURKHEIM (1912) as constituting the defining feature of the religious phenomenon in human society. According to Durkheim, the sacred is that which is both set apart and revered, and he argued that the quality of the sacred stemmed from society itself and the expression of collective solidarity, (*See* RELIGION.)

sacrifice. The offering of a living animal – or in exceptional cases, a human being – to a deity or spirit. The anthropological study of sacrifice has focused on one hand on the symbolic statements which are made about human, animal and spiritual identity and relationships, and on the other on the manner in which sacrifice may be interpreted as reflecting and reinforcing certain aspects of social structure and social solidarity. ROBERTSON-SMITH (1894) proposed that Semitic sacrifice served to produce and reinforce social unity by the sharing of a common meal together with the deity. Other early anthropologists saw TOTEMISM as the origin of sacrifice, though later LEVI-STRAUSS challenged the symbolic logic of this association, claiming that the logic underlying sacrifice is fundamentally different from that underlying totemism (1966). In sacrifice a series of symbolic equivalences acts to establish a series of relationships of contiguity which link two extremes: humans and deities. In totemism however the relation is not of contiguity but of homology between two different series, a natural series of species and a cultural series of groups of persons. As Levi-Strauss points out, the offerer of the sacrifice is first brought into contact with the deity by means of a series of symbolic equivalences, and the sacrificial act itself then breaks this contact by the destruc-

tion of the intermediary term which is the sacrificial victim. Humans and deities are thus brought together to achieve the purpose of the sacrifice, which may be that of expiation or of communion, and then are set apart again.

LEACH has employed the model of a RITE OF PASSAGE in order to interpret the logic of sacrifice (1976). He points out that in a rite of passage the ritual procedure separates the initiate into a 'pure' and 'impure' part, symbolically excluding the impure and incorporating the pure part into the initiate's new status. So in the same fashion he argues that the ritual of sacrifice, by establishing a symbolic equivalence between the donor of the sacrifice and the victim, purifies the donor and creates a new ritual status by means of the purification of the victim. This same logic, he proposes, underlies sacrifice in the many different contexts in which this institution is found.

Sacrifice and human sacrifice have also attracted attention from cultural ecology and from the CULTURAL MATERIALIST perspective, which has focused on this as on other ritual practices in order to demonstrate the thesis that an underlying ecological rationality may be found for even the most apparently non-rational or symbolic customs in human society. Thus M. Harner (1977) argues that Aztec human sacrifice and CANNIBALISM related to population pressure in pre-conquest Mexico. This population pressure and the lack of animal protein, he suggests, generated the adaptive response of large scale cannibalism which was disguised or ideologically justified in terms of religious sacrifice. M. Sahlins among others has challenged this interpretation (1981), criticizing both the ecological evidence upon which Harner rests his case and the underestimation of the importance of the religious motivation underlying sacrifice. In reality the ecological interpretation and the symbolic one are not fundamentally contradictory, provided we are careful to distinguish between the ecological consequences or functions of a given custom, of which its practitioners are either unaware or only partially aware, and the level of conscious motivations, explanations or ideological justifications of the custom. It is legitimate to examine the part played by sacrificial customs in the adaptation of a human group to its environment, but it is also necessary to examine the symbolic values attributed to ritual acts within the logic of a sociocultural system. Harner's suggestion that human sacrifice played a part in reinforcing and justifying the position of the upper classes by means of the assertion of the importance and indispensability of priests is also an important one. Symbolic anthropology occasionally falls into the trap of naïvely assuming that a set of religious practices or dogmas represents the symbolic logic of a culture in general, without taking into account the fact that this set of dogmas may represent and justify the position of a limited group with political power in society. Aztec human sacrifice, as Harner points out, was held to be necessary in order to ensure social, economic and spiritual survival and well-being, and the priests as mediators in sacrifice formed part of a ruling elite which controlled the economic, military and religious activities of the population as a whole and sustained a policy of the Aztec empire's military expansion by means of the complex of warfare and sacrifice. Harris, for example, responds to Sahlins' assertion that Aztec sacrifice represented a 'communion' of priests with victims by stating: 'A ruling class that says it is eating some people out of concern for the welfare of all is not telling the whole story' (1978). It is necessary however to untangle the confusion in Harris' and Harner's own position about the relationship between the ecological and social class basis of sacrifice, as it is to take into account the symbolic logic of sacrifice and the extent to which this constituted part of a common religious and symbolic system accepted throughout society.

Saint-Simon, Comte **Henri de** (1760–1825). French social theorist whose ideas were to influence both COMTE and MARX. Saint-Simon argued that society progressed through three stages of evolution characterized by types of knowledge: the theological, the metaphysical and the positive stages. His evolutionary theory of society and his positivism were to form important elements in the work of Comte, while his study of the emergence of social STRATIFICATION and CLASS relations with the rise of industrial society were important precursors of Marxist social theory.

sanction. The reactions (whether negative or positive) which a social group displays to the conduct of its members. Negative sanctions take the form of punishments, admonishments, deprivations, and so on, and may be organized and codified or informal and diffuse. Positive sanctions include rewards of different kinds such as prestige, material rewards and privileges. (*See* LAW, ANTHROPOLOGY OF; SOCIAL CONTROL.)

Sapir, Edward (1884–1934). US linguist and anthropologist who together with Benjamin Whorf developed the theory of LINGUISTIC RELATIVISM (the Sapir–Whorf hypothesis). This theory, which was influenced by Boasian CULTURAL RELATIVISM as well as by certain trends within linguistics and philosophy, stated that the perception of reality is conditioned by the language of the speaker (e.g. 1921; 1949). (*See* LINGUISTICS AND ANTHROPOLOGY.)

satellite. *See* METROPOLIS-SATELLITE.

Saussure, Ferdinand de (1857–1913). Swiss linguist who is regarded as the founder of the STRUCTURALIST approach to linguistics (e.g. 1916). (*See* LINGUISTICS AND ANTHROPOLOGY.)

savage, savagery. A term in general as well as anthropological use during the 19th century, having been introduced to the social sciences as part of the evolutionary scheme of social types originally proposed by MONTESQUIEU and which consisted of the stages of savagery, BARBARISM and CIVILIZATION. Later the term was questioned by anthropologists because of the pejorative connotations it had acquired, and was replaced in professional usage by the term PRIMITIVE, which was felt to be free of ethnocentric bias. Subsequently 'primitive' itself has been similarly rejected, and the search for a value-free categorization continues, perhaps reflecting a fundamentally uneasy conscience about the professional and ethical commitment of the anthropologist. (*See* CRITICAL ANTHROPOLOGY.)

scapulimancy. A technique of DIVINATION employing the scapula or shoulder bone of an animal.

scarification. The use of scars as part of bodily decoration. (*See* BODY, ANTHROPOLOGY OF.)

schism. Fission or cleavage. The term has been employed in anthropology to describe processes of political and social division, especially in small-scale societies. BATESON extends the concept of schism to form a part of his more general description of social relationships and cultural change. In his account of what he calls 'schismogenesis' Bateson argues that all social relationships and social groups create differences and divergences of opinion, attitudes, NORMS and VALUES. These differences will tend to accumulate and ultimately produce fission or schism in the group, generating new social divisions and units with divergent normative structures. The concept of schismogenesis also forms part of Bateson's account of sociopsychological mechanisms and individual adjustment to society.

science. Views of the relationship between anthropology and science or the scientific method are interesting inasmuch as they throw light on the philosophical and methodological peculiarities and difficulties of the discipline. Our view of the 'scientific' status of anthropology depends upon our view of what science itself is. Some consider it to be the progressive discovery of more and more objective knowledge about reality, while others consider it to be simply the progressive construction of a series of models or paradigms which which have no necessary connection with empirical facts. In the same way, some anthropologists regard the discipline as scientific in the sense that it attempts to uncover the laws of social EVOLUTION or those of the STRUCTURAL organization of human mental and cultural life, while others stress the interpretative and non-scientific nature of anthropological explanation. (*See* EMPIRICISM; ETHNOPHILOSOPHY; HERME-NEUTICS; LINGUISTICS AND ANTHROPOLOGY; MAGIC; PRIMITIVE MENTALITY; RELIGION; VERSTEHEN.)

secondary institution. *See* PRIMARY/SECONDARY INSTITUTION.

sedentarism. Residence in settled communities. (*See* NOMADS.)

segmentary. Used in anthropology to denote LINEAGE systems which define DESCENT groups in terms of identifications with successively more distant APICAL ANCESTORS. The structure of society is thus conceived of as hierarchical or tree-like, in which there are different levels of unity and opposition; segments which are divided at the lowest level are grouped together into larger units at a higher level. EVANS-PRITCHARD's classic account of the segmentary lineage system among the Nuer (1940) relates the segmentary structure to kinship distance, and argues that groups which are opposed at the lowest level will unite at a higher level in opposition to other such groupings which are more distant in terms of unilineal kinship reckoning. The principle of the relativity of social identity described by Evans-Pritchard has been confirmed by anthropologists working not only in unilineal systems but also in societies characterized by other forms of kinship organization. However the segmentary lineage model as formulated by Evans-Pritchard has been criticized by later anthropologists on two main grounds. Firstly, it has been argued that while Evans-Pritchard assumed that conflicts would follow the lines of kinship distance and that the most closely related persons would join together in opposition to more distant groups, conflicts often actually occur more frequently between closely related persons than between distant ones. We thus need to modify the segmentary lineage model to take into account the existence of different types of conflict, rather than taking at face value the assertion that close relatives will always be united against more distant or unrelated persons. It has also been pointed out that the segmentary model is overly static, representing a society conceived of as 'frozen' at one moment in time, and is therefore an inappropriate model for the conceptualization of a real social system as it exists over time. New approaches to the study of lineage systems influenced both by ACTION THEORY and by MARXIST ANTHROPOLOGY thus tend to regard the classic segmentary model as a reflection of native ideology or ideal models and not as a representation of actual social organization.

segregation. *See* APARTHEID; CASTE; RACISM.

Seligman, Charles Gabriel (1873–1940). British ethnologist who taught MALINOWSKI and whose major interests included psychological anthropology and the ethnology of New Guinea and the Sudan.

semantics. The study of meaning in LINGUISTICS. In anthropology the study of semantics has been of central importance in those areas influenced by linguistic theory, including COGNITIVE ANTHROPOLOGY and STRUCTURALISM.

semiology, semiotics. The science of signs and sign-using behaviour. This includes both the study of linguistic and non-linguistic COMMUNICATION and the way in which the patterning of human cultural behaviour constitutes forms of signification which may be interpreted according to common principles, usually by analogy with linguistic behaviour. The notion of semiology as a formalized science originated with SAUSSURE, whose ideas were a principal influence in the shaping of the French STRUCTURALIST movement and are represented principally in the works of LEVI-STRAUSS. The term 'semiotics' was employed by the US philosopher C.S. Peirce and later adopted by C. Morris (1964) in his attempt to formalize a general theory of signs. Semiology or semiotics is a project rather than an established science, but has generated important advances in the anthropological study of communication and SYMBOLISM as well as in the fields of structural and COGNITIVE ANTHROPOLOGY among others.

serf. An agricultural labourer who is bound to the land to such an extent that he may be transferred with the land to another owner. He cannot leave the land or refuse to work. (*See* FEUDALISM.)

Service, Elman R. (1915–). US cultural anthropologist who established the widely accepted EVOLUTIONARY classification of social types into BAND, TRIBE, CHIEFDOM and STATE. His major woks include *Origins of the State and Civilization* (1975).

sex and gender. *See* GENDER.

sexism. *See* GENDER; FEMINIST ANTHROPOLOGY.

sex roles. *See* GENDER; FEMINIST ANTHROPOLOGY; KINSHIP; MARRIAGE; WOMEN AND ANTHROPOLOGY.

sexual division of labour. It has often been argued that the sexual division of labour, especially in simple societies, is a 'natural' phenomenon based on superior male strength and female reproductive functions which led to the distribution of male and female roles in terms of hunter/warrior versus gatherer/mother etc. Molyneux however points out (1977) that apart from any speculation as to how the sexual division of labour may have arisen, it is necessary to examine it as a social and cultural rather than natural phenomenon, since it is a phenomenon organized through and upheld by sociocultural structures including kinship, ritual and mythology. In the same way, while some writers have argued that we should examine male/female complementarity rather than equality, feminist anthropologists have argued that in many cases ideas of complementarity are nothing more than ideological mystifications of what can be objectively seen to be inequalities. Thus Rosaldo (1974) argues that sexual oppression or inequality is universal, and is based on the restriction of women to a private or domestic sphere which is always devalued in relation to the male dominated public sphere. Ortner follows a related argument (1974) based on the universal symbolic association of men with culture and women with nature. Rubin, on the other hand (1975), relates female subordination to the treatment of women as objects in a system of kinship and alliance. Molyneux points out however that these global explanations fail to account for the historical specificity of male/female relations in each social context and within each economic system. The public-private dichotomy and the status of women should thus be explored in each context. (*See* FEMINIST ANTHROPOLOGY; GENDER; WOMEN IN ANTHROPOLOGY.)

shamanism. A Siberian term for a complex of religious and ethnomedicinal beliefs and practices found in widely ranging ethnographic contexts including Asia, Africa and aboriginal America. The shaman is usually defined as a part-time religious specialist, whose abilities are based on direct personal experience. Shamans are usually male but in certain cultures it is possible for a woman to become a shaman. Shamanic experience is generally obtained by means of the use of different kinds of ALTERED STATES OF CONSCIOUSNESS which may be related to the use of HALLUCINOGENS or to other types of exceptional sensory deprivation or stimulation. The shaman thus contrasts with the PRIEST in more formally organized or institutionalized RELIGION, since his or her powers rest on personal abilities and CHARISMA while the power of the priest is that vested in him by the church or the religious organization of which he forms a part.

Shamanism is also similar in certain respects to WITCHCRAFT in that it may involve the use of mystical powers to attack enemies and cause disease. The South American shaman, for example, is both a curer and a sorcerer, and the patterns of accusations and interpretations of sorcery reveal social tensions and structural features in the same manner as in the classic social anthropological studies of witchcraft in African settings.

In the study of shamanism much attention has been paid to the importance of altered states of consciousness, and also to the possible classification of the shaman as a mentally abnormal or disturbed individual. Many observers of shamanism have noted that the signs of shamanic vocation and the behaviour of the shaman are close to symptoms which in our own culture would be defined as psychotic or hysterical. There has been much debate as to whether these behaviours or attributes, which in their cultural context are regarded as normal and essential parts of the shaman's role, are indeed indicators of mental aberration. However the modern anthropological study of shamanism has shown that in many cases the shaman is not regarded as an aberrant or

abnormal individual but as a central figure in culture and society. Amazonian shamans, for example, are often central actors in the political, social and religious system. Not only are they responsible for curing and the magical protection of society, but they are also regarded as repositories of valued cultural and mythical knowledge. The hallucinatory experience or the altered state of consciousness in these cultures is one which the shaman must carefully and gradually control or 'domesticate', bringing society into contact wih powerful and dangerous spiritual forces which he must constantly demonstrate his ability to control and channel in a positive manner. Students of South American shamanism have noted however that there is considerable intra- and intercultural variability in the extent to which the shaman is regarded as a central or a marginal figure, a variability made possible by the fundamental ambiguity of the shaman's role as curer and sorcerer and as intermediary between society and a supernatural world which is both powerful and dangerous.

Some authors such as W. LaBarre (1970) and A.F.C. Wallace (1958) have pointed to the evolutionary aspects of the development of shamanism into institutionalized religion with the process of increasing social complexity and stratification. They point out that vestiges of shamanic experience and power may remain in priestly religions, just as shamanic type specialists may co-exist alongside an established religion, serving different kinds of needs or sectors of the population.

shanty towns. Slum or squatter settlemets which surround the major cities of the Third World. They are the product of rural-urban MIGRATION to cities which are not equipped to deal with the influx of migrants or to provide them with work. In many Third World capital and provincial cities, shanty towns have transformed the social, cultural and economic situations in a brief period of time, presenting urban planners and politicians with a tremendous challenge to provide basic services and at the same time creating a new and massive pool of UNEMPLOYED AND UNDEREMPLOYED labour. Migrants to shanty towns bring with them the cultural and social forms and expectations typical of the rural or provincial areas from which they originate, which, together with the series of new adaptive strategies and organizational forms which are products of their marginal urban experience, constitute the sociocultural profile of the shanty towns.

The anthropological study of shanty towns has focused both on the adaptive and coping mechanisms within them which ensure minimal levels of social organization even in precarious social and economic conditions, and on the relationships between shanty towns and the wider society. As far as such relationships are concerned, it is necessary to examine in more detail the mechanisms by which the urban elite or central urban population manages the relationship with the numerically dominant but socially, economically and politically subordinate marginal population. This centre-periphery relationship in Third World cities reproduces many of the social and class contradictions typical of COLONIALISM and neo-colonialism, but contains these within a single urban context rather than within the context of a rural-urban opposition.

The 'myth of marginality' about shanty towns and squatter settlements which exists in Third World nations portrays them as blights on the landscape, as leftovers from the traditional sector, as disorganized, delinquent and unwilling to develop. In fact they hold much of the urban economy together, providing a source of cheap labour due to unemployment and underemployment and creating much of the total wealth of the city in order to maintain the elite. Views of their culture as pathological and disorganized (CULTURE OF POVERTY) have been challenged by studies showing a high degree of organization, mutual support and cohesion. (*See* CITY, ANTHROPOLOGY OF THE; URBANISM, URBANIZATION.)

sharecropping. A form of share contracting in which the supplier of land receives from the supplier of labour a prearranged proportion of the output. This is a persistent form of agricultural organization in PEASANT economies, in spite of the conventional view of economists and economic historians that it is a transitional stage between tenancy and wage labour or a means of extracting surplus from peasants in quasi-FEUDAL systems. Robertson (1984) examines the positive features of sharecropping, which may have contributed to its persistence. One of these is the fact that it is a free contract which distributes risk equally between landowner and labourer. In fact, the specific characteristics of sharecropping and the degree of exploitation and inefficiency involved (which have generally been assumed to be high) vary from community to community according to the relative scarcity of land and labour and the relationships of social class, kinship ties, and so on which exist between landowner and labourer. It may in certain cases operate to even out differences in land and labour resources within the community.

sharing. *See* RECIPROCITY.

shell money. *See* MONEY.

shifting agriculture. *See* SWIDDEN AGRICULTURE.

shrines. Holy places which are the focus for PILGRIMAGES or acts of devotion. Allegiances to shrines may reflect aspects of local and regional social structure, serving to define local group boundaries or under certain circumstances to obviate these local distinctions in favour of a more inclusive if temporary alliance. (*See* RELIGION.)

sib. A term used by MURDOCK in preference to the term CLAN, in order to describe a maximal unilineal descent group: that is to say, a group which recognizes common ancestry but no longer recalls the exact links. In US anthropology therefore the term is generally employed to refer to two or more LINEAGES related by common descent from a mythological ancestor. In British anthropology such a group is however more commonly referred to as a clan. The term 'clan' in US anthropology is reserved (following MORGAN) for the matrisib, as opposed to the patrisib or GENS.

sick, abandonment of. The practice of abandoning gravely ill persons or those who cannot walk has been reported for a number of HUNTING AND GATHERING and NOMADIC societies. It is found especially among those groups who live close to the margins of survival or in difficult ecological conditions, the best-known case being that of the Eskimo. (*See* DEMOGRAPHY.)

sickness, anthropology of. *See* ETHNOMEDI-
CINE; MEDICAL ANTHROPOLOGY.

sign. A sign in linguistic and SEMIOTIC
theory is defined as a relation between a
signifier, a signified and a given context or
ground. The different kinds of relationship
between signifier and signified give the
different types of sign: INDEX, ICON and
SYMBOL. The relationship between the signifier and signified in the case of an index is
existential, in that of an icon representa-
tional and in that of a symbol conventional.

simple society. One of the terms which have
been employed as a substitute for PRIMITIVE
society, and in explicit or implicit contrast to
COMPLEX society or CIVILIZATION.

sister exchange. *See* ALLIANCE THEORY;
ASYMMETRIC/SYMMETRIC ALLIANCE; ELE-
MENTARY STRUCTURES; MARRIAGE.

sister's daughter marriage. *See* OBLIQUE
DISCONTINUOUS EXCHANGE.

situational analysis. A method of analysis of
social relations which takes as its starting
point a particular situation or moment of
social interaction, and traces out from this
situation the wider context of social NET-
WORKS in which it is embedded. (*See* ACTION
THEORY; ETHNOMETHODOLOGY.)

skewing. A property of KINSHIP TERMINO-
LOGIES such as the CROW and OMAHA
systems which systematically reclassify certain inter-generational relationships as if
they were intra-generational ones.

slash and burn agriculture. *See* SWIDDEN
AGRICULTURE.

slavery. In spite of the importance attached
to slavery by 19th-century EVOLUTIONARY
theorists and within Marx's scheme of the
evolution of SOCIOECONOMIC FORMATIONS,
the topic has been rather marginal to
modern social and cultural anthropology. It
has been in the fields of history and economic history that the topic has been most
exhaustively covered, though there have
also been some significant anthropological
contributions, particularly to the study of
Afro-American and indigenous African

slavery. Many of these have been influenced
by the classic definition of slavery formulated by Nieboer (1900), who viewed it as a
form of property associated with compulsory
labour. Nieboer suggested that slavery arose
where in a situation of open resources and
abundant land it was the only way in which
an entrepreneur could obtain labour. If land
and resources were limited, however, wage
labour would become available and since
this was more efficient it would cause slavery
to disappear. Other authors have stressed
the importance of political factors, arguing
that economic conditions alone are not
sufficient to account for slave systems and
that we should take into consideration the
features of slavery as a system of political
control and social STRATIFICATION.
   Watson (1980) has distinguished two types
of slavery: the 'open' and the 'closed'
modes. In the open, the wealth of the kin
group resides in people, so that slaves are
eventually absorbed into the kin group as
quasi-kinsmen. Indigenous African slavery
predominantly followed this pattern. But in
Asia, because of land scarcity, kin groups
were closed and slaves were treated as
chattels, which Watson terms the 'closed'
mode. Indeed it is important to recognize
that the term 'slavery' covers a wide range of
forms, from those in which slaves themselves
may have or acquire considerable rights and
social position to those where they become
purely an economic element as far as the
dominant group is concerned: hence the
difficulty in defining the concept of slavery
precisely. To define it as a form of property
and compulsory labour, while appearing to
fit the pattern of New World slavery, raises
problems with the anthropological definition
of PROPERTY itself, which is simply a short-
hand term for an unspecified package of
rights in persons or things. Similarly the
element of compulsory labour is difficult to
define and to distinguish from the obligations which 'free' persons may owe to kin
groups, to patrons, and so on (*see* DEBT
SLAVERY). Influenced by the Graeco-
Roman model, many anthropologists in the
past tended to emphasize the role of war and
conquest in creating slave systems, and some
anthropologists today would wish to preserve this as part of the definition of slavery,
though it does not account for situations
where slaves may be purchased or acquired

as payment of debts within the group.

Kopytoff (1977) argues that rather than focusing on questions of definition, we should develop a processual approach to slavery. He views the problem of slavery as one of 'status transformation' (*see* RITES OF PASSAGE). The slave, however acquired, is stripped of his or her old social identity and incorporated into a new one. In extreme chattel slavery this reincorporation is minimal, and the slave remains permanently in a marginal status, but in other systems this reincorporation may be more complex, though rarely reaching the point of complete absorption into the dominant group. Thus the many forms of slavery are forms of 'institutionalized marginality' which the anthropologist may relate to social and historical factors in the wider society. In Afro-American anthropology another important theme in the study of slavery has been the analysis of the social and cultural forms developed within the slave population itself and their continuing effects after the abolition of slavery. (*See* COLONIALISM; ETHNICITY; RACE.)

social action. *See* ACTION THEORY.

social actor. *See* ACTOR.

social anthropology. The dominant tradition in British anthropology has generally been called 'social anthropology', in accordance with the emphasis of British scholars on concepts such as SOCIETY, SOCIAL STRUCTURE, and SOCIAL ORGANIZATION. This predominance of the social is associated with STRUCTURAL FUNCTIONALIST theorists like RADCLIFFE-BROWN and FORTES, who along with other British anthropologists of their time drew heavily upon DURKHEIM's theories of SOCIAL FACTS and the autonomy and independence of the social domain. In North American anthropology of the same period, we may observe a parallel predominance of the CULTURE concept, which paradoxically, although conceptually opposed to British 'social determinism', produced theoretical blind alleys which were similar in many ways, especially in their failure to take into account the historical dimensions of social or cultural systems and the tendency to artificially isolate 'a culture' or 'a society' as a unit of study (*see* CULTURAL RELATIVISM; CUL-

TURAL DETERMINISM.)

In modern anthropology in the USA the term social anthropology is sometimes reserved to indicate the comparative study of societies and cultures, as opposed to the broader field of CULTURAL ANTHROPOLOGY which is considered to include ARCHAEOLOGY, PHYSICAL ANTHROPOLOGY, and LINGUISTIC ANTHROPOLOGY. Many modern writers however prefer to use the term SOCIOCULTURAL SYSTEM or 'sociocultural anthropology' in order to avoid the implications either of cultural or social determinism.

social articulation. This term may have two different senses: it is sometimes employed as an equivalent to INTEGRATION or COHESION, while in Marxist and neo-Marxist writings it refers to the ARTICULATION OF MODES OF PRODUCTION.

social change. *See* CHANGE.

social class. *See* CLASS.

social cohesion. *See* COHESION.

social contract. A concept found in the political theories of LOCKE, HOBBES and ROUSSEAU among others, and with characteristics which vary considerably from author to author. It may be portrayed as an actual historical event or as a desirable state of affairs. It is linked to INDIVIDUALIST theories of the STATE which see the state as the result of the voluntary abdication of certain rights or decision-making processes by individuals in favour of the state, which offers them in return greater physical security and economic and social organization. Social contract theories of the state are opposed both by conflict and class theories and by DURKHEIMIAN and other FUNCTIONALIST theories.

social control. A term sometimes used very widely to refer to all types of forces and constraints which induce conformity to norms and customs in human society. In this sense it is virtually synonymous with social order or SOCIAL ORGANIZATION, since any cultural pattern or code as well as any social institution may be regarded as exercising some form of control by the very fact of its existence as a formalized or codified entity apart from the social ACTOR. The term is also employed in a more restricted sense to refer to the mechanisms of CONFLICT management and the legal system of a society, including informal SANCTIONS as well as formal legal institutions. The study of mechanisms of social control in anthropology has generally employed the term in the broader sense, as an aspect of many different kinds of social institution and cultural code. Thus the anthropological study of social control often includes the analysis of RELIGIOUS and IDEOLOGICAL systems, as in the classic anthropological studies of WITCHCRAFT as a mechanism for regulating deviance and ensuring conformity. Similarly, kinship systems and other areas of social organization such as the educational system may be examined in terms of the coercive or restraining effect which they exercise on members of the group.

The study of social control in FUNCTIONALIST anthropology tended to emphasize – as did DURKHEIM in his theories of deviance and social organization – the pressure to conform as an expression of the interest of the collectivity. Conflict theorists, ACTION THEORISTS and Marxist theorists have been prominent in challenging this emphasis, pointing out that often mechanisms of social control which are presented by a dominant group as being in the interests of all may in fact be acting to preserve the interests of an elite group or a specific social class. It is therefore important to examine critically the ideological underpinnings of social control in terms of the system of political or class relations in the society under study.

Social Darwinism. This term originated with SPENCER (1876) who argued for the application of Darwinian theories of natural selection to the interpetation of human social EVOLUTION. It has subsequently been applied to other theories which employ Darwinian biological evolutionary principles to the analysis of human society. The term is almost always employed as a pejorative one, implying the crude misapplication of biological theory without taking into account the historical, social and cultural dimensions of the organization of human populations. (*See* SOCIOBIOLOGY.)

social differentiation. *See* DIVISION OF LABOUR.

social fact. A concept which formed part of DURKHEIM's sociological and anthropological theory. It refers to the Durkheimian postulate that the social should be explained in terms of the social and not reduced to another level of explanation such as the psychological or the environmental, since social facts have an independent existence and constitute an analytically independent level of reality. This doctrine was widely accepted in the STRUCTURAL FUNCTIONALIST tradition of British social anthropology, and this acceptance led to a failure to explore the interrelations of different dimensions of human behaviour (the biological, the ecological, the psychological and the sociocultural). The philosophical and theoretical implications of this sociological determinism have however come to be increasingly questioned in modern anthropology.

social formation, socioeconomic formation. In Marxist thought, the type of social organization characteristic of a given MODE OF PRODUCTION.

social group. *See* GROUP.

social institution. *See* INSTITUTION.

social integration. *See* INTEGRATION.

socialism. Political philosophies or tendencies which are not always to be clearly distinguished from COMMUNISM. In Marxist thought, the terms 'socialism' and 'communism' are sometimes used interchangeably, and sometimes distinguished. When they are distinguished, 'socialism' is sometimes used to refer to pre-Marxist or non-Marxist political philosophies which are similar in some senses to Marxist 'scientific socialism', while at other times the distinction is based on that between stages of development towards communism. In this latter sense, socialism is an intermediate stage between CAPITALISM and communism, in which the MEANS OF PRODUCTION are taken into social or state ownership, thus creating the conditions for the future emergence of true communal ownership and the withering away of the

state. In its broad sense the term refers to
political philosophies, whether or not they
are classed as 'Marxist', which advocate
state control of the means of production and
the limitation of private property.

socialization. The process of learning to
become a member of society, including both
formal EDUCATION and the informal induc-
tion into social ROLES. In US anthropology
the term ENCULTURATION has been proposed as preferable to 'socialization', in
accordance with the predominant US emphasis on the concept of CULTURE rather
than that of SOCIETY. Studies of child rearing in cross-cultural perspective, and
studies of the correlation between socialization practices and sociocultural patterns,
have been an important element in CULTURE
AND PERSONALITY theory and in PSYCHO-
LOGICAL ANTHROPOLOGY. It should be
emphasized that socialization or enculturation (which actually refer to two aspects of a
single process of learning to participate in a
SOCIOCULTURAL SYSTEM) are not processes
which are confined only to childhood, but
continue throughout adult life as we learn to
adopt new roles and strategies in accordance
with our changing position and circumstances in society.

The nature of socialization processes have
sometimes been invoked by anthropologists
in order to explain phenomena such as the
SEXUAL DIVISION OF LABOUR or other features of sociocultural organization including
KINSHIP TERMINOLOGY (see EXTENSION OF
KINSHIP TERMS) and aspects of RITUAL and
SYMBOLIC systems. However, these interpretations should be treated with caution,
since they do not constitute true explanations of the phenomenon under study. A
child's process of learning of a system
already in existence cannot be held to
explain the origin or functions of that
system.

social mobility. See MOBILITY.

social morphology. In the works of DURK-
HEIM and MAUSS, the study of social
morphology was the study of the relationship between the principles of social organization and the physical distribution and
demographic characteristics of human populations. This tradition of research is carried

on within social anthropology and social
DEMOGRAPHY, and is also an important
influence in certain areas of the work of
LEVI-STRAUSS, where he traces the relationship between the underlying structural logic
of culture and the geographical and physical
expression of a social system.

social movement. A general term covering
political and religious movements, including
SECTS, CULTS and others with varying organizational and structural features. Social
movements are studied as part of social and
cultural CHANGE, both as responses to such
change and as conscious attempts to bring
about change. (See CARGO CULT; MESSIA-
NISM; MILLENARIANISM; REBELLION; REVI-
TALIZATION; REVOLUTION.)

social network. See NETWORK.

social organization. The notion of social
organization was not always clearly distinguished in anthropology from that of SOCIAL
STRUCTURE, until the works of FIRTH established the notion of social organization as a
distinct analytical level (1951). MALINOWSKI
had defined social organization in terms of
the purposive manner in which humans act
upon their environment in order to satisfy
their needs (1948), while RADCLIFFE-
BROWN conceived of social organization as
the arrangement of ROLES associated with
the STATUSES which constituted the social
structure (1952). Firth however criticized the
static and passive conception of role and
social organization implicit in STRUCTURAL
FUNCTIONALIST theory, and was thus a pioneer of ACTION THEORY in anthropology,
examining the dynamic aspects of social
interaction and the importance of choice,
decision and strategy.

Firth distinguished three levels of analysis:
social structure, function, and social organization. Social structure is the set of rules or
principles governing social action, while the
functional aspect is the manner in which
social relations serve individual or collective
ends. Social organization on the other hand
refers to the dynamic, situational and
decision-making, or strategic, aspect of
social relations. This is the domain which
according to Firth should be the principle
area of anthropological enquiry. As he
points out, individuals and groups are

rational decision-makers constantly faced with choices and alternatives in the pursuit of their ends or purposes, and often thrown into conflict or competition with other such groups or persons. The structural functionalist notion of individuals and groups as passively receiving or acting out social roles thus fails to take into account the active and strategic nature of human social action, and the existence of conflicting interests and competitive interactions. All these dimensions have been explored within the field of action theory, which Firth's writing greatly influenced.

social stratification. *See* STRATIFICATION.

social structure. A concept widely used in anthropology, but without a universally accepted definition. In general it is employed to refer to those features of SOCIAL ORGANIZATION including social INSTITUTIONS, ROLES, and STATUSES which ensure the continuity of patterns of behaviour and group relationships over time. 'Social structure' thus refers to the mechanisms which ensure social continuity or conservation, or social REPRODUCTION in Marxist terms. The term is associated in anthropology with the STRUCTURAL FUNCTIONALIST theories of RADCLIFFE-BROWN (1952) and other British social anthropologists, and for this reason is avoided by most anthropologists outside this theoretical tradition because of its implications of a static and ahistorical view of social systems. The structural functionalist approach has often been criticized for assuming that social systems are relatively unchanging and monolithic sets of norms, roles and statuses which the individual passively receives or acts out, and it is consequently felt that the concept of social structure implies both a static conception of society and a sociological determinism which have been increasingly questioned in modern anthropology.

STRUCTURALIST theory in the tradition of LEVI-STRAUSS has also generated extensive criticism of the structural functionalist notion of social structure. Levi-Strauss himself has argued against the empiricist conception of structure as something which is to be observed or abstracted from actual behaviour on the ground. Instead, he argues, the structure of society is to be understood as a series of underlying principles which govern the empirical expression of social systems.

social system. Used generally to describe the orderly and self-perpetuating nature of social relations. A social system may thus be conceived of as a set of ordered relations within or between human groups or communities which tends to perpetuate itself over time. The notion of social system is however not a static one (as that of SOCIAL STRUCTURE is), but implies the possibility that social systems also adapt and evolve over time as a response to internal or external changes and contradictions. The delimitation of a 'social system' by attempting to define the boundaries of a social unit may however pose problems, since interactions and influences often cut across any arbitrary division which we may establish.

society. A term that may have two distinct meanings: that of 'a society' and that of 'society in general'. In the general sense it is synonymous with SOCIAL ORGANIZATION or SOCIAL STRUCTURE, while in its individual sense it is synonymous with SOCIAL SYSTEM. There are as many problems in defining 'a society' as a discrete analytical unit, as there are in defining a CULTURE. A society is generally conceived of as a human group which is relatively large, relatively independent or self-perpetuating in demographic terms, and which is relatively autonomous in its organization of social relations. But it is the relativity of each society's autonomy, independence and self-perpetuating nature which is the crucial factor, and the distinction of one society from another is often arbitrary. It is important in anthropology not to allow these arbitrary divisions to distort our vision of systems of local, regional, national and international social relations. This is precisely what occurred in British social anthropology in the STRUCTURAL FUNCTIONALIST tradition, where the search for the reconstruction of stable and autonomous traditional social structures led to the confusion of analytical levels and the use of local level explanations to account for phenomena which are the product of the interaction of local systems with complex structures of COLONIAL and neo-colonial dependence (*see* DEPENDENCY; WORLD SYSTEMS). A parallel analytical confusion occurred as a result of the US CULTURAL DETERMINIST orientation in cultural anthropology. (*See* CRITICAL ANTHROPOLOGY; MARXIST ANTHROPOLOGY.)

sociobiology. Defined by E.O. Wilson (1975) as dealing with the biological basis of social behaviour. The classic problem which it addresses is that of the mechanisms by which a behaviour may evolve genetically in spite of the fact that it is disadvantageous to the individual engaging in it: that is, the problem of the EVOLUTION of altruistic behaviour. Models for the explanation of this phenomenon fall into the general categories of group selection and kin selection. Theories of kin selection or 'kin altruism' examine the conditions under which natural selection may favour the increase of genes influencing altruistic behaviour, as when (for example) self-sacrificing behaviour favours the survival not of the individual but of his kin, thereby increasing the chances of survival of the gene linked to that behaviour. The Darwinian notion of fitness is therefore modified, introducing the concept of 'inclusive fitness': the individual's genotype and behaviour in the context of that of his neighbours. Theories of group selection argue that among populations with small breeding rates genetic evolution may affect the incidence of socially advantageous traits, thus influencing cultural evolution.

One major problem involved in the application of these theories to the evolution of culture and social behaviour is that they take no account of learned behaviour or cultural transmission, nor of the complexity of human motivation. As Sahlins has pointed out (1976), the use of maximization (cost-benefit) models of human behaviour is not a legitimate extrapolation from genetic concepts of 'fitness maximization'. In other words, individuals do not strive to maximize 'fitness' or reproduction, but are influenced by a wide range of culturally conditioned goals and values in their behaviour. Major difficulties are therefore involved in attempting to use sociobiological models to explain nongenetic (cultural) evolution. (*See* CULTURAL ECOLOGY; PHYSICAL ANTHROPOLOGY.)

sociocultural system. A term adopted as an alternative to 'social system' or 'cultural system' by those anthropologists who wish to avoid sociological or CULTURAL DETERMINISM. The use of the term implies that it is impossible to separate or give priority to either the social or the cultural aspect of human organization. (*See* CULTURE; SOCIETY.)

sociolinguistics. Narrowly defined, this is the study of how a person's speech conveys social information. In this narrow sense sociolinguistics studies the way in which linguistic variables correlate with socioeconomic ones. More broadly, the field includes theories of social INTERACTION concerned with the way in which social reality is constructed and conveyed through communicative behaviour. In this sense it is closely linked to the anthropological study of the ethnography of COMMUNICATION. (*See* ETHNOMETHODOLOGY; LINGUISTICS AND ANTHROPOLOGY.)

sociological paternity, sociological parents. The concept of sociological paternity was originated by MALINOWSKI in his discussion of the Trobriand Islanders' beliefs about CONCEPTION (1922). Since the Trobriand Islanders are a people who deny (at the level of dogma) that copulation is the cause of pregnancy, Malinowski's discussion of sociological paternity is as Leach points out (1959), somewhat confused. Malinowski introduces the concept of sociological paternity to describe the universal sociological recognition of the role of the father, while at the same time depicting a community where it is precisely this sociological recognition which is denied. However the term 'sociological parents' in general anthropological use refers to socially recognized parents (*pater* and *mater*) as opposed to physiological parents (*genitor* and *genetrix*). It is through socially recognized parents that kinship relations from the child to the wider community are traced, even though they may not be the actual physiological parents.

sociology. The science or study of society. The term was coined by COMTE and developed by DURKHEIM who proposed the study of SOCIAL FACTS as the central concern of the discipline. Durkheim did not distinguish sociology from anthropology, though this distinction was to emerge in British and US social scientific circles as the two disciplines developed and drew upon different theoretical, methodological and empirical sources. It was generally considered that sociology was concerned with the study of modern industrial society, employing the methods of analysis and investigation appropriate to large-scale populations (surveys, statistical methods, and so on) while anthropology was concerned with the study of PRIMITIVE, small-scale or FOLK societies and cultures, and was characterized by its HOLISTIC approach and the use of methods appropriate to small populations such as PARTICIPANT OBSERVATION.

In modern sociology and anthropology however there is considerable exchange of ideas between the disciplines, and each discipline has enriched its theoretical and methodological resources by drawing upon the other. Anthropology has also rejected the conventional classification of its subject matter in terms of COMMUNITY STUDIES or the study of 'primitive' culture, and has increasingly turned its attention to problems previously considered to be the province of sociology and to macro-analysis of the historical and social processes affecting local social units. These developments are particularly notable in the field of APPLIED ANTHROPOLOGY, which is often indistinguishable from sociology, and in the application of theories of DEPENDENCY, WORLD SYSTEMS and MARXIST analyses to the problems of DEVELOPMENT and COLONIAL and neo-colonial power structures.

sodality. Types of ASSOCIATION which exist to perform a specific function or special purpose, including such groupings as AGE SETS, secret societies, professional associations etc.

solidarity. Solidarity, or social solidarity, is an important concept in the works of DURKHEIM and other anthropologists within the FUNCTIONALIST and STRUCTURAL FUNCTIONALIST tradition influenced by him. It refers to states of or tendencies towards union and community between members of a given society. Social solidarity is accorded much importance in the Durkheimian theory of RITUAL and RELIGION, and it is interesting to note that although Durkheim's theory of SOCIAL FACTS and their autonomy denies the validity of psychological or other types of

reductionist explanation of social organization, in his emphasis on social solidarity Durkheim is in fact introducing a number of unacknowledged or implicit assumptions of a sociopsychological nature. The concept of social solidarity implies an emotional and VALUE commitment to symbols of common identity and shared culture. In modern anthropology the importance of social solidarity has been more critically assessed, as it is recognized that there is in practice a wide range of variation in individual attitudes, values and emotional commitment towards communal ritual and symbolic expressions. Similarly, we should be aware not only of the strategic manipulation of symbols of social solidarity by individuals and groups, but also of the extent to which these may serve to justify or maintain the position of a dominant group in society (or a dominant class) which monopolizes the control over ritual expressions in the name of the group as a whole.

In Durkheim's theory of the DIVISION OF LABOUR the concept of solidarity recurs in his distinction between two major types of social solidarity: MECHANICAL and organic.

sorcery. *See* WITCHCRAFT.

sororal polygyny. A form of POLYGYNY where the co-wives are sisters.

sororate. A custom by which on the death of a woman her husband is required or has the right to marry her sister. (*See* LEVIRATE; MARRIAGE.)

soul. The idea of the soul is found in all human cultures, though in widely different forms. In general, the soul is regarded as the principle of life or animation which inhabits the body. Souls may be single or multiple, and may take different guises if and when they are separated from the body. Such separation or soul loss is frequently believed to occur during sleep (thus causing dream experiences), during illness, or during ALTERED STATES OF CONSCIOUSNESS or trance. Where there are multiple souls, these may perform different functions in the animation of the body or the psychological and cognitive activities of the individual, and they may also have different destinations or destinies after the death of the individual. The anthropological study of beliefs and statements about the soul has focused on the manner in which they directly or indirectly reveal beliefs or philosophies of individual spiritual identity and destiny, as well as the manner in which they copy or reverse features of normal human life and social structure. (*See* ANIMISM; DEATH; RELIGION.)

Southall, Aidan William (1911–). British social anthropologist whose major theoretical focus was the study of urban anthropology and social CHANGE in East Africa and Malagasy. His works include *Urban Anthropology* (1973).

space. The cultural conception and social use of space, like that of TIME, have been the focus of wide-ranging areas of anthropological enquiry from SOCIAL MORPHOLOGY and cultural ecology to studies of RITUAL, SYMBOLISM, ETHNOPHILOSOPHY and the relatively new field of PROXEMICS. Anthropological studies of space have therefore explored a number of different fields, including the manner in which the use and distribution of space reflects features of social structure, the manner in which it reflects philosophical or cosmological conceptions, its ecological implications, and finally the manner in which space is manipulated intendedly or unintendedly for the purposes of communication. (*See* VISUAL ANTHROPOLOGY.)

species-specific. The concept of species-specific or species-characteristic behaviour is preferred in modern ETHOLOGY to that of INSTINCT. Species-specific behaviour is that which is shared by the majority of members of a species, but is nonetheless subject to modification to some extent by learning or experience.

speech. Actual linguistic behaviour, as opposed to LANGUAGE, the underlying rules or patterns which govern this behaviour.

speech community. A group of persons who share a common code or codes for communication and a common set of rules as to how these codes are to be applied. Such a community need not be monolingual, but may possess a series of languages or variants (dialects or codes) which have generally agreed appropriate contexts and forms of use. Such a speech community may not be easy to identify in practice, since like a CULTURE or a SOCIETY it may be an arbitrary imposition on a system where communication cross-cuts the boundaries which we establish for the purpose of our analysis.

Spencer, Herbert (1820–1903). British social theorist whose ideas regarding 'universal evolution' predated those of Darwin in the field of natural history. Spencer's theory embraced inorganic, organic and superorganic evolution, and he proposed that in all these fields the dominant trend was from homogeneity to heterogeneity and from simpler to more differentiated or complex forms. In his *Principles of Sociology* (1876–96) he used the organic analogy to explain social organization and social evolution. He seized on Darwin's ideas when these were publicized, coining the term 'survival of the fittest' and becoming the founder of SOCIAL DARWINISM which became an ideological support for laissez-faire economics and Victorian liberal individualist social policy.

spheres of exchange. Discrete spheres within which goods and/or services are freely exchangeable, but between which there exist no measures or means of exchange. Such spheres of exchange, or mechanisms to insulate one area of economic activity from another, are commonly found in economies where market exchange is absent or only partially established and where there is no general purpose MONEY. Barth suggests (1966) that this concept, formulated by Bohannan and Dalton in their study of African economies (1965), should be widened to that of 'economic spheres', to include not only exchange relations but all forms of circulation and transformation of value, including inheritance, for example. The notion of spheres of exchange in traditional economies is similar to Salisbury's concept of the 'nexus of economic activity' (1962), which he regards as constituting a functional mechanism for the equitable distribution of resources and power while maintaining social statuses, thereby permitting economic exchanges but preventing them from disrupting the sociopolitical power structure. (*See* ECONOMIC ANTHROPOLOGY.)

spirit. This term may be used as a synonym for SOUL, or in more general terms to refer to supernatural entities – as in Tylor's classic definition of RELIGION as the 'belief in spiritual beings' (1871).

spirit possession. *See* POSSESSION.

spiritualism. Religious and magico-religious beliefs and practices concerned with contact between living human beings and the spirits or ghosts of the dead. The spirits, which are contacted by means of a medium, may be invoked in order to provide guidance and advice or for the purposes of healing. (*See* POSSESSION.)

state. In anthropology the state is usually seen as a stage of sociopolitical EVOLUTION characterized by the existence of a centralized government which has a monopoly on the legitimate use of force by way of conducting public affairs within a specified territory. Definitions of the state in political theory vary widely and have produced much contention and debate, reflecting different political philosophies and the manner in which these conceive of the coercive aspects of state organization as expressions of class domination or as expressions of the collective good or 'sovereign will'. These differences are also evident in the different theories of the origin of the state. The reasons for the emergence of states and the related phenomena of URBANISM and CIVILIZATION from ACEPHALOUS or stateless societies have thus been the focus of considerable debate, both in terms of the evaluation of empirical evidence and the conceptual priority to be accorded to factors such as the ecological, the military, the technological (such as IRRIGATION), the political or the economic.

Anthropologists and archeologists examining the cases of 'pristine' state formation in the Near East, India, China, Mesoamerica and Peru and the secondary state formations which have subsequently occurred have described a set of common recurring features, about which however there is no general agreement as to analytical priorities. These common features include population increases in numbers and density, which are related to increased agricultural production and often to new agricultural technology. The increased population is grouped together in larger communities (towns and eventually cities). At the same time, social and political developments include a more clearly defined division of labour with increasing numbers of specialists, the rise of social STRATIFICATION and social classes, and the emergence of centralized political authorities. Some early states have been characterized as predominantly theocratic, that is to say dominated by priestly control and by the emergence of temples and religious centres as the focus of urban life, while others are predominantly military in character. Most however present a combination of theocratic and militaristic elements, and the interrelations between military and religious power withing the state, and their evolution over time are in themselves important fields of study.

Service (1975) divides theories of state formation in anthropology into two types: conflict theories and integrative theories. Conflict theories, such as those of M.H. Fried (1967), stress the importance of social stratification and the manner in which the state apparatus permits a rising social class to obtain and maintain a dominant position. The political and religious structure of the state is therefore seen as basically a repressive one. Integrative theories on the other hand stress the fact that submission to a centralized authority also brings benefits in terms of the overall growth and increasing complexity of society as a whole. In fact both these approaches have an element of truth, and we should analyse state formation both in terms of its progressive nature in the sense that it integrated larger and more complex social systems, and in its repressive nature in the sense that the cost of this advance was paid primarily by the agricultural producer while the benefits were reaped primarily by the ruling class or the military, theocratic or administrative elite.

Anthropologists and social scientists in general have also addressed themselves to the problem of the stability of state formations in different historical and geographical contexts. Marx had proposed the concept of the ASIATIC MODE OF PRODUCTION to account for the historical stability of many early states which did not follow the European model of development from SLAVERY through FEUDALISM to CAPITALISM but continued instead to reproduce themselves over time without fundamental structural change. The concept of the Asiatic mode of production has however been a controversial one, and modern anthropologists within the Marxist tradition have challenged the assertion that productive forces did not develop in 'Asiatic' type systems, pointing to different kinds of structural instability and change within non-European states, which if not interrupted by the expansion of European IMPERIALISM and COLONIALISM, would have led to the transformation of these systems over time.

statistical model. *See* MECHANICAL/STATISTICAL MODEL.

statistics in sociocultural anthropology. Prior to 1950, the use of statistics in sociocultural anthropology was largely restricted to CROSS-CULTURAL COMPARISON and there was an informal professional resistance to extensive quantification. While numerical data was sometimes collected in fieldwork, analyses of such data rarely went beyond tabular presentations and calculations of means and medians.

In the 1950s and 1960s statistical analyses of field data became more common. Whereas most ethnographers in the earlier part of the century tried to provide HOLISTIC descriptions of many aspects of culture, by the middle of the century research tended to be problem-oriented, emphasizing extensive examinations of particular topics and systematic collection and analysis of quantitative data. Although the statistics used in the 1950s and 1960s tended to be rather simple bivariate tests of significance and measures of association, in recent years computer packages have allowed even anthropologists with limited statistical expertise to use more complex analytic methods such as multiple regression, path analysis and multidimensional scaling.

The types of data collected by sociocultural anthropologists frequently pose problems for statistical analysis. Samples are often too small and causal connections between numerous possibly important variables can be complex. The extent of quantification that is possible for many important

variables is limited. P. and G. Pelto's excellent book on research methods (1978) and Thomas' sensible though unfortunately error-ridden text (1973) discuss the use of bivariate statistics in spite of these problems. Chibnik (1985) has examined multivariate statistical analysis by anthropologists.

The growing interest in intracultural variation and systematic research design, an increased demand for rigour by funding agencies and scholarly journals, and the availability of easily used computer packages all make it likely that sociocultural anthropologists will use statistics more in the future than they do now. The use of bivariate statistical methods to analyse data collected in the field is already routine in North America, if not elsewhere, and the application of multivariate methods is becoming more common. Cross-cultural studies now almost always include statistical analysis.

The eclectic methodology employed by sociocultural anthropologists makes it unlikely that they will ever use statistical methods as much as their colleagues in psychology and sociology. The heavy reliance by psychologists on laboratory experiments and by many sociologists on mass surveys has necessitated extensive and sophisticated use of statistical methods in those fields. Sociocultural anthropologists rarely experiment and use surveys as only one of many research tools. The use of such qualitative methods as case studies and life histories is one way in which sociocultural anthropology is distinct from other social sciences. Almost all sociocultural anthropologists, including those most committed to the use of statistical methods, regard qualitative data analytical procedures as essential. (*See* COMPUTERS IN SOCIOCULTURAL ANTHROPOLOGY; MATHEMATICAL MODELS IN SOCIOCULTURAL ANTHROPOLOGY.)

status. Popularly employed as a synonym for PRESTIGE, but in sociological and anthropological usage it can also mean a position in a SOCIAL STRUCTURE. The fact that these positions are normally arranged in a hierarchical fashion links the two senses of the term. In ROLE theory the distinction between status and role is that between a social position and the behaviour expected of its incumbent. (*See* STRATIFICATION.)

status and contract. An EVOLUTIONARY scheme proposed by MAINE (1861), who argued that primitive societies and primitive legal systems were largely based on status (especially kin status) while modern ones were largely based on contract. (*See* LAW, ANTHROPOLOGY OF.)

stem family. A term coined by Frederic LePlay (1855) to refer to a family form predominating among prosperous landholding rural peoples in parts of Europe. Rights to land or property are handed down from generation to generation and each inheritor becomes the focus for the family organization in that generation.

stem kindred. A term used by W. Davenport (1959) to denote a type of KINDRED organization in which Ego-based personal kindreds coincide with rules of inheritance which make one individual the principal inheritor of corporate property. This individual thus becomes the node around which the kindred is organized. There is thus a genealogical line of title-holders or heirs, each surrounded by his personal kindred. Irish peasant communities typically followed this pattern.

stereotype. An image of or attitude towards persons or groups which is based not on observation and experience but on preconceived ideas. Such stereotypes are often analysed as part of the symbolism of social and group relations, since they both reflect and perpetuate social divisions. Negative stereotypes of the attributes or characteristics of a particular group or category are an important constituent part of different types of DISCRIMINATION and PREJUDICE, including racial, ethnic, gender and class prejudice. In real social interaction among members of stereotyped categories we may perceive both the interaction between mutual stereotypes and the manner in which individuals strategically manipulate, comment upon or negotiate aspects of stereotyped ROLES.

Steward, Julian (1902–72). US cultural anthropologist who was extremely influential in the development of EVOLUTIONARY and ecological theory in modern cultural anthropology. One of his major theoretical contributions was the concept of LEVELS OF SOCIOCULTURAL INTEGRATION. Major works include *The Economic and Social Basis of Primitive Bands* (1936), *Theory of Culture Change* (1957); he also edited *Handbook of South American Indians* (1946–50).

stigma. In the theory of DEVIANCE developed by the sociologist I. Goffman (1967), stigma is an important element in the process of labelling of deviants. It is the identification of an individual as deficient, marginal or in some way excluded from full and normal participation in social life. (*See* ROLE.)

strategy. *See* ADAPTIVE STRATEGY.

stratification. The systematic ranking of persons into categories, particularly in STATE societies where such stratification is institutionalized and is referred to as 'social stratification'. Social stratification both arises from and gives rise to social inequality, and the study of social stratification is linked to those of POLITICAL ANTHROPOLOGY and POWER in cross-cultural perspective. G.D. Berreman suggests (1981) that out of the 'differentiation' of persons, which is a natural and universal phenomenon, inequality, or the social evaluation of differences, arises. The behavioural expression of inequality he terms 'dominance' and he proposes that the combination of inequality and dominance should be called 'social inequality'. In egalitarian or unranked societies the DIVISION OF LABOUR and the distribution of status is based on age, sex and personal attributes. Dominance and status in these groups are often negotiable and contextual. In ranked or inegalitarian societies, however, inequality is institutionalized and embedded in a hierarchy of statuses linked to ranked social entities which transcend individual differences of ability or circumstantial factors. In CHIEFDOMS and pre-state agricultural or pastoral societies ranking may be based on kinship or on specialized roles such as warrior or priest. In state societies ranking is based on social stratification, in which all members of society are ranked according to non-kin characteristics which are employed in turn to allocate access to vital resources (*see* CLASS). The dimensions of social stratification, according to Weber's classic definition, are class, status and power, and all three factors tend to be closely correlated. Status is distinguished from class, according to Weber's formulation, in that status refers to social honour or privilege while class is defined by economic position.

The distinction between ACHIEVED AND ASCRIBED STATUS has proved of some utility in anthropology, though it has been recognized that as a distinction of social types it is overly simplistic. Nevertheless there is a general contrast between the rigid birth-ascribed stratification systems such as the CASTE system or institutionalized RACISM (*see* APARTHEID) and the more open or flexible class based system. However the class system too tends towards status ascription and the naturalization or SACRALIZATION of social divisions by ideologies of natural or divine privilege. Modern studies of caste systems have similarly shown that they include a considerable degree of status negotiation and achievement, often on a group rather than individual basis. Between the caste and class systems generally taken as examples of extreme cases of status ascription and achievement, there are also 'intermediate' types such as the ESTATE system, which ascribes status according to the structural position defined by a legal system and relating to land, office, title, and so on. Berreman suggests a further category: that of ethnic systems, where there are ranked and competing social groups based on cultural heritage.

As far as the origin of social stratification is concerned, it has conventionally been argued that it was related to SURPLUS production, though the difficulty in defining surplus production or what constitutes production over and above SUBSISTENCE level makes this argument difficult to demonstrate. M. Sahlins (1972) and other neo-Marxists have argued that social stratification creates surplus production rather than vice versa, since stratification activates a potential surplus inherent in the productive system. The origin of social stratification is thus seen as the appropriation of domestic production for use outside the household (*see* DOMESTIC MODE OF PRODUCTION). Another approach explains stratification as the product of increasing population size and

density, which make stratified social relations both necessary and feasible. M. Harris (1979) points to the importance of shifts in productive technology (from HUNTING AND GATHERING to SWIDDEN AGRICULTURE to AGRICULTURE) which bring together more people on less land and also increase the workload, thus creating the basis for social stratification.

There are different anthropological approaches to stratification in pre-industrial societies. Some authors seek to identify proto-class relations while others emphasize the lack of clear patterns of stratification, some investigate rank and hierarchy within the community while others explore the position of the community *vis-à-vis* the outside world. MARXIST ANTHROPOLOGY, DEPENDENCY and WORLD SYSTEMS theories have in recent years contributed more sophisticated perspectives on stratification both inside and outside the local community.

structural functionalism. A school of anthropological analysis associated primarily with British social anthropology and with the theoretical influence of RADCLIFFE-BROWN. Other social anthropologists such as MALINOWSKI, FORTES, EVANS-PRITCHARD, FIRTH and GLUCKMAN have also been grouped together as members of the 'structural functionalist' school, though in fact the diversity in theoretical positions among these writers is considerable, and all diverged from the approach of Radcliffe-Brown in important ways. In Radcliffe-Brown's conception (1952), structure was primarily SOCIAL STRUCTURE or the network of social relations and INSTITUTIONS which constituted the enduring framework of society. Function, on the other hand, was the way in which these social relations and institutions contributed to the stable and harmonious functioning of a society conceived of as a self-perpetuating whole.

In response to the basically static and ahistorical nature of Radcliffe-Brown's conception of structure and function, which was unable to deal either with internal conflict or social change, theorists within the structural functionalist tradition itself attempted to modify the conceptual scheme, while those outside it (such as exponents of ACTION THEORY and MARXIST ANTHROPOLOGY) rejected the structural functionalist model in favour of more dynamic or historically sensitive theoretical approaches. The paradox of structural functionalist theory is that this theoretical school which scarcely even existed, since from its origin it was beset by differences and critiques, came to have such a considerable influence on British social anthropology that it has often been termed 'monolithic'. The explanation for this and the parallel ahistoricism of US cultural anthropology during the same period may be in part, as CRITICAL ANTHROPOLOGY has shown, the reluctance of anthropology to come to terms with the ideological and political implications of the historical analysis of Third World communities and their relations with the West.

structuralism. An intellectual movement which began in linguistics and embraces areas as diverse as anthropology, philosophy and literary criticism. In linguistics, structuralism is associated with the pioneering works of SAUSSURE (1916) and Jakobson, and Saussure is regarded as the leader of a revolution in linguistics which established the central concern of the discipline as the study of language as a system of signs and shifted the focus from the study of 'surface structures' to that of DEEP STRUCTURES or underlying structural principles. In the anthropological structuralism pioneered by LEVI-STRAUSS (1963) the linguistic model has been taken as a basis for the understanding of human culture and the human mind. Levi-Strauss proposes that culture is to be understood as a surface phenomenon which reveals the universal human tendency to order and classify perceived phenomena and experience. While the surface phenomena vary, the underlying ordering principles are the same. From the analysis of KINSHIP and MARRIAGE systems in his early works, Levi-Strauss has increasingly shifted towards the analysis of MYTH and SYMBOLISM as domains in which the free operation of the mind is more easily examined.

As is the case also in structural linguistics, the principle of BINARY OPPOSITIONS is of great importance in structural anthropology. It is argued that just as sound systems function in terms of systems of contrasts, so too do mental and cultural systems. No term is therefore to be understood in isolation, but instead as part of a contrasting system built up from elementary or binary oppositions. Typical binary oppositions regarded by Levi-Strauss as universal elements in the cultural vocabulary include right-left, raw-cooked, nature-culture, centre-periphery, and man-woman. He makes no radical distinction between behavioural systems (social institutions, ritual) and ideational ones (myth, symbolism). According to his theory, each may be a manner of commenting upon or resolving contradictions inherent in the other. However his works are perhaps contradictory in this sense, since at some moments he asserts his adherence to the Marxist doctrine of the primacy of infrastructures, while reserving the right to devote his attention to the analysis of the formation and transformation of superstructures.

Structuralism has been immensely influential, especially in the analysis of kinship and marriage and that of myth and symbolism, which as we have seen have been the main areas of analysis pioneered by Levi-Strauss. However we have not seen the general application of structuralist principles in other fields (for example in economic or political anthropology) which would be necessary in order to substantiate the claim that structuralism constitutes a general science of communication and sociocultural behaviour. Criticisms of structuralist theory have focused on its static and essentially ahistorical nature, suggesting the need to modify the concept of structure to take into account not only the active role of the individual in creating sociocultural systems, but also the historical and dynamic nature of such systems. Many anthropologists accordingly incorporate elements of structuralist methodology for the study of the underlying logic of communicative or symbol systems, without necessarily embracing all of the implications of the Levi-Straussian conception of structure. At the same time, it is important to recognize that many of the criticisms of Levi-Strauss's theories are anticipated or dealt with in his own works, though ultimately without an overall synthesis which confronts all their contradictions and implications.

structure. *See* SOCIAL STRUCTURE; STRUCTURALISM.

subculture. A group culture which diverges in part from the dominant culture of the wider society. If it is characterized by systematic opposition to dominant cultural values it may be termed a COUNTER-CULTURE.

subincision. The cutting of the penis along the underside. This form of genital mutilation may occur together with CIRCUMCISION or alone. (*See* INITIATION.)

subsistence. The notion of subsistence, and those of 'subsistence economy' or 'subsistence agriculture' are frequently employed, yet often without sufficient awareness of the theoretical difficulties involved in defining subsistence or SURPLUS. The use of the term implies that the economy or technological system under question is limited to the satisfaction of basic or primary needs of the producers, though in order to define these primary needs we must take into account the social and cultural criteria which enter into the definition of a minimal level of consumption for each individual or family. As ECONOMIC ANTHROPOLOGY has shown, there is no such thing as a true subsistence economy, since in every type of economic system there is surplus production over and above immediate family needs which may be devoted to ritual or prestige consumption, to communal use or for exchange. This surplus production serves in part to insure the group against temporary productive difficulties affecting some or all of its members, and constitutes also a vital element in the creation and expression of social and political relationship as well as in many cases in the acting out of religious, ceremonial and ritual obligations.

substantivism. *See* FORMALISM/SUBSTANTIVISM; ECONOMIC ANTHROPOLOGY.

suicide. Anthropological studies of suicide have been influenced profoundly by DURKHEIM's pioneering study (1897), which distinguished two types of suicide: the altruistic and the anomic. The former, which is more common in traditional societies, is an expression of commitment to social and cultural norms, since it represents the reaction of the individual in the face of strong social pressures. Suicide may be in these terms a prescribed or expected response to extreme situations of shame, social disapproval, bereavement, defeat in war, and so on. Anomic suicide, on the other hand, is characteristic of modern society and represents the response of an individual who is so poorly integrated into his or her culture and its norms that he or she feels that 'life has no meaning' and therefore commits suicide. (*See* ANOMIE.)

Sumner, William Graham (1840–1910). US social theorist who advocated the application of the principles of natural selection and survival of the fittest to human society (SOCIAL DARWINISM). Sumner's major work of influence in anthropology is *Folkways* (1906) which is a comparative study of customs and mores in the light of his evolutionary theory of society. He popularized the term ETHNOCENTRISM.

supernatural. *See* RELIGION.

superorganic. The superorganic view of CULTURE (or of SOCIETY) which argues that cultural or social phenomena should be explained in terms of cultural or social theories, and not reduced to other levels of explanation such as the psychological or the ecological. This view, which was first put forward by DURKHEIM (*see* SOCIAL FACT) was also adopted by US cultural anthropologists such as KROEBER, LOWIE and WHITE and in British social anthropology by the STRUCTURAL FUNCTIONALIST school. One critique of the superorganic theory argues that since cultural phenomena actually occur in association with other types of phenomena such as the psychological or the ecological, it is therefore untenable to separate them analytically. This argument has been advanced by some anthropologists who suggest that cultural phenomena do not have an independent existence and therefore cannot be studied as if they had. There is a risk involved in this view however in that it may lend itself to reductionism. Another critique associates superorganicism with CULTURAL DETERMINISM, though as D. Kaplan points out (1965) cultural explanations are not necessarily any more deterministic than any other kind of scientific explanation.

superstructure. In Marxist social theory there is an important analytical distinction between INFRASTRUCTURE or base and superstructure. The infrastructure is the economic base of society, and the superstructure the social relations and institutions which develop around this base and act to reproduce it. Much controversy surrounds the Marxist thesis of the determination 'in the last instance' of superstructure by infrastructure. (*See* MARXIST ANTHROPOLOGY.)

surface structure. *See* DEEP AND SURFACE STRUCTURE.

surplus. The concept of surplus in economics and ECONOMIC ANTHROPOLOGY is related to that of SUBSISTENCE, since surplus is generally defined as production over and above immediate subsistence needs. Like subsistence, the concept of surplus raises immediate theoretical difficulties, due to the relative nature of definitions of subsistence needs. Surplus production has often been cited as one of the root causes of social STRATIFICATION, URBANIZATION and the rise of social classes, the STATE and CIVILIZATION. However several authors have pointed to difficulties in this formulation, arguing that it is not the surplus which generates stratification, but stratification which generates surplus by activating an unrealized potential for surplus in the productive system. It should also be noted that the concept of surplus may lead us to assume that the producer 'does not need' what he exchanges or renders in tribute, thus disguising the obligatory or even coercive nature of some redistributive and market economies which extract from the producer goods which are not surplus to his or her requirements. The uncritical use of the term 'surplus production', like that of 'subsistence economy', leads us to fail to analyse the extremely complex mechanisms of political, social and economic dominance and dependency which act to maintain marginal or peasant producers in a relationship of unequal exchange with the dominant regional, national and international economic system.

In Marxist social theory the use of the term 'surplus' is related to Marx's concept of surplus value, which is the value of the labour extracted from the producer over and above that which is necessary to reproduce labour power itself (wages). This surplus value is appropriated by the class which owns or controls the means of production.

survival. In 19th- and early 20th-century EVOLUTIONARY theories of society, this concept was employed to refer to customs or traits which were regarded as leftovers from an earlier evolutionary stage (*see* ARCHAISM). The FUNCTIONALIST anthropologists led by MALINOWSKI challenged the use of this concept, arguing that all customs and features of a society or culture should be interpreted in terms of their contemporary meaning and function.

swidden agriculture/swidden horticulture. A form of cultivation, also referred to as 'slash and burn' or 'shifting' agriculture, characterized by the clearing and burning of existing vegetation (typically tropical forest) in order to plant. Such fields are cultivated for a brief period and then left to lie fallow for a longer period or abandoned altogether. This type of cultivation is generally associated with traditional societies of low population density in regions of low soil fertility such as the Amazon rainforest, though recent theorists have suggested that the system of shifting agriculture combined with HUNTING AND GATHERING strategies may in fact permit much greater population densities and a greater degree of sedentarism than was previously believed. In ecological terms, swidden cultivation is characterized by its high degree of integration into the natural tropical forest ecosystem, whose characteristics it conserves to a considerable extent. It has thus been described as a 'mimetic' system, with principles radically different from those of intensive agricultural strategies which act to transform totally the natural landscape. However it is the only ecologically viable agricultural strategy to have been developed thus far on a large scale in the tropical rainforest, and attempts to apply intensive agricultural techniques brought from other regions have generally been dismal failures, resulting only in the destruction of the ecological balance of the natural rainforest. National DEVELOPMENT strategies for tropical forest regions (such as those in Latin America) are usually beset by ethnocentric and centralistic prejudice against swidden cultivation and its practitioners, presenting the tropical forest region as virtually 'uninhabited'. As a result ETHNO-CIDAL and ecocidal policies are the rule.

symbolism, symbolic anthropology. The terms 'symbol' and 'symbolism' have been subject to widely varying uses and interpretations in anthropology, and those anthropologists who are linked together by a common concern for SEMIOTICS, symbolism or symbology by no means share a common theoretical orientation or even a common vocabulary. We may point to several different trends within the anthropological study of symbolism: the STRUCTURALIST approach pioneered by LEVI-STRAUSS, the 'symbolic anthropology' of D. Schneider (1970) which develops out of COGNITIVE ANTHROPOLOGY, the 'interpretative anthropology' practised by Geertz (1971), TURNER's focus on symbols as part of the social process (1967), to name but a few. The modern study of symbolism in anthropology also draws from diverse interdisciplinary sources including linguistics and sociolinguistics, microsociology, influenced by Goffman (1967), the study of folklore, literary criticism and semiotics or semiology.

A common interest in all these approaches however is a concern for meaning and COMMUNICATION. Thus Turner and others (M. Douglas (1966), for example) who advocate the study of symbols 'in action' centre on questions of the motivation of symbols and signs. This approach focuses on the natural relations between signs, symbols, the world and experience. Turner distinguishes between sign and symbol in that the former refers to indexical relations with the world while the latter refers to iconic relations with inner experience. The distinction between INDEX and ICON is thus used by Turner as equivalent to that between metonym and metaphor, where the former is a simple substitution and the latter is a complex representation. However the use of the terms index, icon, metonym and metaphor varies somewhat from author to author, which may cause considerable confusion if the particular usage is not specified.

The distinction between sign and symbol is a similar point of controversy. In C.S. Peirce's terminology, which is widely employed in semiotics, index, icon and symbol are all types of sign, the symbol being

distinguished from the others by the fact that the relationship between signifier and signified is purely arbitrary. Turner however distinguishes sign and symbol in terms of indexical and iconic relations: 'we master the world through signs...we master...ourselves through symbols'. A key characteristic of symbols for Turner is their 'motivated' nature or their link to natural and emotional meanings, in other words their non-arbitrariness. D. Sperber however (1975) criticizes Turner's criterion of 'motivation' as the distinguishing feature of symbols, and argues for the abolition of the separable category of symbolism, retaining only the cognitive and interpretative processes performed by various sign relations.

In general the Anglophone approach to the study of symbols has been, as Sperber points out, to emphasize the ACTOR rather than the message and the message rather than the code. This emphasis on performance and the neglect of competence has been modified to some extent since the critiques of STRUCTURAL FUNCTIONALISM have created general awareness of the need to study symbolic form as well as symbolic function, but is still a dominant trend in much British and US anthropology. Geertz has, for example, criticized Levi-Strauss' 'cerebral savage' and his 'cryptological' approach, since Levi-Strauss analyses symbols as closed structures and not as Geertz proposes as 'texts' built out of social materials. Geertz thus advocates (1971) the textual and interpretative approach which he terms the 'thick description' of culture as an 'acted document'. Like Turner, he argues that meaning comes from purpose and not from formal structures, and that the emphasis on internal relations among symbolic elements in such structures distracts from the proper object of enquiry which is the informal logic of actual life. Sperber argues on the contrary that this cannot replace the first order analysis of semiotic structures. In this he is in agreement with Sahlins (1981) who also points out that much of anthropology deals with the relationship between signs without first of all examining the constitution of symbolic order and meaning.

Sahlins also examines the issue of the relationship between symbolism in modern and traditional society. He argues that in bourgeois society the economic system does not escape symbolic determination as is sometimes asserted. It is rather that 'economic symbolism is structurally determining'. But not all cultures have this same arrangement of semiotic domains. Our own dominant symbolic grid creates notions and oppositions of nature/culture, work/play, expressive/practical, and so on, based on our own symbolically constituted practical interest in production. D. Schneider also argues (1970) against the received notion of the distinction between expressive and practical domains, a distinction which has shaped the anthropological interpretation of symbolism. He advocates the study of culture as a total system of meanings and symbols, rather than the accretion of isolated studies of cultural symbols. He also diverges from the sociological approach to symbolism, since he argues that symbolic systems should not be separated out into bits linked to aspects of social organization but rather should be studied as wholes.

BATESON's early formulations of the concept of culture as a mechanism for the generation and transmission of information (*see* CYBERNETICS) anticipated many of the concerns of modern symbol studies (1972). His emphasis on PLAY and his notion of METACOMMUNICATION have also been extremely influential. In modern symbol studies a new emphasis has emerged on play and creativity in symbolism and RITUAL, in which they are seen as activities through which humans expand and reorganize their consciousness. Turner also anticipates this development in his theory of symbolism as the key to access to the primal ground or creative impulse of culture which he terms 'communitas'.

symmetric alliance. *See* ASYMMETRIC/SYM-METRIC ALLIANCE.

sympathetic magic. *See* MAGIC.

synchronic. Studies, analyses or theoretical approaches may be said to be synchronic when they are characterized by the examination of data at a single moment in time or without regard for DIACHRONIC or HISTORICAL process.

syncretism. A term usually applied to religious phenomena or movements, though it may be applied to cultural CHANGE in general. Syncretism is the combination or blending of elements from different religious (or cultural) traditions. This is a general feature of the development of religious and cultural systems over time, as they absorb and reinterpret elements drawn from other traditions with which they are in contact. The term is however particularly employed to refer to situations of culture contact which generate religious systems which are a mixture of Christian and native or traditional beliefs and practices. It has therefore been extensively used as a description of the religious systems of colonial and post-colonial Africa, of Afro-American populations etc. The dynamic reinterpretation of Christian doctrine in terms of local beliefs and practices is one of the ways in which populations subject to missionizing within colonial and neo-colonial systems demonstrate their continuing cultural creativity, and may also become a way of expressing their political dissent. (*See* CULT; MILLENARIANISM; SECT.)

syntax. The rules by which morphemes (the smallest units of meaning in language) are permitted to be sequentially ordered. The study of the meaning (as opposed to the formal rules of ordering) of linguistic elements is called SEMANTICS.

systems analysis, systems theory. A system is a set of interconnected variables, change in any one of which will affect all the others. Systems theory is the thesis which holds that variables should not be analysed in isolation but rather for their interrelation as part of a system, and systems analysis is the study of the manner in which and degree to which each variable within a system affects the others under given conditions of internal or external instability or change. While anthropologists frequently employ some form of systems analysis or systems model in order to analyse their data, the theoretical implications of a systems approach are complex. The definitions of the boundaries of a given system are extremely problematic, since social and cultural systems are not closed but open ones, which affect and are affected by variables in what we may for any given analytical purpose define as the 'environment'. Similarly, the assumption of EQUILIBRIUM inherent in systems theory is extremely problematic for the study of sociocultural systems and sociocultural evolution. The key to the productive use of systems analysis models in anthropology is the recognition that such systems do not exist in reality but are analytical devices which we may impose in order to investigate our data more fruitfully.

T

taboo, tabu. Derived from the Polynesian *tapu* (or *tafoo*), and first described by Captain Cook in his account of the Polynesian customary AVOIDANCE of certain persons, places or objects. The original Polynesian term may be translated as SACRED, and implies the combination of ritual power and ritual danger. Subsequently the term was extended outside its original context to cover a wide variety of ritual avoidances or prohibitions in different ethnographic environments, including prohibitions on eating certain foods (*see also* TOTEMISM), on contact with certain kinsmen or persons in special ritual states, and also to the universal prohibition on INCEST. FREUD incorporated taboo as part of his psychoanalytical theory of human psychosocial development, and characterized it as a mixture of attraction or desire and repulsion or fear which reflected a primitive psychological conflict.

In modern anthropology the most influential treatment of taboo has been that of Mary Douglas (1966), who interprets different kinds of ritual prohibitions as the product of systems of CLASSIFICATION, which generate social, psychological and intellectual responses of rejection towards phenomena which cut across or threaten their classificatory order. However the modern study of SYMBOLISM and RITUAL does not attempt to retain taboo as a unitary concept, nor to seek a universal explanation of all the different forms of ritual avoidance which occur in different ethnographic contexts. Instead, each form of avoidance or prohibition is related to the symbolic and sociocultural context in which it occurs.

tabula rasa. Literally 'blank slate' in Latin; used to refer to theories of mental development or psychology which maintain that hereditary or inbuilt influences are minimal and that learning or experience is entirely responsible for shaping the development of the individual.

Tax, Sol (1907–). US cultural anthropologist who undertook research in Mesoamerica. He founded the journal *Current Anthropology*.

taxonomy. A CLASSIFICATORY scheme of objects or phenomena. The taxonomic paradigm has been of immense importance in modern linguistics, psychology and anthropology and has been used to model fields like language, KINSHIP and systems of classification of natural phenomena (*see* COGNITIVE ANTHROPOLOGY). The study of the classificatory principles of such schemes may also be referred to in itself as taxonomy: 'folk taxonomy', for example, is the study of native or folk systems of classification.

technoenvironmental. The complex of factors related to the environment, and the exploitation of that environment by a human group possessing a given level and type of technological development. (*See* TECHNOLOGY.)

technology. The technology of a human group is the total system of means by which the group interacts with its environment. This includes the use of tools, the pattern of WORK, the information or knowledge employed and the organization of resources for productive activity. Technology is thus a broader term than MATERIAL CULTURE which refers to the inventory of material artifacts characteristic of a given population. It is inseparable from economy and social organization, and is also dependent on the cultural classification of relevant resources in the natural environment. Theories of sociocultural evolution which place emphasis on the importance of certain innovations or discoveries in the field of technology or material culture (such as the use of fire, the origin of agricultural or irrigation technology, the plough, metals, the wheel and writing) may be termed 'technological determinist' theories, and should be distinguished from economic determinism, which places emphasis rather on the total organization of the economy (including the social organization of productive relations) as opposed to simply technological innovation.

Technology is linked on one side to social organization and economy and on the other to the environment. As the modern anthropological notion of technoenvironmental systems suggests, it is an error to regard technology and environment as separable and mutually interacting systems. The interpenetration of technology and environment is in fact so great that they form a single system. This system is not bounded in space, since technological elements are constantly and readily diffused from one population to another, changing the ecosystem everywhere that they are used. (*See* CULTURAL ECOLOGY; ENERGY; EVOLUTION.)

teknonymy. The practice of naming which refers to a person according to his or her relationship with a child. J. Overing Kaplan has interpreted this practice (1976) as a feature of systems of KINDRED organization, which stress consanguineal ties by emphasizing ties to children. A woman who refers to her husband, for example, as 'father of x' or 'father of my child' is stressing the kinship which is created by the birth of the child, thus avoiding the specification of an affinal tie ('husband').

temperament. *See* CULTURE AND PERSONALITY.

temple. A building which acts specifically as a centre for religious activity. Temples are associated with the rise of PRIESTS and URBANIZATION.

tenancy. *See* LAND TENURE.

terminology, kinship. *See* KINSHIP TERMINOLOGY.

territory. The principle of territory was opposed by social scientists, following MAINE and MORGAN, to that of KINSHIP as principles of social organization characteristic of modern and primitive society respectively. Over the course of time this simple opposition has been modified, as it has been recognized that in any social system there is an interaction and interrelation between the principles of territory and kinship.

text. Any sample of speech, writing or communicative behaviour which we take as an object of study or analysis. Anthropologists such as C. Geertz (1971) have proposed the study of cultural systems in terms of 'texts' or 'acted documents'. (*See* SYMBOLISM.)

thanatomia. *See* VOODOO DEATH.

Thanatos. In the PSYCHOANALYTICAL theory of FREUD, this is the death or destructive instinct, as opposed to EROS, the life or sexual instinct.

thaumaturgy. Having to do with miracles. Some CULTS and SECTS where miracles are an important element have been called thaumaturgical. (*See* MAGIC; WITCHCRAFT; RELIGION, ANTHROPOLOGY OF.)

theodicy. The theological problem of the existence of suffering and evil in the world, and the religious or theological solutions or resolutions which are proposed to reconcile this problem. (*See* RELIGION, ANTHROPOLOGY OF.)

theory. A theory in the strict sense of the term is a set of lawlike generalizations which is employed to explain and predict empirical phenomena. However few such theories (if any) exist in the social sciences, where the term is usually employed interchangeably with MODEL.

Third World. A term which is often loosely employed to refer to the nations of Asia, Africa and Latin America. In economic terms it refers to the nations which are regarded as underdeveloped or developing (*see* DEVELOPMENT) and politically to those which are not aligned with the Western capitalist First World or the Eastern socialist Second World; these countries are described generally as the 'non-aligned movement'. Some writers now also define a Fourth

World, constituted by those nations within the Third World which display least economic development or possess the fewest exploitable resources.

thought. See CLASSIFICATION; COGNITIVE ANTHROPOLOGY; LINGUISTICS AND ANTHROPOLOGY; PRIMITIVE MENTALITY; PSYCHOLOGICAL ANTHROPOLOGY; STRUCTURAL ANTHROPOLOGY.

time. It is an anthropological commonplace to state that perceptions of time, like those of space, are culturally relative and culturally conditioned, and the study of systems of cyclical (repetitive) and linear time reckoning has attracted the attention of several anthropologists. Conceptions of time and calendar not only reflect patterns of work and relationships with the environment, but also religious and ideological concerns. All societies grapple with the problems of the conservation and reproduction of the social order in the face of the linear passage of time, imposing upon this linear passage different kinds of cyclical model which assert the recreation and transcendence of given social, ideological and/or religious categories.

Tonnies, Ferdinand (1855–1936). German sociologist whose formulation of the distinction between GEMEINSCHAFT and GESELLSCHAFT was an important influence on the works of DURKHEIM and REDFIELD among others (e.g. 1887).

tools. See TECHNOLOGY.

totemism. The word 'totem' is derived from Ojibwa, an Algonquin language, where it denotes clan membership. It was extended in anthropological usage at one time to include a range of customs in which human groups were associated with animal species, among them the belief that the animal is the mythological ancestor of the clan and the associated observance of special ritual procedures or AVOIDANCES (typically the avoidance of eating the flesh of the animal concerned). Totemism as a theoretical topic stimulated much anthropological discussion and debate in the 19th century. McLENNAN (1865) affirmed that totemism derived from the combination of fetishism (the worship of

objects) with exogamous unilineal descent groups. FRAZER (1910) on the other hand associated totemism with a stage of development in which humans were ignorant of physiological paternity (see CONCEPTION) and regarded totemism as the origin of SACRIFICE. He thus attempted to establish the existence of a complex involving clan organization, exogamy and animal or plant emblems, placing this complex in its evolutionary context. In 1924 RIVERS defined totemism as a combination of a social element (the exogamous group linked to a given species) with a psychological one (the belief in descent from the totem species) and a ritual one (respect or prohibition with regard to the totem species). Subsequent discussion questioned the empirical validity of the association between exogamy, food prohibitions and the existence of animal or plant emblems, and developed new functional as opposed to evolutionary interpretations. MALINOWSKI (1954) linked totemism to the desire to control magically the fertility of animal species by linking each species to a ritual specialist and thus to his family and kin. RADCLIFFE-BROWN (1952), following DURKHEIM (1912), stressed the SACRED or ritual relationship between social groups and their totems as emblems of group membership and foci of social solidarity.

In his famous demolition of the concept of totemism, Levi-Strauss (1962) argues that it is an 'illusion', or an arbitrary conjunction of features which have a much wider significance. Animal or plant symbolism, which is as he points out the central feature of so-called totemic systems, is to be explained in his view as a product of the construction of correspondences between human groups and natural species in terms of oppositions. The human group is not seen to resemble the animal species; it is the differences between human groups which resemble the differences between animal species. Natural species are chosen, he affirms, because they are 'good to think', not because they are 'good to eat' as in the functionalist explanation. The differences between natural species thus form a model for the conceptualization of the differences between human groups, and 'totemism' is seen as nothing more than one example or set of examples of a universal tendency to classify one domain by modelling it on another.

tourism. Many of the regions and peoples studied by anthropologists are affected by tourism to a greater or lesser degree, and in some cases it has radically transformed their economic and social circumstances. Tourism to 'exotic' regions may include a visit to the 'primitive' inhabitants as part of the package, and these are often presented as part of tourism promotions at a national and international level. But a great many of the ordinary peasant communities of the Third World are also affected by tourism to some extent. It brings apparent immediate economic benefits in terms of cash income and/or possibilities of employment, but upon closer analysis many have concluded that the disadvantages outweigh the advantages. Such disadvantages or negative aspects of tourism – as far as the majority of the local people are concerned – include the distortion of the economy by the tourist trade (raising prices and rents, for example), the fact that the income from tourism is often concentrated in the hands of commercial tourist enterprises and does not filter down to the population in general, and the cultural and artistic distortion which may be introduced by the creation of a market for exotic handicrafts and customs. Many have concluded that tourism as a means of economic development is no substitute for the creation of economic growth and employment opportunities which are more organically linked to the region and its productive potential.

towns. See CITY, ANTHROPOLOGY OF THE; URBANISM/URBANIZATION.

trade. The exchange of goods between persons or groups, where the parties enter into the transaction on more or less equal terms. The use of the term implies that the economic aspect of the transaction is paramount, though the limit between trade and other forms of EXCHANGE or RECIPROCITY is not always easy to define. Some forms of ceremonial exchange might also be interpreted as forms of trade, where the negotiation of prices or values is nonetheless latent or hidden. In the same way, exchanges which are apparently free trading transactions may in fact be disguised relations of unequal exchange, as in the case of relationships with BROKERS and PATRONS, where one party has more power than the other to determine the terms of the transaction. The study of trading relationships is an important element of ECONOMIC ANTHROPOLOGY, and the formal and symbolic aspects of trade have also been studied as expressions of the forms of integration and reciprocity which link local groups to one another. Different forms of trade express the social relationships which exist between the parties: silent trade, for example, is a form of trading relationship between potentially hostile or socially distant groups, and where the dangers of negotiation are avoided by avoiding all direct contact. In many traditional economies there is a tendency to buffer or mitigate the direct economic nature of trade by establishing different kinds of social relationships involving mutual obligations with regard to the exchange of goods and services. The institution of trading partnerships, found in many areas of the world, is an example of this tendency.

Trading relationships are not studied in anthropology purely in the strict economic sense, that is, as exchanges of goods. They are placed instead in the context of the total system of circulation and distribution of values, both material and symbolic. The exchange of goods in itself may seem meaningless unless we place it in the context of the total system of exchanges, which may include ceremonial valuables, knowledge and expertise, human capital, and so on, which constitutes the economic and social organization of the group. Trade is simply one form or modality of exchange among many others. Nevertheless we should not underestimate its importance, as it is often a vital factor in systems of regional socioeconomic integration. As such, trading relations may also be studied in terms of their historical and evolutionary consequences, as means of the distribution of culture traits across linguistic and ethnic boundaries. The archaeological study of trade relationships in this sense is of great interest for the tracing of the mutual interrelations and interchanges between different geographical regions and different cultural traditions.

tradition. In archaeology, a set of interrelated cultural elements or traits which persists over a relatively long time span is called a tradition. In anthropology, the word is used instead for patterns of BELIEFS, CUSTOMS,

VALUES, behaviour and knowledge or expertise which are passed on from generation to generation by the socialization process within a given population. The term has sometimes been used as a synonym for CULTURE itself, particularly in ETHNOLOGY, where the study of 'traditional everyday culture' or FOLK culture was the dominant concern. Modern anthropologists and ethnologists however tend not to place so much emphasis on the centrality of the concept of tradition, since it does not allow for the essentially dynamic and adaptive nature of sociocultural systems. As these writers have pointed out, the uncritical use of the concept of tradition may make us fail to examine the key problem of the relationship between cultural persistence or continuity and cultural change, a problem which is to be approached not only in terms of cultural elements in themselves but also in terms of the historical process of social reproduction and social change in the population concerned. (*See* ORAL TRADITION; GREAT/ LITTLE TRADITION.)

trait, cultural. *See* CULTURAL TRAIT.

trance. *See* ALTERED STATES OF CONSCIOUSNESS.

transactionalism. In anthropology, a type of ACTION THEORY approach pioneered by F. Barth in his study of the political system of the Swat Pathans (1959). Barth sees the ACEPHALOUS political organization of the Swat Pathans as a formal framework of society constituted by a network of kinship and locality, against the background of which DYADIC ties link individuals to one another in relations of dominance and submission. Primary political groups are composed of clients linked to leaders by dyadic contractual ties, and these leaders in turn align their groups within a wider political system. Political action is therefore seen as the manipulation of dyadic ties in order to create followings. Critiques of this approach have focused on Barth's failure to analyse the overall class structure of Swat Pathan soiety, and on the application of a 'market' or 'rational' model which is felt by some to be inappropriate. (*See* INTERACTION THEORY.)

transculturation. Used as a synonym for ACCULTURATION to refer to the processes of cultural CHANGE resulting from culture contact.

transfer of technology. The transfer of technology from one nation or one type of economic system to another is a major factor in economic DEVELOPMENT. The manner in which technology is transferred may also distort this development in characteristic ways, maintaining forms of DEPENDENCY on more developed economies among the receiving nations. (*See* APPROPRIATE TECHNOLOGY; INTERMEDIATE TECHNOLOGY.)

transformational linguistics, transformational-generative linguistics. Linguistic theories associated with the US linguist Noam Chomsky (1965), who opposed BEHAVIOURIST theories which attempted to account for language in terms of learning theory and observable speech behaviour. Chomsky argued that it was necessary to account for linguistic PERFORMANCE in terms of linguistic COMPETENCE, and his theories attempt to uncover the underlying rules which govern the human ability to learn and employ speech, to create new utterances, and to distinguish meaningful utterances from meaningless ones. Transformational theory assumes that there exists a DEEP STRUCTURE and a surface structure in language, and the transformational rules are those which operate or mediate between the two, giving rise to the production or GENERATION of a potentially infinite variety of meaningful utterances. The theories of Chomsky were extremely influential in the development of STRUCTURAL and COGNITIVE anthropology. (*See* LINGUISTICS AND ANTHROPOLOGY.)

transhumance. *See* NOMADS; PASTORAL NOMADS.

translation. The problems of anthropological interpretation have been likened by some anthropologists, among them EVANS-PRITCHARD, as akin to those of linguistic translation. He suggested that the task of anthropology, like history, was essentially humanistic and interpretative. The problems involved in 'translating culture' have been prominent in discussions of CULTURAL RELATIVISM and the related theory of

LINGUISTIC RELATIVISM. These issues have been extensively debated within COGNITIVE ANTHROPOLOGY which has moved away from an initial position of relativism towards the assertion of universal underlying frameworks of CLASSIFICATION (*see* COLOUR TERMS). The view of anthropology as translation has been challenged by those theorists who regard it as idealist and who prefer to stress the search for the discovery of laws or regularities in human social organization and development in terms of its material base. (*See* CULTURAL ECOLOGY; EVOLUTION; MARXIST ANTHROPOLOGY).

transnational. *See* MULTINATIONAL AND TRANSNATIONAL CORPORATIONS.

tribe. This term has been widely used in anthropology, but there is no general consensus as to its precise definition or appropriate application. The Roman word *tribua* meant a political unit, and was used to refer to social groups defined by the territory they occupied. MORGAN (1877) defined the tribe as a group which possessed social institutions but not political ones. MAINE (1861) characterized it as a group in which legal relations were based on the principle of status rather than that of contract. In this sense of a prepolitical or pre-contract society, the term passed into general usage as a synonym for a PRIMITIVE social group.

The term is used as part of the EVOLUTIONARY scheme of social types which has been widely adopted in US anthropology and which consists, in ascending order, of BAND, tribe, CHIEFDOM and STATE. Of these categories that of tribe has been the most widely debated and questioned. When it is employed in this evolutionary sense to indicate a level or type of sociopolitical organization, it generally refers to groupings which consist of more than one local community and which are united by common cultural characteristics and some form of political leadership or political organization at a supralocal level. Where such supralocal leadership is more accentuated and there is a development of greater occupational specialization in crafts, military and religious activities together with a REDISTRIBUTIVE economy we may speak of the emergence of chiefdoms.

There is another use of the term tribe, linked especially to the history of Africa, which has different implications from those outlined above. 'Tribe' in the context of colonial and post-colonial Africa has been the subject of considerable debate and disagreement, as it has been shown that the concept of tribe was largely a colonial creation, a creation which was then attributed by colonial powers to the pre-existing characteristics of African populations and in turn became a 'problem' which was held to stand in the way of independence and self-government. Tribal divisions and tribal consciousness were largely a creation of the efforts of colonial rulers to impose order and supralocal unity upon previously largely autonomous local communities, and where there was previously a loose and contextually relative sense of ethnic identity, colonial rule often imposed a tribal division which then acquired increasing concreteness due to the need to adapt to the administrative and political demands of colonial rule.

Anthropological study of African peoples showed that the colonial concept of the tribe as an ethnically, linguistically, culturally and politically autonomous and self-conscious unit was a gross oversimplification of the complex panorama of inter-ethnic and regional social relations of pre-colonial Africa. The realization of the artificial nature of the concept of tribe generated a rejection among anthropologists and also among African politicians and intellectuals, who began more and more to question the relevance of the concept for the interpretation of contemporary African social and political organization. Thus modern anthropologists prefer to employ the notion of ETHNICITY and inter-ethnic relations in order to analyse and interpret what are indeed very real problems of inter-group conflict but which are not fruitfully conceived of in terms of 'tribalism'. Similarly the notion of 'detribalization' or the loss of tribal loyalties which was supposed to accompany modernization and urbanization has also been questioned as an oversimplification of the historical process of conflict, competition and adaptation between different racial and ethnic groups.

Turner, Victor W. (1920–83). Anthropologist who has made important contributions to the study of RITUAL and SYMBOLISM. Major works include *Schism and Continuity in an African Society* (1957), *The Forest of Symbols* (1967), *The Drums of Affliction* (1968), *The Ritual Process* (1969), *Dramas, Fields and Metaphors* (1972) and *Revelation and Divination in Ndembu Ritual* (1975).

twins. Twin births are accorded special magical or RITUAL significance in many different cultures, and their anomalous nature may be interpreted on the one hand as dangerous and defiling or on the other as especially powerful and sacred. Twin births may be symbolically interpreted as similar to animal births (which are multiple, while human ones are normally single) or alternatively as evidence of spiritual intervention. The killing or abandoning of one or both twins is reported for some traditional societies, while in others the twins may be revered and accorded deferential treatment.

two-line terminology. *See* ASYMMETRIC/SYMMETRIC EXCHANGE; DRAVIDIAN KINSHIP SYSTEM.

Tylor, Sir **Edwin Burnett** (1832–1917). British anthropologist who travelled to Mexico and other tropical regions and, upon the basis of his observations and written accounts, formulated his theories of ancient and primitive society. His *Primitive Culture* (1871) proposed three stages of social EVOLUTION, which he conceived of as stages in the evolution of RELIGION from ANIMISM through polytheism to monotheism. He also formulated the concept of CULTURE as it was later to be employed in US anthropology. Another concept which originated with Tylor was that of SURVIVAL, which was adopted by many social evolutionary theorists. He pioneered the field of CROSS-CULTURAL ANALYSIS, investigating ADHESIONS or sets of associated cultural traits, taking into account both parallel and independent evolution and DIFFUSION.

U

ultimogeniture. The rule of INHERITANCE or SUCCESSION which favours the last-born child, or last-born son in those societies where inheritance or succession is solely or preferentially by males.

unconscious. In the PSYCHOANALYTICAL theories of FREUD and his followers it is supposed that mental functioning may be divided into three realms: the conscious mind, of which we are aware, the subconscious, of which we are not aware but which we may call into consciousness, and the unconscious mind whose content is not normally available to consciousness.

underdevelopment. *See* DEVELOPMENT.

undifferentiated. A term sometimes used as a synonym for BILATERAL or cognatic kinship or descent.

unemployment and underemployment. Situations in which the total productive potential of the workforce is not taken up by the formal sector of the economy. In underemployment, even though workers may not be employed in the formal sector, they are occupied in some form of economic activity whether full or part time, and such activity in the informal sector often makes a substantial though officially unrecognized contribution to the economy as a whole. However the category of underemployment covers a wide range of different types of economic activity, and we should be careful to distinguish each of these and its consequences both for the domestic and the wider economy.

unilineal. *See* DESCENT; LINEAGE THEORY; MATRILINEAL; PATRILINEAL.

untouchables. An English term used to describe those CASTES, subcastes and individuals who are considered to be most impure, and certain contacts with whom are polluting. Gandhi called these people *Harijan* (sons of God) but in India generally untouchables are referred to by the name of the caste to which they belong. Untouchables are themselves divided into castes and subcastes which are ranked and restrict intermarriage and commensal relations. The post-Independence Indian constitution has abolished caste untouchability but caste POLLUTION continues to play an important role at village level. (*See* JAJMANI.)

urban anthropology. *See* CITY, ANTHROPOLOGY OF THE.

urbanism, urbanization. The concepts of urbanism and urbanization denote the predominance and the growth of urban centres in society. Like other concepts, such as those of CIVILIZATION, DEVELOPMENT, or INDUSTRIALIZATION, the concept of urbanism is beset by ETHNOCENTRIC bias and theoretical and analytical confusions. The definition of the CITY in itself is a point of considerable controversy, with different authors focusing on such varied aspects as the ecological, the demographic, the economic or the political, according to their theoretical orientation. We should distinguish the study of cities as such from the study of the phenomenon of urbanism and its consequences for the entire social system. Urbanism transforms rural or FOLK life as well as creating city life, since the growth of the city and the shaping of its economic and political relations with the rural areas are inseparable. The consequences of urbanism thus include the changing patterns of demographic composition and social, political and economic organization of rural communities in response to their evolving interdependence with urban centres.

use value. Production in small-scale traditional societies is generally directed to use value, not EXCHANGE VALUE. In the capitalist economy however the criterion of use value is suppressed in favour of ALIENATED production for exchange value. (*See* DOMESTIC MODE OF PRODUCTION; SUBSISTENCE; SURPLUS).

uterine. In KINSHIP studies, may be used as a synonym for MATRILINEAL or MATRILATERAL kinship.

uxorilocal. From the Latin, meaning 'in the woman's place'. This is a RESIDENCE rule or pattern whereby on MARRIAGE the couple goes to live with or near the woman's family or kin group. This pattern is often found among HORTICULTURALISTS and has been linked to the solidarity of the female working group. It also relates to the custom of BRIDESERVICE and in some systems to the political importance of the relationship between father-in-law and son-in-law. It is generally preferred in modern anthropology to the term MATRILOCAL, which suggests a link to MATRILINEAL descent that is not always present.

V

value. *See* EXCHANGE VALUE; LABOUR VALUE; SURPLUS VALUE.

values. The notion that cultural and social INTEGRATION are based on shared fundamental value orientations has been an important one in many anthropological theories. Both FUNCTIONALIST and STRUCTURAL FUNCTIONALIST theories tended to assume EQUILIBRIUM or group unity to be an ultimate collective value expressed through culture. US and German culture theorists in particular have pursued the notion that cultures are integrated by distinctive value emphases or orientations. The CULTURE AND PERSONALITY school accordingly links culture types to the selection of temperamental or psychological types, or the Freudian or neo-Freudian perspectives which link the psychodynamics of personality to the structure of culture. Both of these approaches within PSYCHOLOGICAL ANTHROPOLOGY place importance on the notion of shared values as factors in cultural integration. KLUCKHOHN (1952) has probably made one of the most notable uses of the value concept, which he defines as 'a conception, explicit or implicit, distinctive of an individual or characteristic of a group, of the desirable which influences the selection from available modes, means and ends of action'. Kluckhohn formulated the concept of 'value orientations', which are organized complexes of values which apply to broad segments of life and are a key factor in cultural integration. Similarly REDFIELD and others pursued the approach which stressed values and WORLD VIEW as a central anthropological concern.

Like British structural functionalists, US culture theorists tended to assume both integration and equilibrium as the norm, postulating as a result monolithic value systems supposedly applying to all members of society at all times. Critics of these perspectives have stressed the existence of multiple, internally contradictory and conflicting values and value systems, and have tended to disagree with the notion that values in themselves are a powerful organizational or cohesive force in society or in culture, tending to see them rather as expressions of other forces.

Van Gennep, Arnold (1873–1957). Dutch-born scholar who was a prolific contributor to French folklore studies and ethnology, but who is principally remembered for his classic study of RITES OF PASSAGE (1909; trans. 1960) which has profoundly influenced the study of RITUAL and SYMBOLISM. Van Gennep was a critic of DURKHEIM in his time, especially of the latter's 'canonization' of the social and his disregard for the individual.

Veblen, Thorsten B. (1857–1929). US sociologist and economist who coined the term 'conspicuous consumption' as part of his theory of the 'leisure class' in modern industrial society. Veblen analysed economic institutions as expressions of values, attitudes and mores in society. In his *Theory of the Leisure Class* (1899) he argued that conspicuous consumption existed in order to create an impression rather than meet a need. He also focused on conflict as a central feature of modern industrial society, particularly the conflict between the owners of capital and the technical and labour element.

Verstehen. 'Understanding' in German. Associated in the social sciences with the theories of WEBER who argued that *Verstehen* was a necessary part of explanation in the social sciences. For Weber *Verstehen* was both a method of apprehension of social reality and an intrinsic feature of that reality, since human beings act in society according

285

to motivations and values and not in a mechanistic fashion.

violence. *See* CONFLICT; LAW, ANTHROPOLOGY OF; WARFARE.

virilocal. From the Latin, meaning 'in the man's place'. This term is used to denote a RESIDENCE pattern or rule in which after MARRIAGE a couple resides with or near the man's family or kin group. The term is usually preferred in modern anthropology to PATRILOCAL, though this latter term may be employed where the kinship system is also patrilineal. Virilocal residence has been linked to the solidarity of the male work group or property holding and political unit.

visions. *See* ALTERED STATES OF CONSCIOUSNESS; SHAMANISM.

visual anthropology. This relatively recent area of anthropological specialization includes different aspects of the study of visual dimensions of human behaviour, as well as the development of increasingly sophisticated visual methods for anthropological research, teaching and cultural interchange. It thus combines fields such as the anthropology of ART, the use of photography and ethnographic film in anthropology, the field of PROXEMICS or the study of the sociocultural use of space, and the study of perception and visual SYMBOLISM in crosscultural perspective. It is only in recent years that anthropologists have begun to submit visual categories and visual structuring to careful scrutiny whether within the cultures we study or within our own methodological toolkit. For example, the use of photography and ethnographic film as research tools and educational media has been examined more carefully in terms of the implicit messages which these methods may imply regarding their subject matter, and in terms of the manner in which by unthinkingly imposing our own visual and sequential ordering we may be distorting the categories of the culture we attempt to present. An interesting development in this field is the training of informants to handle photographic and filming equipment in order to allow them to express through these media their own conceptual ordering of their reality.

voluntary/involuntary associations. *See* ASSOCIATIONS.

voodoo (vudu). A term probably derived from the Yoruba *vodu* (god, spirit, sacred object) and employed to refer to the SYNCRETISTIC religious cult practised by the peasant and proletarian population of Haiti, and by elements of the black population of the Caribbean, Brazil and the southern United States. Much of the vocabulary and the beliefs and rites associated with voodoo are of African origin, mixed with elements from the Catholic religion. Worshippers are possessed by anthropomorphic spirits who take part in feasting and dancing, give advice and perform cures. (*See* POSSESSION.)

'voodoo death' (thanatomia). Death by magical (psychosomatic) causes following sorcery or taboo violation. This is due to a combination of psychological and physical causes, the immediate cause of death probably being dehydration, since the person who is socially 'dead' does not eat or drink.

W

warfare. War is a form of CONFLICT characterized by the use of armed aggression between groups. This ranges from the raiding and feuding typical of small-scale societies to the full-scale armed conflict of a technologically equipped war between modern nations. The anthropological study of war has been characterized by continuing debate between those who wish to relate it to underlying psychological tendencies (innate human aggression) or to an implicit ecological rationality, and those who reject this type of explanation as reductionist. Those who argue that warfare is an expression of innate human aggression and territoriality fail to take into account the fact that there are very many culturally variable forms of conflict and conflict management in human societies, and that warfare is only one of a set of possible aggressive and non-aggressive responses to such stimuli as stress and overcrowding. In many societies there is no tradition of warfare or organized violence, and conflicts may be managed without recourse to physical aggression. In other societies however such aggression is the norm, whether in individual or group form. There is no evidence however that such societies are more subject to stress, overcrowding or other factors which would stimulate the expression of innate aggressive tendencies.

The ecological approach to the explanation of warfare has been adopted by many anthropologists, who relate warfare in traditional societies to the maintenance of equilibrium between population, resources and territory. Thus it is argued for example by R. Rappaport, who employs a systems theory approach in order to interpret culture as an adaptive mechanism (1968), that among the Tsembaga Maring of New Guinea warfare may be understood as one element in a complex system of CYBERNETIC interconnections between culture and ecosystem.

The Tsembaga Maring ritual cycle, which involves the raising and sacrifice of pigs, feasting and trading, marriage negotiations and sporadic warfare, acts according to Rappaport to preserve the balance of the ecosystem, to order intergroup relations and to redistribute land, resources and population in relation to one another.

Critics of the ecological approach have pointed out that the assumption of an underlying ecological rationality may lead us to ignore the symbolic, political and ideological dimensions of warfare. They have also argued that the assumption of a system in equilibrium is not necessarily applicable to all cases of warfare, since warfare is often an expression of imbalance, change and internal and external contradiction. Some anthropologists indeed link warfare to the emergence of social CLASSES and the formation of STATES, stressing its conflictory rather than integrative functions. Indeed it seems fair to object that the FUNCTIONALIST approach to warfare is often over-stretched, finding an underlying integrative logic to a custom which is *par excellence* the expression of conflict and which often leads to the destruction of human groups and the disintegration of their social system. However we should seek a balance between the conflict and integration views, since it is evident that in some cases the primary function of war is the symbolic demarcation of group boundaries and the expression of group solidarity. Such is the case of 'wars' which are largely ceremonial in nature and do not involve serious injury or widespread killing. But different social groups vary in the extent to which they take the symbolism of war literally, and it is also necessary to recognize that there are groups where the expression of boundaries and solidarity does involve a high degree of violence and extra-group aggression. In the case of the Yanomamo of Brazil, for example, both intra- and extra-group levels of aggressive behaviour are extremely high, conflict, violence and group fission being the norm, see Chagnon (1968). Some anthropologists have nevertheless attempted to find an underlying ecological rationality for the Yanomamo and other such cases involving warfare and female INFANTICIDE. Nevertheless there is no evidence that groups such as the Yanomamo represent systems in equilibrium, and it is perhaps more probable that the situation among them represents instead a crisis in social reproduction, produced at least in part by the indirect and direct effects of external pressures by settlers, colonizers and the national society.

In the case of modern large-scale warfare it is even more difficult to sustain explanations in terms of psychological tendencies, ecological balance or symbolic social integration. Modern warfare should be analysed instead in the total context of international relations (*see* COLONIALISM; DEPENDENCY; IMPERIALISM; WORLD SYSTEMS) and while it may manipulate sociopsychological factors such as aggression and solidarity, its underlying rationality is above all to be understood in economic and historical terms.

Warner, William Lloyd (1898–1970). US anthropologist who studied Australian aboriginal social and kinship systems and also pioneered areas of urban anthropology (e.g. 1937).

Weber, Max (1864–1920). German sociologist who together with DURKHEIM and MARX is acknowledged as one of the founding fathers of the social sciences. Weber's work has been of considerable influence in anthropology, especially his investigation of religion, his theories of STRATIFICATION and his methodological contributions. He argued that under certain circumstances belief systems could be decisive factors in social and economic change, thus contesting Marx's theory of the universal primacy of infrastructures. His famous study of the Protestant ethic (1958) demonstrates the importance of the beliefs and values associated with Protestantism in creating the conditions for the rise of European capitalism. Weber also made important contributions to the study of the differences between traditional and modern society, creating a typology of forms of AUTHORITY and arguing that

BUREAUCRACY was the expression of the dominant rational–legal mode of authority in modern society (*see* CHARISMA; ROUTINIZATION; RATIONALIŻATION). In his writings on methodology Weber explored the nature of sociological understanding (VERSTEHEN) and the possibilities of a value-free stance for social scientific explanation. Major works include *Economy and Society* (1968), *The Protestant Ethic and the Spirit of Capitalism* (1958), and *From Max Weber: Essays in Sociology (1958).*

Weltanschauung. See WORLD VIEW.

Westermarck, Edward (1853–1936). Philosopher and social theorist who studied human sexual and marriage customs and the history of human morality (e.g. 1914; 1926). (*See* INCEST.)

Western society, the West. A term used loosely to refer to the nations of Europe and North America or to the capitalist 'developed' world. May be contrasted with 'the East' (socialist societies) or with 'underdeveloped' nations. (*See* DEVELOPMENT; THIRD WORLD.)

White, Leslie Alvin (1900–75). US cultural anthropologist whose theories of cultural EVOLUTION were of great influence in stimulating the development of neo-functionalist evolutionary and ecological approaches in modern US anthropology. White placed particular emphasis on the importance of ENERGY use as a measure of sociocultural evolution. Major works include *The Evolution of Culture* (1959).

Whiting, John Wesley Mayhew (1908–   ). US cultural anthropologist who is an important pioneer of CROSS-CULTURAL ANALYSIS in PSYCHOLOGICAL ANTHROPOLOGY.

Whorf, Benjamin Lee (1897–1941). US anthropologist and linguist who is best-known for the 'Sapir–Whorf hypothesis' of LINGUISTIC RELATIVITY, which held that every language represents and creates a distinct reality (e.g. 1956). (*See* LINGUISTICS AND ANTHROPOLOGY.)

widow inheritance. The practice of extending or continuing the MARRIAGE alliance by passing a widow on to her dead husband's brother (LEVIRATE), son or other male relative. This may be interpreted both as an expression of the structural importance of the marriage alliance as a relationship between two kin groups and as one of a number of ways in which men attempt to control female sexuality by limiting the options open to a woman and avoiding situations where she would be able to exercise free choice.

Wilson, Monica (1908–82). British social anthropologist who studied rituals and age organization among the Nyakyusa of Central Africa (e.g. 1963).

Wissler, Clark (1870–1947). US anthropologist who contributed much to the promotion and popularization of anthropological and ethnographic research. As a theorist he introduced the CULTURE AREA concept, and also postulated a set of nine cultural universals in terms of which he ordered his lists of CULTURE TRAITS (e.g. 1923). (*See* AGE-AREA HYPOTHESIS.)

witchcraft. In EVANS-PRITCHARD's classic definition, witchcraft is the inherent power to harm other persons by supernatural means (1937). This power is distinguished by Evans-Pritchard from sorcery, which is learned and is the harmful or aggressive use of MAGIC. This distinction between witchcraft and sorcery was widely adopted by many Africanists, but outside Africa 'witchcraft' may be used indiscriminately to refer to mystical aggression whether or not magical means are employed. In the case of the Zande, among whom Evans-Pritchard carried out his classic study, witchcraft is believed to be a hereditary power, though this is not universally the case in African witchcraft or in other ethnographic regions. Following his work, witchcraft and sorcery have been studied – especially within British social anthropology – as mechanisms of social control and for the expression and resolution of social tensions and conflicts. Evans-Pritchard also explored the religious and philosophical aspects of witchcraft beliefs as part of a system which explains personal fortune and misfortune. In many traditional and small-scale societies witchcraft or sorcery beliefs are a common part of the idiom of interpersonal and intergroup

relationships, revealing structural as well as momentary or purely personal contradictions, in addition to embodying conceptions of the intervention of supernatural agencies in human existence. (*See also* SHAMANISM.)

wizard. A term which has been proposed to cover both 'witch' and 'sorcerer', in order to avoid Evans-Pritchard's classic distinction between WITCHCRAFT and sorcery in contexts where this is not appropriate.

women and anthropology. Anthropological studies of the status and role of women have been influenced, as N. Quinn points out, both by FEMINISM and by different political views of the role of women in US and European society. The studies which have been carried out into the cross-cultural comparison of women's status have mainly been undertaken by women anthropologists, and many of the pioneers in this field have been US women. Their studies are often linked to feminist discussions of the role of women, of PATRIARCHY and of male dominance in general terms. Some anthropologists for example put together a number of superficially similar ethnographic cases of female subordination in order to argue that there is a universal sexual asymmetry in human society based on the division of public and domestic spheres and the limitation of women to the domestic sphere, or based on the symbolic association of women with nature and men with culture. However as Quinn points out such studies are oversimplifications of the complex nature of female status, which is composed of different elements some of which may be classed as 'high' and others 'low', while others still are 'equal' with those of men. She suggests that although we should not entirely reject the hypothesis of universal female subordination we should explore its dimensions more carefully and demonstrate in more detail the interdependencies which exist between different aspects of female status and their relation to political, economic, social and ideological systems.

An important strand in the anthropological study of women has been the study of male bias in ethnography, and of how female viewpoints in culture and society are not communicated to, or not understood by, male (or male-oriented) ethnographers.

These studies have sometimes stressed that female status is not always low, but may be perceived as such by male-biased ethnography. Some feminist anthropologists have argued that in pre-colonial societies women are not always subject to male domination or patriarchal structures, which are in fact introduced with male-oriented colonial power structures. Some critics have detected a contradiction between feminist anthropologists who argue for the universality of male dominance and others who attempt to demonstrate that in certain pre-colonial contexts there is considerable sexual equality.

A number of different theories have been advanced to explain the regularities – or the variability – in women's status in cross-cultural perspective. Some theorists argue that greater male levels of aggression are responsible for universal female subordination, though this theory has been largely rejected as a crude oversimplification of the social and ideological nature of gender relations. Others emphasize the importance of the female childbearing and childrearing role which limits women's mobility and restricts them to the domestic sphere, though it can be argued that if nature assigns to women the role of bearing children, it is culture and society which assigns them exclusive responsibility for raising and caring for them. Many writers have focused on the socialization process, showing how this differentiates male and female role expectations, though this cannot be regarded as a causal explanation of structures of male dominance.

In accounting for the cross-cultural variability of female status, many writers have focused on economic factors. For example, it has been pointed out that in some HUNTING AND GATHERING societies there is very little male-female status differentiation and correspondingly little separation of the domestic and public spheres. Draper has shown that the seminomadic !Kung follow this pattern, whereas among the settled !Kung male-female status differential increases. Other writers have pointed to the high contribution of women in HORTICULTURAL economies and their reduced participation in agriculture, and to the concomitant changes in female status and in such factors as POLYGYNY. It has been suggested accordingly that monogamous nuclear families tend to develop with the emergence of agriculture, with women being restricted to the domestic sphere. Other writers link the low status of women to the rise of the STATE and the consequent devaluation of kinship ties and the relegation of women to the domestic sphere, since men are the focus of property holding, production and political relations.

Sanday, examining the female role in production and female status cross-culturally (1973), found that in societies where the productive contribution of women is low their status also tends to be low, and that equal status is more often correlated with an evenly balanced SEXUAL DIVISION OF LABOUR. However in some societies where female productivity is important the status of women is low, since their production is ideologically devalued in comparison with that of men (as in the case of hunting versus gathering in some band societies, or the common definition of female domestic and childrearing tasks as 'non-work' in spite of the fact that they play an essential part in the reproduction of the labour force). In terms of women's political participation, Sanday found the degree of such participation to be correlated with a number of factors including the physical absence of men and the economic power and independence of women.

WARFARE has been cited by some as a reason for the development of ideologies of male dominace, despite the important economic contribution of women in times of war. Another factor which may be important is the creation by men of spheres of ceremonial activity or exchange from which women are excluded. Other writers have seen the root of female subordination in the manipulation of women as objects in a system of MARRIAGE alliances, which also generates the dominant male concern for the control over female sexuality. However it should be noted that there may be some ethnographic male bias operating here in the failure to recognize the extent to which women themselves may actively participate in marriage exchanges, and that the effects of different marriage practices vary in the extent to which they involve female subordination. Finally, it has been frequently suggested that MATRILINY creates high female status since it makes women central to social continuity, though again this depends on the degree of domestic and public authority accorded to women, as in some matrilineal systems the emphasis is on relationships between men traced through women but not controlled by them. UXORILOCALITY or MATRILOCALITY may have some effect in creating and perpetuating solitary female groups which are not easily dominated by men who are dispersed by the uxorilocal residence rule. (*See* DOMESTIC GROUP; FAMILY; FEMINIST ANTHROPOLOGY; GENDER.)

world systems. The world systems paradigm was developed by Wallerstein (1974), who defines it as a social system based on an international division of labour mediated through trade exchanges without the need for a unified political structure. This system creates 'core', 'periphery' and 'semiperiphery' zones with differential participation in the overall economy and with differing internal class and economic organization. This is a model which together with DEPENDENCY theory challenges conventional models of economic DEVELOPMENT. Wallerstein opposes the Marxist model of multiple MODES OF PRODUCTION ordered in lineal (evolutionary) succession. Instead, he states that in the modern world the economy is to be understood in terms of a single unitary model, which is the capitalist world system. Marxists on the other hand see the world capitalist economy as made up of distinct modes of production found empirically in diverse SOCIAL FORMATIONS and united by their ARTICULATION to capitalist modes of exchange. The advantage of the unitary model is that one avoids reifying modes of production as separate entities, and is thus better able to perceive the dynamic of interacting spheres. On the other hand the model of the coexisting variety of modes of production may be more appropriate to certain ethnographic contexts, and avoids too the tendency in the unitary theory to regard the periphery as passive and the centre as the determining force. (*See* METROPOLIS-SATELLITE.)

world view. The system of VALUES, attitudes and BELIEFS held by a specified group. The German term *Weltanschauung* may also be employed with the same meaning. The concept has been important in the study of FOLK and PEASANT societies (*see* COMMUNITY STUDIES) and is associated in particular with the work of REDFIELD (1956). The stress on the importance of world view and ideological factors in influencing responses to CHANGE found in Redfield's work among others prefigured the interests of COGNITIVE ANTHROPOLOGY, which however differentiates more carefully aspects of world view such as cognitive systems, affective and attitude systems, and action systems. The stress on the importance of world view has been associated with CULTURAL RELATIVISM and has been criticized for its assumption that systems of values, beliefs and attitudes are unitary and shared by all members of the group.

writing. *See* LITERACY.

Selective Bibliography and Further Reading

Abbreviations of Periodicals

AA	American Anthropologist	JFR	Journal of Folkloristic Research
ARA	Annual Review of Anthropology		
		MAQ	Medical Anthropology Quarterly
BJS	British Journal of Sociology		
CA	Current Anthropology	NYRB	New York Review of Books
HO	Human Organization	SWJA	Southwestern Journal of Anthropology
JAR	Journal of Anthropological Reasarch		

R.L. Abel: 'A Comparative Theory of Dispute Institutions in Society', *Law and Society Review* (1973)

R.D. Abrahams: 'Introductory Remarks to a Rhetorical Theory of Folklore', *Journal of American Folklore* (1968)

J.B. Aceves: *Aspects of Cultural Change* (New York, 1972)

J.M. Acheson: 'Anthropology of Fishing', *ARA* (1981)

J.W. Adams: 'Recent Ethnology of the Northwest Coast', *ARA* (1981)

R.N. Adams and R.D. Fogelson: *The Anthropology of Power* (New York, 1977)

R.N. Adams *et al*, eds: *Social Change in Latin America Today* (New York, 1960)

M.H. Agar: 'Whatever Happenned to Cognitive Anthropology?', *HO* (1982)

L. Althusser and E. Balibar: *Reading Capital* (1966; Eng. trans., London, 1970)

R. Ardrey: *The Territorial Imperative* (London, 1966)

W. Arens: *The Man-eating Myth* (New York, 1979)

C.M. Arensberg: *Family and Community in Ireland* (Cambridge, Mass., 1968)

T. Asad: *Anthropology and the Colonial Encounter* (London, 1973)

R.A. Austen: *Modern Imperialism* (Lexington, Mass., 1969)

J.L. Austin: *How to do Things with Words* (Oxford, 1962)

J.J. Bachofen: *Myth, Religion and Mother-Right* (1861; Eng. trans., New York, 1967)

G. Baer and E.J. Langdon: *South American Shamanism* (in press)

F. Bailey: *Stratagems and Spoils* (Oxford, 1969)

P.T. Baker and W. Sanders: 'Demographic Studies in Anthropology', *ARA* (1972)

T. Baker: *Über die Musik der nordamerikanischen Wilden* (Leipzig, 1882)

G. Balandier: *Political Anthropology* (Harmondsworth, 1970)

E. Banfield: *The Moral Basis of a Backward Society* (Chicago, 1958)

M. Banton, ed.: *Anthropological Approaches to the Study of Religion* (London, 1966)

——: *Political Systems and the Distribution of Power* (London, 1965)

P. Baran: *The Political Economy of Growth* (New York, 1957)

G.W. Barlow and J. Silverberg, eds: *Sociobiology: Beyond Nature/Nurture?* (Boulder, 1980)

J.A. Barnes: *Networks in Social Anthropology* (Reading, Mass., 1972)

——: 'Kinship Studies', *Man* (1980)

R.H. Barnes: 'Number and Number Use in Kedang', *Man* (1982)

H.G. Barnett: *Innovation: the Basis for Cultural Change* (New York, 1963)

S. Barnett, ed.: *Concepts of Person* (Cambridge, Mass., 1932)

F. Barth: *Political Leadership among the Swat Pathans* (London and New York, 1959)

——: *Nomads of South Persia* (London, 1961)

——: *Models of Social Organization* (London, 1966)

——: *Ritual and Knowledge among the Baktaman of New Guinea* (Oslo, 1975)

——: *Process and Form in Social Life* (London, 1981)

M.A. Bartolome *et al*: *Declaration of Barbados: for the Liberation of the Indians* (Copenhagen, 1971)

R. Basham: *Urban Anthropology* (Palo Alto, 1978)

A. Bastian: *Der Mensch in der Geschichte* (Leipzig, 1860)

R. Bastide: *Applied Anthropology* (London, 1973)

G. Bateson: *Steps to an Ecology of Mind* (San Francisco, 1972)

R. Beals: 'Towards an Ethics for Anthropologists', *CA*, (1971)

J. Beattie: *The Bunyoro: an African Kingdom* (New York, 1960)

——: 'Checks on the Abuse of Political Power in the African State', in Cohen and Middleton, eds (1967)

T.O. Beidelman: *A Comparative Analysis of the Jajmani System* (New York, 1959)

C. Belshaw: *Traditional Exchange and Modern Markets* (Englewood Cliffs, 1965)

R.F. Benedict: *Patterns of Culture* (New York, 1934)

——: *The Chrysanthemum and the Sword* (Boston, 1967)

J.W. Bennett: 'Further Remarks on Foster's Image of the Limited Good', *AA* (1966)

B. Berlin and P. Kay: *Basic Color Terms* (Berkeley, 1969)

H.R. Bernard: 'The Power of Print', *HO* (1985)

H. Bernstein: 'African Peasantries: a Theoretical Framework' *Journal of Peasant Studies* (1979)

G.D. Berreman: 'Ecology, Demography and Domestic Strategies in the Western Himalayas', *JAR* (1978)

——: *Social Inequality* (New York, 1981)

A. Beteille: *Social Inequality* (London, 1969)

B. Bettelheim: *Symbolic Wounds* (Glencoe, Ill., 1954)

D. Bickerton: 'Pidgin and Creole Studies', *ARA* (1976)

D. Bidney: 'Cultural Relativism', *International Encyclopaedia of the Social Sciences* (1968)

L.R. Binford: *An Archeological Perspective* (New York, 1972)

R.E. Blanton: 'Anthropological Studies of Cities', *ARA* (1976)

P.M. Blau: *Exchange and Power in Social Life* (New York, 1964)

T. Blick, ed.: *The Comparative Reception of Darwinism* (1974)

M. Bloch: *Feudal Society* (1949; Eng. trans., London, 1961)

——: *Placing the Dead* (London, 1971)

——, ed.: *Marxist Analyses in Social Anthropology* (London, 1975)

——, ed.: *Political Language and Oratory in Traditional Society* (London, 1975)

—— and S. Guggenheim: 'Compadrazgo, Baptism and the Symbolism of a Second Birth', *Man* (1981)

—— and J. Parry: *Death and the Regeneration of Life* (London, 1985)

L. Bloomfield: *Language* (New York, 1933)

F. Boas: *The Kwakiutl of Vancouver Island* (New York, 1909)

——: *The Mind of Primitive Man* (New York, 1911)

——: *Primitive Art* (New York, 1927)

——: *Anthropology in Modern Life* (New York, 1928)

——: *Race, Language and Culture* (New York, 1940)

P.K. Bock, ed.: *Peasants in the Modern World* (Albuquerque, 1969)

P.J. Bohannan and G. Dalton, eds: *Markets in Africa* (Evanston, Ill., 1965)

——, ed.: *Law and Warfare* (New York, 1967)

J. Boissevain: *Friends of Friends* (Oxford, 1974)

E. Bott: *Family and Social Network* (London, 1971)

C. Bougle: *Caste in India* (Cambridge, 1971)

K.E. Boulding and M. Tappan, eds: *Economic Imperialism* (Ann Arbor, 1972)

E. Bourguignon: *Psychological Anthropology* (New York, 1979)

J. Breman: *Patronage and Exploitation* (Berkeley, 1974)

I.R. Buchler and H.A. Selby: *Kinship and Social Organization* (New York, 1968)

R. Burling: 'Cognition and Componential

Analysis', *AA* (1966)

J. Burrow: *Evolution and Society* (Cambridge, 1966)

K.N. Cameron: *Marxism: the Science of Society* (1985)

F. Cancian: *Economics and Prestige in a Maya Community* (Stanford, Cal., 1965)

——: 'Social Stratification', *ARA* (1976)

R.W. Casson: *Language, Culture and Cognition* (New York, 1981)

C. Castaneda: *Teachings of Don Juan* (Harmondsworth, 1970)

N. Chagnon: *Yanomamö, the Fierce People* (New York, 1968)

E.J. Chambers and P.D. Young: 'Mesoamerican Community Studies', *ARA* (1979)

C.H. Chase: 'Infant Mortality and its Concomitants', *Medical Care* (1977)

M. Chibnik: 'The Use of Statistics in Sociocultural Anthropology', *ARA* (1985)

V.G. Childe: *Man Makes Himself* (London, 1941)

——: *What Happened in History* (London, 1942)

N. Chomsky: *Aspects of the Theory of Syntax* (Cambridge, Mass., 1965)

J.A. Clifton, ed.: *Applied Anthropology* (Boston, 1970)

——: 'Human Organization', *Journal of the Society for Applied Anthropology*

R.B. Coats and A. Perkin: *Computer Models in the Social Sciences* (London, 1977)

H. Codere: *Fighting with Property* (New York, 1950)

——: 'Money Exchange Systems and a Theory of Money', *Man* (1968)

A. Cohen: 'Political Anthropology: the Analysis of the Symbolism of Power Relations', *Man* (1969)

——: *Two-dimensional Man* (London, 1974)

P.S. Cohen: 'Theories of Myth', *Man* (1965)

R. Cohen and J. Middleton, eds: *Comparative Political Systems* (New York, 1967)

—— and E. Service: *Origins of the State* (Philadelphia, 1978)

S. Cohen: *Folk Devils and Moral Panics* (London, 1972)

N. Cohn: *The Pursuit of the Millennium* (London, 1957)

S. Cole: *The Neolithic Revolution* (New York, 1969)

J.F. Collier: 'Legal Processes', *ARA* (1975)

E. Colson: *The Plateau Tonga of Northern Rhodesia* (Manchester, 1962)

J. Comaroff: *The Meaning of Homage Payments* (London, 1980)

A.C. Comte: *System of Positive Polity: Course of Positive Philosophy* (1830–42; Eng. trans., London, 1877)

H.C. Conklin: *Hanuno Agriculture* (Rome, 1957)

F. Cottrell: *Energy and Society* (New York, 1955)

R. Coulborn, ed.: *Feudalism in History* (Princeton, 1956)

D. Cushman and G. Marcus: 'Ethnographies as Texts', *ARA* (1982)

G. Dalton: 'Primitive Money', *AA*, (1965)

——, ed.: *Primitive, Archaic and Modern Economies* (New York, 1968)

W. Davenport: 'Non-unilinear Descent and Descent Groups', *AA*, (1959)

T. David: *Figuring Anthropology* (1976)

E.G. Davis: *The First Sex* (New York, 1971)

S.H. Davis: *Victims of the Miracle* (Cambridge, 1977)

W.L. d'Azevedo: 'A Structural Approach to Aesthetics', *AA* (1958)

L. Degh and A. Vazsonyi: 'Does the Word "Dog" bite?', *JFR* (1983)

I. Devore and R.B. Lee, eds: *Man the Hunter* (Chicago, 1968)

S. Diamond: *In Search of the Primitive* (New Brunswick, 1974)

G.W. Dimbleby and P.J. Ucko, eds: *The Domestication and Exploitation of Plants and Animals* (London, 1969)

——, R. Tringham, P.J. Ucko, eds: *Man, Settlement and Urbanism* (London, 1972)

W.T. Divale and M. Harris: 'Population, Warfare and Male Supremacist Complex', *AA* (1976)

M. Dobb: *Studies in the Development of Capitalism* (London, 1945)

R.M. Dorson: *Folklore and Traditional History* (The Hague, 1972)

M. Douglas: *Purity and Danger* (London, 1966)

——: *Natural Symbols* (London, 1970)

——: *Implicit Meanings* (London, 1975)

J. Dow and R. Halperin: *Peasant Livelihood* (New York, 1977)

——: 'The Image of Limited Production', *HO* (1981)

Draper: '!Kung Women', in Reiter, ed. (1975)

H.E. Driver and K.E. Schnessler: 'Componential Analysis of Murdock's Ethnographic Sample', *AA* (1967)

P. Drucker and R.F. Heizer: *To Make my Name Good* (Berkeley, 1967)

C. Dubois: *The People of Alor* (Cambridge, Mass., 1960)

J. Dubois: *A Description of the Character, Manners and Institutions of the People of India* (Madras, 1862)

J.P. Dumont: *Knowledge and Passion* (1980)

L. Dumont: 'The Dravidian Kinship Terminology as an Expression of Marriage', *Man* (1953)

——: 'Marriage in India', *Contributions to Indian Sociology* (1964)

——: 'Descent or Intermarriage?', *SWJA* (1965)

——: *Homo Hierarchicus* (London, 1970)

——: *Affinity as a Value* (London, 1983)

A. Dundes: *The Study of Folklore* (Englewood Cliffs, 1965)

W. Dupré: *Religion in Primitive Cultures* (The Hague, 1975)

E. Durkheim: *The Elementary Forms of Religious Life* (1912; Eng. trans., London, 1915)

——: *The Division of Labor in Society* (1933; Eng. trans., New York, 1947)

——: *Suicide* (Eng. trans., London, 1952)

——: *Moral Education* (London, 1961)

—— and M. Mauss: *Primitive Forms of Classification* (1903; Eng. trans., London, 1963)

K. Dwyer: 'The Dialectic of Ethnology', *Dialectical Anthropology* (1979)

N. and R. Dyson-Hudson: 'Nomadic Pastoralism', *ARA* (1980)

D. Easton: 'Political Anthropology' in B. Siegel, ed. (1959)

——: *A Systems Analysis of Political Life* (New York, 1965)

M.W. Edelman: 'We already know why black Babies die', *Washington Post* (February, 1984)

F. Eggan: *Essays in Social Anthropology and Ethnology* (New York, 1975)

P. Ekman: *Expressions of Emotion in Man and Animals* (New York, 1972)

S. Elgin and J. Grinder: *A Guide to Transformational Grammar* (New York, 1973)

P. Eliade: *Cosmos and History* (New York, 1959)

H. Ellis: *Selected Essays* (London, 1940)

R.M. Emerson: *Contemporary Field Research* (1983)

F. Engels: *The Origins of Family, Private Property and the State* (1884)

A.L. Epstein: *Contention and Dispute* (Canberra, 1974)

T.S. Epstein: 'Productive Efficiency and Customary Systems of Rewards in Rural South India' in R. Firth, ed. (1967)

E.E. Evans-Pritchard: *Witchcraft, Magic and Oracles among the Azande* (Oxford, 1937)

——: *The Nuer* (Oxford, 1940)

——: *The Divine Kingship of the Shilluk of the Nilotic Sudan* (Cambridge, 1948)

——: *Anthropology and History* (Manchester, 1961)

——: *Essays in Social Anthropology* (London, 1962)

——: *Theories of Primitive Religion* (Oxford, 1965)

—— and M. Fortes: *African Political Systems* (London, 1940)

H.J. Eysenck: *Race, Intelligence and Education* (London, 1971)

L.A. Fallers: *Inequality* (Chicago, 1973)

F. Fanon: *The Wretched of the Earth* (Harmondsworth, 1965)

Feminist Anthropology Collective: *No Turning Back: Writings from the Women's Liberation Movement, 1975–80* (1981)

A. Ferguson: *An Essay on Civil Society* (1767)

K. Finkler: *Spiritualist Healers in Mexico* (1985)

R. Firth: *We, the Tikopia* (London, 1936)

——: *Malay Fishermen: their Peasant Economy* (London, 1946)

——: *Elements of Social Organization* (London, 1951)

——: *Economics of the New Zealand Maori* (Wellington, 1959)

——: *Social Change among the Tikopia* (London, 1959)

——: *Essays on Social Organization and Values* (London, 1964)

—— ed.: *Themes in Economic Anthropology* (London, 1967)

D. Forde: *Marriage and Family among the Yako* (1941)

——: *The Context of Belief* (1958)

——: *Habitat, Economy and Society* (1963)

——: *Yako Studies* (1964)

—— and A.R. Radcliffe-Brown, eds: *Afri-*

can Systems of Kinship and Marriage (London)

A. Forge: Primitive Art and Society (London, 1973)

M. Fortes: The Dynamics of Clanship among the Tallensi (London, 1945)

——: The Web of Kinship among the Tallensi (London, 1949)

——: Oedipus and Job in West African Religion (Cambridge, 1959)

——: Kinship and the Social Order (Oxford, 1969)

——: 'Time and Social Structure' in M. Fortes, ed. (1970)

——, ed.: Social Structure (Oxford, 1970)

R.F. Fortune: Sorcerers of Dobu (London, 1932)

G. Foster: 'The Dyadic Contract', AA (1961)

——: 'Peasant Society and the Image of the Limited Good', AA (1965)

——: Traditional Societies and Technological Change (New York, 1973)

N.D. Foustel de Coulanges: The Ancient City (1864; Eng. trans., New York, 1955)

R. Fox: Kinship and Marriage (Harmondsworth, 1967)

A.G. Frank: Capitalism or Underdevelopment in Latin America (New York, 1967)

——: Latin America, Underdevelopment or Revolution (New York, 1969)

J.G. Frazer: The Golden Bough (London, 1926–36)

——: Totemism and Exogamy (London, 1910)

D. Freeman: Margaret Mead and Samoa (Cambridge, Mass., 1983)

P. Freire: Pedagogy of the Oppressed (London, 1972)

S. Freud: The Interpretation of Dreams (London, 1900)

——: Totem and Taboo (London, 1913)

——: The Future of an Illusion (London, 1927)

——: Civilisation and its Discontents (London, 1929)

M.H. Fried: The Evolution of Political Society (New York, 1967)

——et al, eds: War: the Anthropology of Armed Conflict and Aggression (New York, 1968)

B. Friedan: The Feminine Mystique (Harmondsworth, 1965)

J. Friedman: 'Marxism, Structuralism and Vulgar Materialism', Man (1974)

—— and M.J. Rowlands: The Evolution of Social Systems (London, 1977)

C. Fry: Aging in Culture and Society (New York, 1980)

J.S. Furnivall: Netherlands Society (Cambridge, 1967)

P. Furst, ed.: Flesh of the Gods (London, 1972)

H.G. Gadamer: Truth and Method (London, 1979)

C. Geertz: 'The Changing Role of the Cultural Broker', Comparative Studies in Society and History (1960)

——: Pedlars and Princes (Chicago, 1963)

——, ed.: Old Societies and New States (New York, 1966)

——: 'Religion as a Cultural System' in M. Banton, ed. (1966)

——, ed.: Myth, Symbol and Culture (New York, 1971)

——: 'Deep Play: Notes on the Balinese Cockfight', Daedalus (1972)

——: The Interpretation of Cultures (New York, 1973)

L.P. Gerlach and V.H. Hine: Lifeway Leap (Minneapolis, 1973)

R. Geuss: The Idea of a Critical Theory (Cambridge, 1981)

M.J. Giovannini and C.S. Holzberg: 'Anthropology and Industry', ARA (1981)

M. Gluckman: Custom and Conflict in Africa (Oxford, 1955)

——: Order and Rebellion in Tribal Africa (London, 1963)

——: The Ideas in Barotse Jurisprudence (New Haven, 1965)

——: Politics, Law and Religion in Tribal Society (London, 1965)

——, ed.: Essays in the Ritual of Social Relations (Manchester, 1962)

M. Godelier: Perspectives in Marxist Anthropology (London, 1977)

——: 'Infrastructures, Society and History', CA (1978)

Goffman: Interaction Ritual (New York, 1967)

——: The Presentation of Self in Everyday Life (London, 1969)

I. Goldman: 'Status Rivalry and Cultural Evolution in Polynesia', in R. Cohen and J. Middleton, eds (1967)

N.L. Gonzalez: 'Towards a Definition of Matrifocality', in N.E. Whitten and J. Szwed, eds (1970)

W.H. Goodenough: 'Componential Analysis and the Study of Meaning', *Language* (1956)

——: *Description and Comparison in Cultural Anthropology* (Chicago, 1970)

——: *Culture, Language and Society* (1971)

J. Goody: 'Religion and Ritual', *BJS* (1961)

——: *Death, Property and the Ancestors* (Stanford, 1962)

——: *Production and Reproduction* (Cambridge, 1976)

——: *The Domestication of the Savage Mind* (Cambridge, 1977)

——: *Cooking, Cuisine and Class* (Cambridge, 1982)

——, ed.: *The Developmental Cycle in Domestic Groups* (Cambridge, 1958)

——, ed.: *Kinship: Selected Readings* (Harmondsworth, 1971)

—— and Tambiah, eds: *Bridewealth and Dowry* (Cambridge, 1973)

T.F. Gossett: *Race: The History of an Idea in America* (Dallas, 1963)

A. Gramsci: *Selections from the Prison Notebooks* (London, 1971)

C.J. Greenhouse: 'Anthropology at Home: Whose Home?', *HO* (1985)

S. Gudeman: *The Demise of a Rural Economy* (London, 1978)

G. Guterriez: *Teología de la liberación*

J. Habermas: *Communication and the Evolution of Society* (London, 1979)

P. Hage: 'On Male Initiation', *Man* (1981)

E.T. Hall: *Handbook of Proxemic Research* (1974)

A.E. Hammel, ed.: 'Formal Semantic Analysis', *AA* [special publ.] (1965)

I. Hamnett: *Chieftainship and Legitimacy* (London, 1975)

——, ed.: *Social Anthropology and Law* (London, 1977)

M. Harner: *Hallucinogens and Shamanism* (New York, 1973)

——: 'The Ecological Basis for Aztec Sacrifice', *Ethnology* (1977)

M. Harris: *Cows, Pigs, Wars and Witches* (New York, 1967)

——: *Cannibals and Kings* (London, 1978)

——: *Cultural Materialism* (New York, 1979)

M.J. Herskovits: *Dahomey* (New York, 1938)

——: *Man and his Works* (New York, 1941)

——: *The New World Negro* (Indiana, 1966)

R. Hertz: *Death and the Right Hand* (New York, 1960)

M. Herzfeld: *Ours Once More* (Austin, 1981)

E.J. Hobsbawm: *Primitive Rebels* (Manchester, 1959)

A.M. Hocart: *Caste* (London, 1950)

R. Hofstader: *Social Darwinism in American Thought* (New York, 1935)

M. Hollis and S. Lukes, eds: *Rationality and Relativism* (Oxford, 1982)

A. Holmberg: 'Changing Community Attitudes and Values', in R. Adams, ed. (1960)

L. Holy and Stuchlik, eds: *The Structure of Folk Models* (London, 1981)

J.J. Honigmann, ed.: *Handbook of Social and Cultural Anthropology* (Chicago, 1974)

D. Horowitz: *Imperialism and Revolution* (London, 1969)

R. Horton: 'African Traditional Thought and Western Science', *Africa* (1967)

A. Howard: 'Interactional Psychology', *AA* (1982)

R. Howell: *Teasing Relationships* (1973)

G. Huizer and B. Mannheim: *The Politics of Anthropology* (The Hague, 1979)

J. Huizinga: *Homo ludens* (London, 1949)

D. Hume: *An Enquiry concerning the Principles of Morals* (1752)

D.E. Hunter and P. Whitten, eds: *Encyclopaedia of Anthropology* (1976)

J.H. Hutton: *Caste in India* (Cambridge, 1946)

D. Hymes, ed.: *Reinventing Anthropology* (New York, 1973)

I. Illich: *Deschooling Society* (New York, 1971)

R.B. Inden: *Marriage and Rank in Bengali Culture* (Berkeley, 1976)

N. Islam, ed.: *Agricultural Policy in Developing Countries* (London, 1974)

J.A. Jackson: *Migration* (Cambridge, 1969)

——, ed.: *Role* (Cambridge, 1972)

N.W. Jerome *et al*, eds: *Nutritional Anthropology* (1980)

E. Johnson and R.F. Spencer: *Atlas for Anthropology* (Dubuque, 1960)

J.G. Jorgensen: *Comparative Studies by Harold E. Driver* (1974)

——: *Cross-cultural Comparisons* (1979)

A.L. Kaeppler: 'Dance in Anthropological Perspective', *ARA* (1978)

R.M. Kanter: *Commitment and Community* (Cambridge, Mass., 1972)

K.M. Kapadia: *Industrialisation and Rural Society* (Bombay, 1972)

B. Kapferer, ed.: *The Power of Ritual* (Adelaide, 1979)

D. Kaplan: 'The Superorganic: Science or Metaphysics?', *AA* (1965)

A. Kardiner: *The Psychological Frontiers of Society* (New York, 1945)

——: *Culture and Personality* (New York, 1945)

—— and E. Prebble: *They Studied Man* (London, 1962)

C.W. Keefer: 'Psychological Anthropology', *ARA* (1977)

A. Keesing: 'Shrines, Ancestors and Cognatic Descent', *AA* (1970)

——: *Kin Groups and Social Structure* (New York, 1975)

——: *Elota's Story* (New York, 1978)

——: 'Linguistic Knowledge and Cultural Knowledge', *AA* (1979)

J. Keith, ed.: *Age and Anthropological Theory* (Ithaca, 1980)

A.J. Kelso: *Physical Anthropology* (1974)

Kleinman: *Patients and Healers* (London, 1980)

C.K.M. Kluckhohn: *Mirror for Life* (London, 1950)

—— and A. Kroeber: *Culture: Peabody Museum Papers* (1952)

I. Kopytoff: 'Classification of Religious Movements', *Proceedings of the Meeting of the American Ethnological Society* (1964)

——: 'Ancestors as Elders in Africa', *Africa* (1971)

——, ed.: *Slavery in Africa* (Madison, 1977)

F. Korn: *Elementary Structures Reconsidered* (Berkeley, 1973)

A.L. Kroeber: *Anthropology* (New York, 1923)

——: *Handbook of the Indians of California* (Washington, DC, 1925)

——: *Configurations of Culture Growth* (Berkeley, 1944)

T. Kuhn: *The Structure of Scientific Revolutions* (Chicago, 1962)

D. Kumar: *Land and Class in South India* (Cambridge, 1965)

A. Kuper: *Anthropologists and Anthropology* (London, 1983)

H. Kuper, ed.: *Urbanization and Migration in West Africa* (California, 1965)

G.P. Kurath: *Dances of Anahuac* (New York, 1960)

W. LaBarre: 'The Cultural Basis of Emotions and Gestures', *Journal of Personality* (1947)

——: *The Ghost Dance* (New York, 1970)

J.S. La Fontaine: 'Ritualization of Women's Life Crises in Bugisu', in J.S. La Fontaine, ed. (1972)

——, ed.: *The Interpretation of Ritual* (London, 1972)

R.O. Lagace: *Nature and Use of the Human Relations Area Files (HRAF)* (1974)

R.T. Lakoff: *Language and Women's Place* (New York, 1975)

J.B. Lamarck: *Zoological Philosophy* (1809; Eng. trans., London, 1914)

L. Lamphere and M.Z. Rosaldo, eds: *Women, Culture and Society* (Stanford, 1974)

L.L. Langness: *Life History in Anthropological Science* (New York, 1965)

C. Lasch: *The Culture of Narcissism* (New York, 1979)

P. Lawrence: *Road Belong Cargo* (Manchester, 1964)

E. Leach: *The Political Systems of Highland Burma* (Cambridge, 1954)

——: 'Concerning Trobriand Class and the Kinship Category Tabu' in J. Goody, ed. (1959)

——: *Pul Eiya* (London, 1961)

——: *Rethinking Anthropology* (London, 1962)

——, ed: *The Structural Study of Myth and Totemism* (London, 1967)

——, ed: *Dialectic in Practical Religion* (1968)

——: *Genesis as Myth* (London, 1969)

——: *Levi-Strauss* (London, 1970)

——: *Culture and Communication* (London, 1976)

L.S. Leakey: *Human Origins* (Menlo Park, Cal., 1976)

W.P. Lebra: *Culture-bound Syndromes, Ethnopsychiatry and Alternate Therapies* (1976)

A. Leeds: 'Some Preliminary Considerations Regarding the Analysis of Technologies', *Kroeber Anthropological Society Papers* (1965)

——: 'Institutions', in D.E. Hunter and P. Whitten, eds (1976)

V.I. Lenin: *Imperialism, the Highest Stage of Capitalism* (1915)

M.B. Leons and F. Rothenstein: *New Directions in Political Anthropology* (1979)

F. LePlay: *Les ouvriers européens* (Paris, 1855)

W.A. Lessa and E.Z. Vogt, eds: *Reader in Comparative Religion* (New York, 1965)

R.A. Levine: 'Anthropology and the Study of Conflict', *Journal of Conflict Resolution* (1961)

G. Levitas: 'Fasts, Feasts, Famine and Fitness', *MAQ* (1983)

C. Levi-Strauss: *The Elementary Structure of Kinship* (1949; Eng. trans., London, 1969)

——: *Tristes Tropiques* (1955; Eng. trans., London, 1968)

——: *Structural Anthropology*, 2 vols (1958–63; Eng. trans., London, 1968–9)

——: *Totemism* (1962; Eng. trans., London, 1963)

——: *The Savage Mind* (1962; Eng. trans., London, 1969)

——: *Mythologiques* (Paris, 1964–72)

——: 'The Future of Kinship Studies', *Proceedings of the Royal Anthropological Institute* (1965)

——: 'The Concept of Primitiveness', in I. Devore and R.B. Lee, eds (1968)

L. Levy-Bruhl: *The Primitive Mentality* (London, 1923)

T. Lewellen: *Political Anthropology* (South Hadley, Mass., 1983)

I.M. Lewis: *A Pastoral Democracy* (London, 1961)

——: *Ecstatic Religion* (London, 1971)

O. Lewis: *The Children of Sanchez* (New York, 1961)

——: 'The Culture of Poverty', *Scientific American* (1966)

R. Linton: *The Study of Man* (New York, 1936)

——: *The Cultural Background of a Personality* (New York, 1945)

——: *The Tree of Culture* (New York, 1955)

M. Llewelyn-Davies: 'Women, Warriors and Patriarchs', in S.B. Ortner, ed. (1981)

P. Lloyd: 'The Political Structure of African Kingdoms', in M. Banton, ed. (1965)

A. Lomax: *Folksong Style and Culture* (Washington, DC, 1968)

——: *Cantometrics* (New York, 1977)

N. Long: *Family and Work in Rural Societies* (London, 1984)

K. Lorenz: *On Aggression* (New York, 1966)

F.G. Lounsbury and H. Scheffler: *A Study in Structural Semantics* (Englewood Cliffs, 1971)

A.O. Lovejoy: *The Great Chain of Being* (Cambridge, Mass., 1937)

R.H. Lowie: *Primitive Society* (New York, 1920)

——: *The Crow Indians* (New York, 1935)

——: *History of Ethnological Theory* (New York, 1937)

P. Lubbock: *The Origin of Civilization and the Primitive Condition of Man* (London, 1870)

S. Lukes: *Emile Durkheim* (London, 1973)

——: *Individualism* (Oxford, 1973)

L. and J.S. Macdonald: 'The Black Family in the Americas', *Sage Race Relations Abstract* (1978)

D. McLellan, ed.: *Selected Works of Marx and Engels* (1968)

D.C. McLelland: *The Achieving Society* (Princeton, 1961)

J.F. McLennan: *Primitive Marriage* (London, 1865)

——: *Studies in Ancient History* (London, 1886)

N. McLeod: 'Ethnomusicological Research and Anthropology', *ARA* (1974)

——: 'Ethnomusicology', in B.J. Siegel, ed. (1974)

P. Magnarella: 'Cultural Materialism and the Problem of Possibilities', *AA* (1982)

H.S. Maine: *Ancient Law* (London, 1861)

L. Mair: *Primitive Government* (Harmondsworth, 1962)

——: *Anthropology and Social Change* (London, 1969)

B.K. Malinowski: *Argonauts of the Western Pacific* (1922)

——: *Crime and Custom in Savage Society* (1926)

——: *Sex and Repression in Savage Society* (1927)

——: *The Sexual Life of Savages* (1929)

——: *Coral Gardens and their Magic* (1935)

——: *Magic, Science and Religion* (1948)

——: *The Family among the Australian Aborigines* (1963)

——: *A Diary in the Strict Sense of the Term* (1967)

T.R. Malthus: *Essay on Population* (1798)

D.G. Mandelbaum: 'Alcohol and Culture', *CA* (1965)

W.P. Mangin: *Peasants in Cities* (Boston, 1970)

G.E. Marcus: *Anthropology as Cultural Critique* (Chicago, 1986)

R.R. Marrett: *The Threshold of Religion* (London, 1900)

M. Marriott: 'Hindu Transactions', in B. Kapferer, ed. (1976)

K. Marx: *The Poverty of Philosophy* (1847)

——: *The Communist Manifesto* (1848)

——: *Grundrisse* [1857–8] (Harmondsworth, 1973)

——: *Contribution to the Critique of Political Economy* (1859)

——: *Capital* (1867–94)

—— and F. Engels: *The Holy Family* (1845)

——: *The German Ideology* (1845–6)

A. Mattelart: *Transnationals and the Third World* (South Hadley, Mass., 1983)

M. Mauss: *The Gift* (1925; Eng. trans., London, 1954)

Maybury-Lewis: 'Prescriptive Marriage Systems', *SWJA* (1965)

E. Mayo: *The Human Problems of an Industrial Civilisation* (Harvard, 1933)

M. Mead: *Coming of Age in Samoa* (New York, 1928)

——: *Growing up in New Guinea* (New York, 1930)

——: *Sex and Temperament in Three Primitive Societies* (New York, 1935)

——: *Male and Female* (New York, 1956)

——: *New Lives for Old* (New York, 1956)

——: *Culture and Commitment* (New York, 1970)

C. Meillassoux: 'From Production to Reproduction', *Economy and Society* (1972)

——, ed.: *The Development of Indigenous Trade and Markets in West Africa* (London, 1971)

A. Merriam: *The Anthropology of Music* (Chicago, 1964)

R.K. Merton: *Social Theory and Social Structure* (New York, 1949)

——: *The Sociology of Science* (New York, 1973)

D.A. Messerschmidt, ed.: *Anthropologists at Home in North America* (Cambridge, 1981)

A. Métraux: *The Ethnography of Easter Island* (Honolulu, 1940)

——: *Les Incas* (Paris, 1962)

J. Middleton, ed.: *Myth and Cosmos* (New York, 1967)

Missionaries, Anthropologists and Cultural Change, Studies in Third World Societies, no. 25 (1984)

M. Molyneux: 'Androcentrism in Marxist Anthropology', *Critique of Anthropology* (1977)

J. Monney: *The Ghost Dance Religion* (1896)

A. Montagu: *The Concept of Race* (New York, 1964)

——: *Man and Aggression* (New York, 1972)

C.L. de Montesquieu: *L'Esprit des lois* (1748)

J. Montgomery: *Appropriate Technology and Social Values* (New York, 1982)

R. Moore and S.L. Washburn: *Ape into Human: A Study of Human Evolution* (1980)

L.H. Morgan: *League of the Iroquois* (1851)

——: *Systems of Consanguinity and Affinity* (Washington, DC, 1870)

——: *Ancient Society* (New York, 1877)

O. Morgenstern and J. von Neumann: *Theory of Games and Economic Behaviour* (1947)

C. Morris: *Signs, Language and Behavior* (New York, 1946)

——: *Signification and Significance* (Cambridge, Mass., 1964)

G.P. Murdock: *Social Structure* (New York, 1949)

——: *The Ethnographic Atlas: A Summary* (1967)

——: *Outline of World Cultures* (New York, 1972)

P. Murphy: 'Oral Literature', *ARA* (1979)

G.K. Myrdal: *Economic Theory and Underdeveloped Regions* (London, 1958)

——: *The Asian Drama* (Harmondsworth, 1968)

J. Nash: 'Anthropology of the Multinational Corporations', in M.B. Leons and F. Rothenstein (1979)

——: 'Ethnographic Aspects of the World Capitalist System', *ARA* (1981)

R. Needham: *Structure and Sentiment* (Chicago, 1962)

——: 'Terminology and Alliance, Parts 1 and 2', *Sociologus* (1966–7)

——, ed.: *Rethinking Kinship and Marriage* (London, 1971)

C. Nelson, ed.: *The Desert and the Sown* (Berkeley, 1973)

R.W. Nicholas: 'Factions, a Comparative

Analysis', in M. Banton, ed. (1965)

Nieboer: *Slavery as an Industrial System* (The Hague, 1900)

A. Oakley: *Sex, Gender and Society* (London, 1972)

G. Obeyeskere: *Medusa's Hair* (Chicago, 1981)

H.T. Odum: *Environment, Power and Society* (New York, 1971)

B. O'Laughlin: 'Marxist Approaches to Anthropology', *ARA* (1975)

M.E. Opler: 'The Themal Approach in Cultural Anthropology', *SWJA* (1968)

——: 'An Outline of Chiricahua Apache Social Organization', in F. Eggan, ed. (1964)

M.K. Opler: *Culture and Social Psychiatry* (New York, 1967)

——, ed.: *Culture and Mental Health* (New York, 1959)

H. Orenstein: *Gaon* (Princeton, 1966)

S.B. Ortner: 'Is Female to Male as Nature is to Culture', in L. Lamphere and M.Z. Rosaldo, eds (1974)

——, ed.: *Sexual Meanings* (Cambridge, 1981)

K. Overing: *The Piaroa* (Oxford, 1976)

R.E. Park: *Race and Culture* (Glencoe, 1950)

J.P. Parry: *Caste and Kinship in Kangra* (London, 1979)

T. Parsons: *The Structure of Social Action* (1937)

——: *Toward a General Theory of Action* (1951)

——: *The Social System* (1957)

L. Peattie: *The View from the Barrio* (New York, 1970)

C.S. Peirce: *Collected Papers* (Cambridge, Mass., 1935–58)

R. Peltazoni: *Essays on the History of Religion* (1954)

P. and G. Pelto: *Anthropological Research* (New York, 1970)

W.J. Perry: *Children of the Sun* (London, 1923)

——: *The Origin of Magic and Religion* (London, 1923)

J. Piaget *et al*: *The Moral Judgement of the Child* (London, 1960)

K. Pike: *Language in Relation to a Unified Theory of the Structure of Human Nature* (The Hague, 1967)

J. Pitt-Rivers: *The People of the Sierra* (Chicago, 1971)

L. Plotnicov and A. Tuden: *Essays in Comparative Social Stratification* (New York, 1970)

D. Pocock, ed.: *The Hypergamy of the Patidars in Kapadia* (1972)

——: 'Notes on Jajmani Relationships', *Contributions to Indian Sociology* (1972)

K. Polanyi: *Trade and Markets in the Early Empires* (Boston, 1957)

——: *Primitive, Archaic and Modern Economies* (New York, 1968)

S. Polgar: *Population, Ecology and Social Evolution* (1975)

K. Popper: *The Poverty of Historicism* (London, 1957)

——: *The Open Society and its Enemies* (London, 1966)

D.A. Posey *et al*: 'Ethnoecology as Applied Anthropology in Amazonian Development', *HO* (1984)

L. Pospisil: *Anthropology of Law: A Comparative Theory* (New York, 1974)

G.T. Prance *et al*: 'The Ethnobotany of Paumiri Indians', *Economic Botany* (1977)

N. Quinn: 'Anthropological Studies on Women's Status', *ARA* (1977)

A.R. Radcliffe-Brown: *The Andaman Islanders* (1922)

——: 'On Joking Relationships', *Africa* (1940)

——: *Structure and Function in Primitive Society* (1952)

——: *Method in Social Anthropology* (1958)

P. Radin: *Primitive Man as Philosopher* (New York, 1927)

——: *Method and Theory of Ethnology* (New York, 1933)

R. Rappaport: *Pigs for the Ancestors* (New Haven, Conn., 1968)

——: 'Ritual, Sanity and Cybernetics', *AA* (1971)

R. Redfield: *The Folk Culture of Yucatan* (Chicago, 1941)

——: *The Little Community* (Chicago, 1955)

——: *Peasant Society and Culture* (Chicago, 1956)

G. Reichel Dolmatoff: *Amazonian Cosmos* (Chicago, 1971)

P. Reining, ed.: *Kinship Studies in the Morgan Centennial Year* (1972)

R. Reiter, ed.: *Toward an Anthropology of*

Women (New York, 1975)

P.P. Rey: *Colonialisme, neo-colonialisme et transition au capitalisme* (Paris, 1971)

A.I. Richards: *Land, Labour and Diet in Northern Rhodesia* (London, 1939)

——: *Chisungu* (London, 1956)

——: *Chisungu: A Girl's Initiation Ceremony among the Bemba of Northern Rhodesia* (1956)

M.A. Rinkiewich and J.P. Spradley, eds: *Ethics and Anthropology* (1976)

H.H. Risley: *The Ethnology, Language, Literature and Religion of India* (London, 1907–09)

W.J.H. Rivers: *Social Organization* (London, 1924)

A.F. Robertson: *People and the State* (Cambridge, 1984)

W. Robertson-Smith: *Kinship and Marriage in Early Arabia* (Cambridge, 1885)

——: *Lectures on the Religion of the Semites* (London, 1894)

C.G. Rossetti: 'The Ideology of Banditry', *Man* (1982)

T. Roszack: *The Making of a Counter-Culture* (New York, 1969)

J.J. Rousseau: *Le Contrat social* (1762; Eng. trans., London, 1955)

C. Sachs: *The Wellsprings of Music* (The Hague, 1962)

M. Sahlins: 'Poor Man, Rich Man, Big Man, Chief', *Comparative Studies in Society and History* (1963)

——: *Culture and Practical Reason* (Chicago, 1971)

——: *Stone Age Economics* (Chicago, 1972)

——: *The Use and Abuse of Biology* (Ann Arbor, 1976)

——: 'Reply to Marvin Harris', *NYRB* (28 June, 1979)

R.F. Salisbury: *From Stone to Steel* (Melbourne, 1962)

M. Sallnow: 'Comunitas Reconsidered: the Sociology of Andean Pilgrimage', *Man* (1981)

P.R. Sanday: 'Toward a Theory of the Status of Women', *AA* (1973)

——: *Female Power and Male Domination* (London, 1981)

E. Sapir: *Language* (New York, 1921)

——: *Selected Writings* (Berkeley, 1949)

M.F. de Saussure: *Course in General Linguistics* (1916; Eng. trans., New York, 1959)

I. Schapera: *A Handbook of Tswana Law and Custom* (London, 1955)

H.W. Scheffler: 'Kinship, Descent and Alliance', in J.J. Honigmann, ed. (1974)

—— and F.G. Lounsbury: *A Study in Structural Semantics* (Englewood Cliffs, 1971)

N. Scheper Hughes: 'The Margaret Mead Controversy', *HO* (1984)

D.M. Schneider: 'Some Muddles in the Models', in M. Banton, ed. (1965)

L. Schneider: *Sociological Approaches to Religion* (New York, 1970)

E.F. Schumacher: *Small is Beautiful* (New York, 1973)

M. Schwartz, V. Turner and A. Tuden: *Political Anthropology* (Chicago, 1966)

H.B. Schwartzmann: 'The Anthropological Study of Children's Play', *ARA* (1976)

J.R. Searle and D. Vanderveken: *Foundations of Illocutionary Logic* (Cambridge, 1985)

D. Seddon, ed.:*Relations of Production* (London, 1978)

C.R. Seligman: *Melanesians of British New Guinea* (Cambridge, 1910)

E. Service: *Origins of the State and Civilization* (New York, 1975)

W.B. Shaffir, R.A. Stebbins and A. Turowetz, eds: *Fieldwork Experience* (1980)

T. Shanin: 'Defining Peasants', *Sociological Review* (1982)

M. Shubik: *Game Theory and Related Approaches to Social Behavior* (New York, 1964)

B.J. Siegel, ed.: *Biennial Review of Anthropology* (Stanford, 1959)

H.R. Silver: 'Ethnoart', *ARA* (1979)

G.E. Simpson: *Melville Herskovits* (1973)

G. Sjoberg: *The Pre-industrial City* (New York, 1960)

B.F. Skinner: *About Behaviourism* (London, 1974)

A.G. Smith: *Communication and Culture – Readings in the Codes of Human Interaction* (1966)

M.G. Smith: *Government in Zazzau* (London, 1960)

——: *Kinship and Community in Caniacon* (New Haven, 1962)

A.W. Southall: *Urban Anthropology* (London, 1973)

H. Spencer: *Principles of Sociology* (London, 1876–96)

D. Sperber: *Rethinking Symbolism* (Cambridge, 1975)

G.D. Spindler, ed.: *The Making of Psychological Anthropology* (1978)

M.E. Spiro: 'Religion: Problems of Definition and Explanation', in M. Banton, ed. (1966)

——: *Kinship and Marriage in Burma* (Berkeley, 1978)

B. Spooner: *Population Growth* (Cambridge, Mass., 1970)

——: *The Cultural Ecology of Pastoral Nomads* (1973)

M.N. Srivnas: *Caste in India* (Berkeley, 1962)

R. Stavenhagen: *Social Classes in Agrarian Societies* (New York, 1975)

——: *Indian Ethnic Movements and State Policies in Latin America* (1983)

J.H. Steward: *The Economic and Social Basis of Primitive Bands* (1936)

——: *Handbook of South American Indians* (1950)

——: 'Levels of Socio-Cultural Integration: an Operational Concept', *SWJA* (1951)

——: *Theory of Cultural Change* (Urbana, 1955)

G.W. Stocking: *Race, Culture and Evolution* (New York, 1968)

B. Stoll: *Fishers of Men or Founders of Empire?* (London, 1982)

M. Strathern: *Women in Between* (Cambridge, 1972)

W.G. Sumner: *Folkways* (Boston, 1906)

C. Suret: *French Colonialism in Tropical Africa* (London, 1971)

Sutton-Smith: *The Folkgames of Children* (Austin, 1972)

G. Swanson: *The Birth of the Gods* (1960)

J.F. Szwed and N.W. Whitten: 'The Social Organization of a Movement of Revolutionary Change', in N.W. Whitten and J.F. Szwed, eds (1970)

E. Terray: *Marxism and 'Primitive Society'* (New York, 1972)

J.J. Thomas: *An Introduction to Statistical Analysis for Economists* (London, 1973)

J.C. Thrupp: *Millenial Dreams in Action* (New York, 1970)

N. Tinbergen: *The Animal in its World*, 2 vols (Cambridge, Mass., 1932–72)

M. Todaro: *International Migration in Developing Countries* (New York, 1976)

F. Tonnies: *Community and Association* (1887; Eng. trans., New York, 1955)

C.M. Turnbull: *The Forest People* (New York, 1961)

R. Turner, ed.: *Ethnomethodology* (Harmondsworth, 1974)

V.W. Turner: *Schism and Continuity in African Society* (New York, 1957)

——: *The Forest of Symbols* (Ithaca, 1967)

——: *The Drums of Affliction* (Oxford, 1968)

——: *The Ritual Process* (1969)

——: *Dramas, Fields and Metaphors* (New York, 1974)

——: *Revelation and Divination in Ndembu Ritual* (1975)

S. Tyler: *Cognitive Anthropology* (New York, 1969)

E.B. Tylor: *Primitive Culture* (New York, 1871)

——: *Anthropology* (New York, 1894)

C.A. Valentine: *Culture and Poverty* (Chicago, 1968)

Van den Berghe: *Race and Ethnicity* (New York, 1970)

A. Van Gennep: *The Rites of Passage* (1909; Eng. trans., 1960)

J. Vansina: *The Tio Kingdom of the Middle Congo* (London, 1973)

J. Van Willigen: 'Truth and Effectiveness', *HO* (1984)

——: *Applied Anthropology* (1986)

S. Varese: *The Forest Indians in the Present Political Situation of Peru* (Copenhagen, 1972)

S. Vatuk: 'A Structural Analysis of Hindi Kinship Terminology', *Contributions to Indian Sociology* (1969)

A. Vayda: *Environment and Cultural Behavior* (New York, 1969)

F.W. Vogel: *A History of Ethnology* (1975)

A.F.C. Wallace: 'Revitalization Movements', *AA* (1958)

——: *Religion: an Anthropological View* (1967)

——: *Culture and Personality* (New York, 1970)

I. Wallerstein: *The Modern World System* (1974)

——: *The Capitalist World Economy* (Cambridge, 1979)

W.L. Warner: *A Black Civilization* (New York, 1937)

S.L. Washburn and R. Moore: *Ape into Human* (1980)

J.B. Watson: *Behaviorism* (Chicago, 1924)

W. Watson: *Asian and African Systems of Slavery* (Oxford, 1980)

M. and R. Wax: 'The Notion of Magic', *CA* (1963)

M. Weber: *The Methodology of the Social Sciences* (1949)

——: *The Protestant Ethic and the Spirit of Capitalism* (New York, 1958)

——: *Economy and Society* (New York, 1968)

S. Weisner *et al*: 'Concordance between Ethnographer and Folk Perspective', *HO* (1982)

E. Westermarck: *Marriage Ceremonies in Morocco* (London, 1914)

P. Wheatley: *Nagara and Commandery* (Chicago, 1983)

D.R. White: 'Mathematical Anthropology' in J.J. Honigmann, ed. (1974)

L.A. White: *The Evolution of Culture* (1959)

W.H. Whiteley: *Language Use and Social Change* (Dar es Salaam, 1968)

B.B. Whiting: *Children of six Cultures* (New York, 1963)

J.W.M. Whiting: *Becoming Kwoma* (New Haven, 1941)

—— and I.L. Child: *Child Training and Personality* (New Haven, 1953)

N.E. Whitten and J. Szwed, eds: *Afro-American Anthropology* (New York, 1970)

N.E. Whitten and D.M. Wolfe: 'Network Analysis', in J.J. Honigmann, ed. (1974)

N.E. Whitten, ed.: *Cultural Adaptations and Ethnicity in Contemporary Ecuador* (1982)

B.L. Whorf: *Language, Thought and Reality* (Cambridge, Mass., 1956)

W.H. Whyte, ed.: *Industry and Society* (New York, 1946)

B.J. Williams: 'A Critical View of Models in Sociobiology', *ARA* (1981)

B. Wilson: *Sects and Society* (London, 1961)

E.O. Wilson: *Sociobiology* (Cambridge, Mass., 1975)

M. Wilson: *Good Company* (Boston, 1963)

P. Wilson: *The Promising Primitive* (1980)

W.H. Wiser: *The Hindu Jajmani System* (Lucknaw, 1958)

C. Wissler: *Man and Culture* (New York, 1923)

K. Wittfogel: *Oriental Despotism* (New Haven, 1957)

J. Woddis: *New Theories of Revolution* (London, 1972)

E. Wolf: *Peasants* (Englewood Cliffs, 1966)

——: *Peasant Wars of the Twentieth Century* (New York, 1969)

D.M. Wolfe: *Organizational Stress* (New York, 1964)

P. Worsley: *The Trumpet Shall Sound* (London, 1957)

S.I. Yanigasako: 'Family and Household', *ARA* (1979)

J. Yoors: *The Gypsies* (1967)